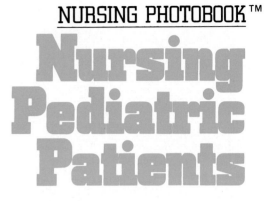

NURSING PHOTOBOOK™

Nursing Pediatric Patients

NURSING83 BOOKS™
INTERMED COMMUNICATIONS, INC.
SPRINGHOUSE, PENNSYLVANIA

NURSING83 BOOKS™

NURSING PHOTOBOOK™ SERIES
Providing Respiratory Care
Managing I.V. Therapy
Dealing with Emergencies
Giving Medications
Assessing Your Patients
Using Monitors
Providing Early Mobility
Giving Cardiac Care
Performing GI Procedures
Implementing Urologic Procedures
Controlling Infection
Ensuring Intensive Care
Coping with Neurologic Disorders
Caring for Surgical Patients
Working with Orthopedic Patients
Nursing Pediatric Patients
Helping Geriatric Patients
Attending Ob/Gyn Patients
Aiding Ambulatory Patients
Carrying Out Special Procedures

NURSING SKILLBOOK® SERIES
Reading EKGs Correctly
Dealing with Death and Dying
Managing Diabetics Properly
Assessing Vital Functions Accurately
Helping Cancer Patients Effectively
Giving Cardiovascular Drugs Safely
Giving Emergency Care Competently
Monitoring Fluid and Electrolytes Precisely
Documenting Patient Care Responsibly
Combatting Cardiovascular Diseases Skillfully
Coping with Neurologic Problems Proficiently
Using Crisis Intervention Wisely
Nursing Critically Ill Patients Confidently

NURSE'S REFERENCE LIBRARY®
Diseases
Diagnostics
Drugs
Assessment
Procedures

Nursing83 DRUG HANDBOOK™

NURSING PHOTOBOOK™ Series

PUBLISHER
Eugene W. Jackson

EDITORIAL DIRECTOR
Jean Robinson

CLINICAL DIRECTOR
Barbara McVan, RN

ART DIRECTOR
Lisa A. Gilde

Intermed Communications Book Division

DIRECTOR
Timothy B. King

DIRECTOR, RESEARCH
Elizabeth O'Brien

DIRECTOR, PRODUCTION AND PURCHASING
Bacil Guiley

Staff for this volume

BOOK EDITOR
Katherine W. Carey

SENIOR CLINICAL EDITOR
Paulette J. Strauch, RN

CLINICAL EDITOR
Mary L. Clements, RN, CCRN

ASSOCIATE EDITOR
Dario F. Bernardini

SPECIAL ASSIGNMENTS EDITOR
Patricia R. Urosevich

PHOTOGRAPHER
Paul A. Cohen

ASSOCIATE DESIGNERS
Linda Jovinelly Franklin
Scott M. Stephens
Carol Stickles

ASSISTANT PHOTOGRAPHER
Thomas Staudenmayer

EDITORIAL/GRAPHIC COORDINATOR
Doreen K. Stowers

CLINICAL/GRAPHIC COORDINATOR
Evelyn M. James

COPY EDITOR
Sharyl D. Wolf

EDITORIAL STAFF ASSISTANT
Cynthia A. O'Connell

PHOTOGRAPHY ASSISTANT
Frank Margeson

ART PRODUCTION MANAGER
Robert Perry

ARTISTS
Virginia Crawford
Diane Fox
Donald G. Knauss
Robert H. Renn
Louise Stamper
Joan Walsh
Ron Yablon

RESEARCHER
Vonda Heller

TYPOGRAPHY MANAGER
David C. Kosten

TYPOGRAPHY ASSISTANTS
Janice Auch Haber
Ethel Halle
Diane Paluba
Nancy Wirs

PRODUCTION MANAGERS
Wilbur D. Davidson
Robert L. Dean, Jr.

PRODUCTION ASSISTANT
Terry Gallagher

ILLUSTRATORS
Jack Crane
Len Epstein
Russell Farrell
Jean Gardner
Robert Jackson
Bob Jones
Don Kruzinski
Jamin Morse
John Murphy
Dennis Schofield
Bud Yingling

SERIES GRAPHIC DESIGNER
John C. Isely

COVER PHOTO
Photographic Illustrations

Clinical consultants for this volume

Martha Underwood Barnard, RN, BSN, MN, MA
Nurse Clinician/Nurse Practitioner/Faculty
University of Kansas Health Center School of Medicine and School of Nursing
Kansas City, Kan.

Karen E. Roper, RN, BSN, MSN
Assistant Director of Nursing Education
Children's Hospital of Philadelphia
Philadelphia, Pa.

PB-021282

Library of Congress Cataloging in Publication Data

Main entry under title:

Nursing pediatric patients.

(Nursing photobook)
"Nursing82 books."
Bibliography: p.
Includes index.
1. Pediatric Nursing—Handbooks, manuals, etc.
I. Intermed Communications, inc.   II. Series.   [DNLM:
1. Pediatric nursing.   WY 159 N9746]
RJ245.N883   1982   610.73'62   82-6273
ISBN 0-916730-47-6   AACR2

Contents

Contributors

At the time of original publication, these contributors held the following positions.

Martha Underwood Barnard is a nurse clinician/nurse practitioner specializing in ambulatory pediatrics and pediatric endocrinology at the University of Kansas Health Center School of Medicine and School of Nursing. She is also a faculty member there, and an advisor for this PHOTOBOOK. She holds a BSN degree from the University of Missouri in Columbia and an MN degree from the University of Florida, Gainesville. An MA degree graduate of the University of Kansas, Lawrence, she is a doctoral candidate in child development and child psychology there. Ms. Barnard's memberships include the American Nurses' Association, Sigma Theta Tau, the American Diabetes Association, the Council of Nurse Practitioners, and the National Association of Pediatric Nurse Associates and Practitioners.

Kimberly Karch Biby is a pediatric staff nurse at Dallas County Hospital District-Parkland Memorial Hospital in Dallas. She holds a BSN degree from the University of Florida in Gainesville.

Elizabeth Billet is a pediatric clinical nurse specialist at UCLA Medical Center in Los Angeles. She is a BSN degree graduate of Marquette University, Milwaukee, and an MA degree graduate of the University of California, Los Angeles. She is a member of the American Association of Critical-Care Nurses and the Association for the Care of Children in Hospitals.

Jeanne Fitzpatrick is a clinical nurse specialist in pediatric cardiology at UCLA Hospital in Los Angeles. She earned a BS degree at Mount St. Mary's College in Los Angeles, and an MN degree at the University of California, Los Angeles. Ms. Fitzpatrick is a certified critical-care registered nurse, and a member of the American Association of Critical-Care Nurses and the American Hospital Association.

Leslie Mayrand Hutton is a clinical nursing supervisor at Nemours Children's Hospital in Jacksonville, Florida. She holds a BSN degree from Incarnate Word College in San Antonio, Texas, and an MSN degree from the University of Texas Health Science Center at San Antonio.

Janet Kandra-Dix is a head nurse at Children's Hospital of Philadelphia. She holds both BSN and MS degrees from the University of Delaware in Newark. Ms. Kandra-Dix is a member of Sigma Theta Tau.

Kristy Kiel is an instructor in ambulatory pediatrics at the University of Florida's College of Nursing in Gainesville, Florida. She earned a BSN degree at Florida State University in Tallahassee, and an MSN degree at the University of Florida in Gainesville. She holds memberships in the American Nurses' Association and Sigma Theta Tau, and is certified in Florida as an advanced registered nurse practitioner.

Debra K. Miller, a staff education instructor at Children's Hospital of Philadelphia, holds a BSN degree from Temple University, Philadelphia. Ms. Miller also has an MSN degree from the University of Pennsylvania in Philadelphia.

Lynne B. Picus is a head nurse on a medical unit at Children's Hospital of Philadelphia. She graduated with a BSN degree from Temple University, Philadelphia.

Karen E. Roper, an advisor for this PHOTOBOOK, is assistant director of nursing education at Children's Hospital of Philadelphia. Ms. Roper earned a BSN degree at Cornell University in Ithaca, N.Y., and an MSN degree at the University of Pennsylvania in Philadelphia.

Katherine Soss is a unit supervisor at St. Francis Medical Center in Trenton, New Jersey. She earned a nursing diploma at St. Francis Medical Center School of Nursing, Trenton. Ms. Soss is working toward a BSN degree at Trenton (N.J.) State College.

hat do you consider the greatest challenge of pediatric nursing? Relating successfully to a frightened child who may be in pain? Evaluating medication dosages quickly and accurately? Helping distraught parents?

As a pediatric nurse, you face all these challenges—and more. This PHO-TOBOOK is designed to give you the know-how you need to deal confidently with young patients and their parents, whether you're an experienced pediatric nurse, or a newcomer to the field.

In this book, we'll focus on the age-group ranging from toddler to preteen. We won't deal with newborns (a specialty itself), or with the distinctive problems of adolescence. From time to time, however, we'll provide information and special tips that apply specifically to these two pediatric age groups.

If you consider communicating with a child and his parents to be one of your greatest challenges, you'll find plenty of helpful suggestions throughout this book. The first section in particular is packed with information on how to relate to a youngster, in both outpatient and hospital settings. In addition, you'll find a wealth of information on basic assessment techniques and procedures, including how to obtain blood and urine specimens.

As you know, a child isn't just a small adult. His distinctly different anatomy and physiology profoundly affect such varied nursing responsibilities as giving medications and administering cardiopulmonary resuscitation (CPR). So, in the book's second section, we'll provide detailed information on giving medications (as well as tips for encouraging a child's compliance). Throughout the book, where appropriate, we'll give you information on specific medications the doctor may order for a child.

For clear, step-by-step information on identifying respiratory and cardiac problems and dealing with life-threatening emergencies, turn to the third section. There, you'll find detailed instructions on clearing a child's airway and giving CPR. You'll also learn how to care for the seizure-prone child. And, because poisoning, burns, and multiple trauma are common pediatric emergencies, we'll tell you how to cope with these injuries.

In the fourth section, you'll learn about some special nursing challenges—cleft lip and palate and orthopedic problems. You'll also gain insight into two of the most heartbreaking problems a pediatric nurse ever faces—child abuse and terminal illness.

As you'll quickly discover, this is a book you can rely on. We on the PHOTOBOOK staff hope that you'll enjoy using it as much as we enjoyed putting it together. As we discovered while taking photographs, a child's unpredictability can occasionally cause problems. But as you'd surely agree, his spontaneous nature also provides some of pediatric nursing's greatest joys.

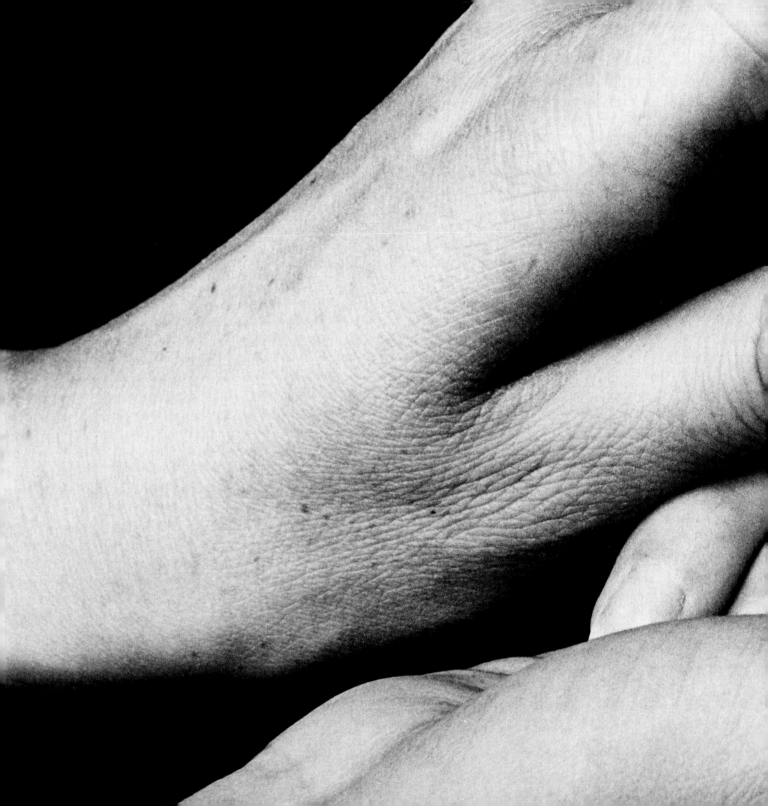

Understanding Pediatric Basics

Assessment
Procedures
Hospitalization
Restraints

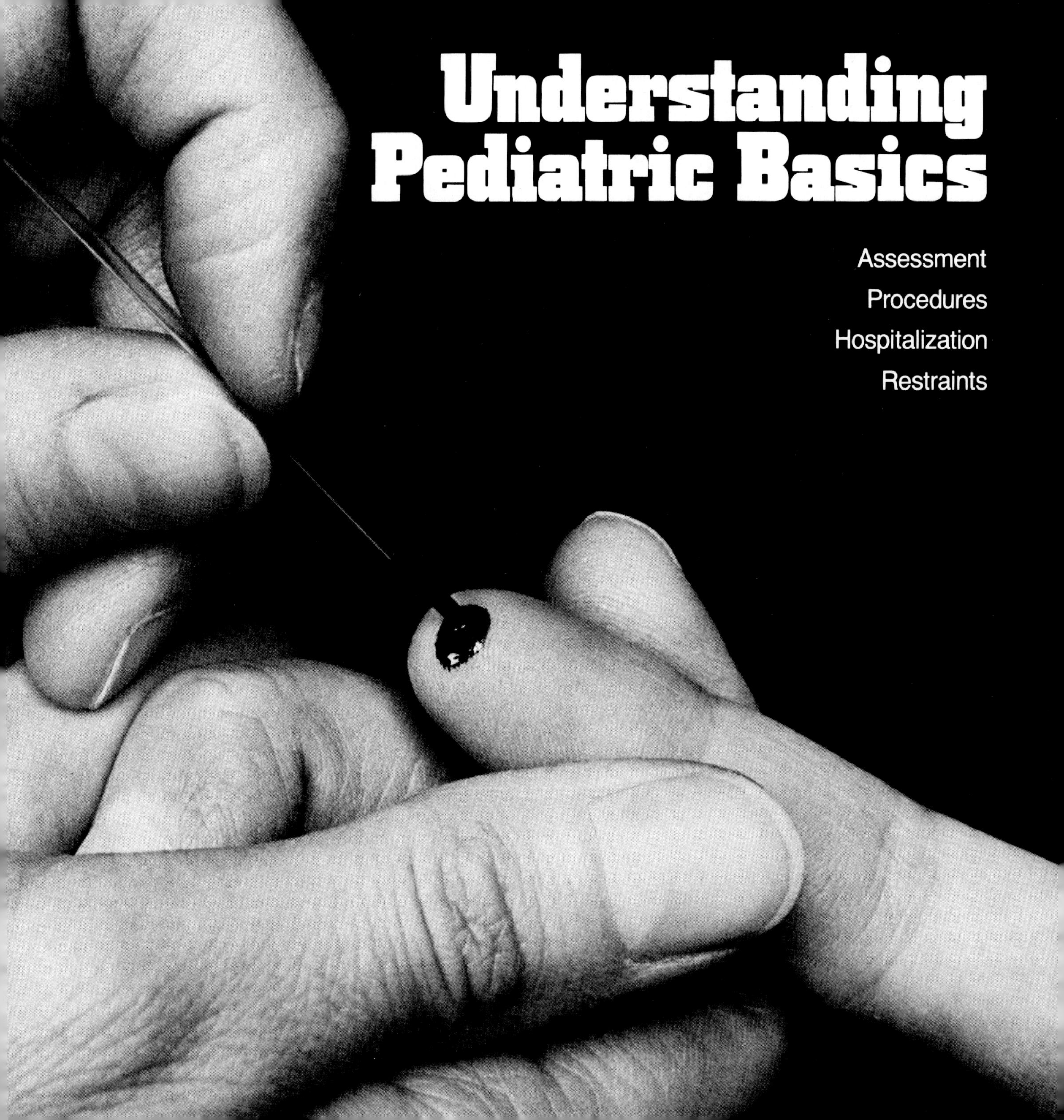

Assessment

How to make friends

"I'm worried about my daughter Jenny," Mrs. Lang confides. "She's almost 2 years old, and she's not talking yet. She was always a quiet baby, so I wasn't worried at first. But now..." As a nurse, what would you advise?

Of course, you'd recommend a physical assessment for Jenny, including tests for possible hearing impairment. And the sooner she gets it, the better. Like vision impairment, a hearing loss can profoundly affect a child's development. That's why, in this section, we'll place special emphasis on both vision and hearing assessment.

What other potential problem areas do you need to explore? That depends. Are you an office nurse? A hospital floor nurse? Does the child's health history suggest a particular problem? Your answers determine the extent of your examination. But for now, let's assume that your patient appears healthy. Use the following guidelines to decide if further investigation is needed.

1 *You'd like to talk with 4-year-old Alan Wolfe, and encourage his cooperation with your pediatric assessment. But when you approach him, he sits silently, staring up with his big brown eyes. You're afraid he'll cry. What's he thinking?*

If you can remember how it felt to be a child, you may gain some insight into Alan's behavior. From his viewpoint, most people are bigger than he is. What's more, strange people—like you—make him feel shy and uncertain. Uniforms and equipment may look scary. How can you put him at ease?

Let's start at the beginning. Read this photostory for tips that work wonders with many young patients.

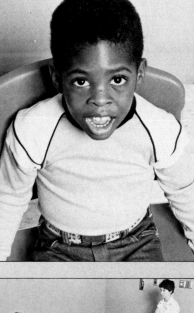

2 When you enter the room, move to the corner farthest from the child. By doing so, you allow the child to size you up from a safe distance.

Give the child a chance to make the first move toward you—when *he's* ready. But if you must make the first move, avoid scaring the child with sudden movements, or over-enthusiasm.

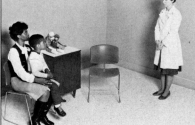

3 Place yourself at the child's eye level or lower, and introduce yourself. But avoid prolonged eye contact, since the child may feel that you're staring at him.

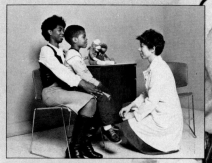

4 When the child's at ease, offer to shake his hand. This nonthreatening physical contact may break the ice between you. *Nursing tip:* Take this opportunity to assess the child's grasp and skin temperature.

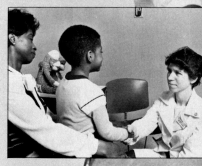

SPECIAL CONSIDERATIONS

5 Use play techniques and toys, such as puppets and dolls, to communicate with the child. Remember, because play is familiar to the child, he'll find it reassuring. Talk to him about toys, hobbies, pets, or other subjects he's interested in, and encourage his friendship with compliments. Use toys to help him describe symptoms; for example, ask him to show you where it hurts by pointing to a specific spot on a doll. If possible, let the child play with assessment equipment before you use it. Continue to use play techniques throughout the assessment procedure.

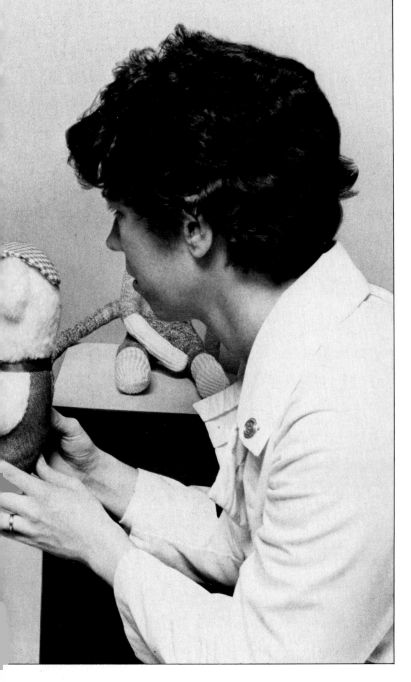

Communicating effectively: Some tips

What's the first step toward providing complete care for your pediatric patient? Compiling an up-to-date patient history, of course. Sure, it sounds elementary—but as a pediatric nurse, you know what a challenge it can be. Not only must you establish rapport with your young patient, but you must communicate effectively with his parents or other care-givers as well. Your success—or lack of it—can set the tone for all future interactions. So, before you take another pediatric history, take a moment to review these tips.

• Provide a private, quiet setting for the child and his family. Also, provide toys, games, or books to distract the child. He may become restless or anxious during a long interview.

Nursing tip: Note how the child plays with toys. Your observations can give you insight into his coordination and motor development.

• Introduce yourself to the whole family. Sit down to conduct the interview, to avoid giving them the impression that you're rushed. Also, by being closer to the child's level, you appear less threatening to him. Address family members individually, by name, throughout the interview. Try to establish a warm, relaxed atmosphere.

• Tell the parents why you need a nursing history. They may wonder why they must repeat some of the same information they've already given the doctor. Explain that your nursing history will help you tailor nursing care for the child's individual needs.

• Determine the identity of the child's primary care-giver. Don't just assume that his mother has this role—in some families, the father, a grandparent, or an older sibling assumes this responsibility. Try to elicit most of your information from the primary care-giver, since he or she probably knows the child best.

• Address yourself to the child as well as to his parents. If he's age 4 or older, he probably can supply some reliable information himself. But, even if he can't, don't ignore him. By showing interest in him, you can begin establishing rapport.

• No matter whom you're addressing, use a quiet, unhurried tone of voice and simple, direct language. Use everyday words instead of medical terms.

• Use open-ended questions whenever possible, rather than questions requiring only a simple yes or no. This technique encourages the family to provide more detailed information. For example, don't say, "Has Johnny had all his vaccinations?" Instead, say, "What vaccinations has Johnny had?"

• Keep the interview as informal as possible. But don't let the conversation stray too far off the track. If necessary, redirect the conversation with a tactful comment like this: "Tell me some more about Johnny's nosebleeds. When do they usually occur?"

• Be a good listener. Don't interrupt, and encourage the parents and child to elaborate on their answers, when appropriate. Whenever possible, document their exact words.

• Stay alert for nonverbal clues to meaning; for example, nodding, looking down suddenly, nervous hand gestures, or restlessness. *Note:* If parents seem reluctant to answer a particular question, explain why you need the information. But if they continue to resist, don't pressure them. You may discourage them from providing future health care for the child. Clearly document which aspects of health history they're reluctant to discuss.

• When documenting information about the child's development, ask specific, concrete questions. Remember, affectionate parents sometimes exaggerate their child's abilities. Don't say, "Does Maggie talk much yet?" Instead say, "What words and phrases does Maggie use regularly?"

• Give parents a chance to express their concerns. Keep in mind that they may have questions they're embarrassed to broach. If you perceive an unexpressed concern, try to draw them out with a statement like this: "Many parents have difficulty toilet training their child. Has this been a problem for you?"

• Remain open, accepting, and nonjudgmental throughout the interview. Avoid offering advice or expressing opinions until you've documented as much information as possible about the child and his health.

Assessment

DOCUMENTING

Taking a child's history

Chances are, your doctor's office, clinic, or hospital has an interview form for you to follow when you document your patient's history. Make sure it covers these major points:

Identity: Document the child's name, age, address, religion, and sex. Also, document the name and relationship of others who have provided information, and the date of the interview.

Chief complaint: What's the reason for this visit? Does the child have a specific problem, or is he here only for a routine checkup? If he currently has a health problem, describe it thoroughly, including how long he's had the problem, what its signs and symptoms are, whether any actions or treatment makes the symptoms better or worse, and whether the parents have been giving the child any medications for it. (Don't forget to document home remedies and over-the-counter medications, as well as any the doctor's prescribed.) Ask the child to describe his symptoms; document his exact words or gestures.

Medical history: Include prenatal and birth complications, postnatal problems, and early feeding difficulties. These facts can provide clues to current problems. Also, document all illnesses the child's had (for example, chicken pox, mumps, measles, tonsillitis, earaches, and flu), and ask the parents to estimate how often he gets minor colds. Note any accidents (including burns and poisoning), surgeries, or hospitalizations. Of course, you'll also document any chronic problems, such as a heart defect or diabetes. Finally, document all the vaccinations the child's received. *Note:* Confirm this information with the child's medical records, if available. If the family's new to the community, stress the importance of having a copy of their medical records transferred.

Medications and allergies: Is the child currently taking medication? If so, document its name and dosage and the reason he needs it. Then, find out if the child has any chronic allergies, including hay fever and asthma, and if he's ever had any allergic reactions to medication (particularly penicillin), food (including milk and fruit juices), insect stings, or anything else. (If necessary, describe signs of possible allergic reaction to the parents.) Document allergies on your interview form and document medication allergies in red on the child's Kardex and chart cover. If the parents are unaware of any possible allergies, write "No allergies known" on your interview form.

Habits: Find out about the child's eating, sleeping, and elimination patterns. Does he have any specific eating or bedtime routines? Does he have frequent nightmares? Does he wet his bed? If the answers you get reveal anything abnormal (for example, if the child's chronically constipated), ask for more information about his eating and drinking habits. Also, inquire about the child's play habits, and his relationship with his peers.

Systems review: Working from head to toe, inquire about any possible problems. Use open-ended questions, unless you repeatedly receive negative answers. In that case, ask more specific questions. For example, if the parents insist that the child's always healthy, you might ask whether he ever has a runny nose. Use the parents' responses to guide you when you conduct a physical examination.

Family history: Does anyone in his family have a chronic illness, such as diabetes, hypertension, asthma, a birth defect, a severe or unusual allergy, heart or kidney disease, or cancer? Are any members of the child's immediate family dead? (If so, document the cause of death.) Note any major illnesses of the child's siblings. (Consider using a genotype or pedigree chart to document this information.)

Developmental history: Document the child's growth and development. When did he first roll over, sit alone, stand up, and walk? When did he begin talking? When did his first tooth erupt? Pay particular attention to his interactions with you and his family. Note whether he seems older or younger than his age. (For guidelines on assessing development, see the appendices to this book.)

Other considerations: Briefly describe your overall impression of the child, including any physical, emotional, or developmental problems you've noticed or suspect. Ask yourself if his balance, coordination, and cognitive ability seem normal for his age. If appropriate, consider referring the child to a child psychologist for developmental testing.

Pediatric assessment: Some guidelines

Little Sammy Tilden's one of your favorite patients. When you examined him 6 months ago, at age 18 months, he was a cheerful, cooperative toddler. But today, to your dismay, he seems like a different child. Cranky and withdrawn, he resists you at every step of the physical assessment procedure. What's gone wrong?

Maybe nothing. A child's personality can change dramatically, in even 6 month's time. As he changes, his view of the world changes, too. That's why careful preparation, geared to the child's current stage of development, is essential—no matter how many times the child's experienced a particular procedure in the past.

Of course, because each child's an individual, you can never predict exactly how he'll behave simply by noting his age. But by understanding the approaches and techniques that work best for each age group, you can make the examination proceed as smoothly as possible.

For example, let's say that your patient's between 6 and 12 months old. You can expect him to be upset if you separate him from his parent. So, to minimize problems, ask the parent to hold the infant during the examination, and to distract him with toys or quiet talk. If the infant's quiet, auscultate his chest and abdomen first. Then, because he may become upset when you examine his head, follow a toe-to-head format to complete the examination.

Nursing tip: When assessing an infant, speak to him and observe his responses. Expect him to acknowledge your voice by exhibiting the blink or startle reflex, turning his head toward the sound, and/or lying still, as though listening.

In the following chart, you'll find tips for assessing other pediatric age groups. For any pediatric assessment, keep these basic guidelines in mind:
• Wash your hands before beginning.
• Don't undress the child yourself; instead, ask his parent to do it. The child will feel less threatened if his parent undresses him.
• Before performing auscultation, percussion, and palpation, warm both your hands and your equipment (including the stethoscope's diaphragm).

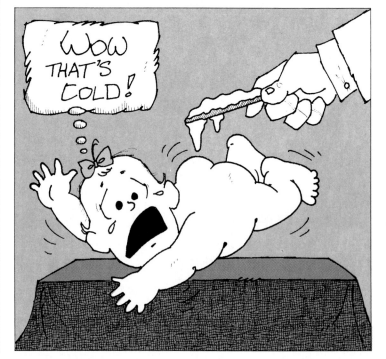

1-3 Toddler

May be shy around strangers and resist being undressed or touched by you. Learning to explore and manipulate his environment.

Assessment guidelines
• Take advantage of the child's growing curiosity about his surroundings. Attract his attention with dolls, puppets, and other toys, and use them to acquaint him with the equipment you'll use (for example, the otoscope, stethoscope, and blood pressure cuff). Give him a toy to play with during the examination. *Important:* Keep in mind that a toddler's attention span is very short, and that he may be too shy or frightened to play. Use your own judgment about how long to play with him.
• Allow the child to sit in his parent's lap, or to stand next to his parent, throughout the examination. Placing the child on an examination table will probably frighten him. *Note:* If a procedure requires a reclining position, have the child lie on his parent's lap.
• Ask the parent to remove the child's clothing as you examine each body part, and then to replace his clothing. Minimizing the time the child remains undressed will reduce his anxiety.
• If the child's quiet, auscultate his chest and abdomen first. Leave until last those procedures the child may find upsetting; for a toddler, these include the ear and mouth examination.

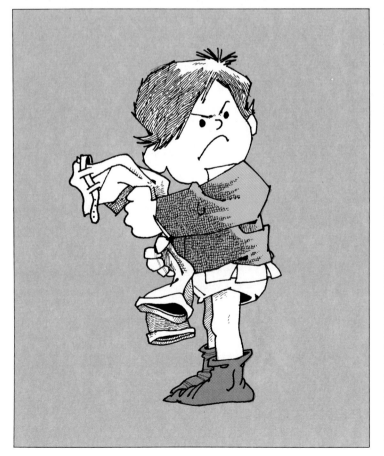

4-6 Preschooler

Eager to please when put at ease; enjoys being the center of attention. Beginning to develop a sense of initiative.

Assessment guidelines
• Allow the child to choose where to sit during the examination. He may prefer to sit on his parent's lap, on a chair next to his parent, or on the examination table. (A preschooler may enjoy the feeling of being on stage while sitting on the table.)
• Use play and explanation to prepare the child, as suggested for the toddler. Explain that the stethoscope helps you "hear how things are working inside." If the child seems to enjoy friendly teasing (many children do at this age), explain that you're going to examine his ears "to see if an elephant or giraffe's inside." When auscultating his abdomen, say that you're listening to what he had for breakfast.
• Encourage the child's cooperation with flattery and frequent praise. Tell (rather than ask) him what he can do to help you; for example, say, "Now, hold up your T-shirt so I can listen to how your heart sounds."
• Allow the child to undress himself, if he can. Permit him to leave on his underwear.
• Since a well-prepared preschooler is usually cooperative and unafraid, follow a head-to-toe format. *Note:* Younger preschoolers may fantasize about mutilation when around strangers; this may make them anxious about assessment procedures. Provide additional support and reassurance if you suspect you are assessing such a child.

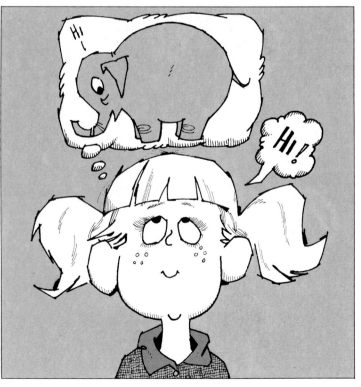

Assessment

Pediatric assessment: Some guidelines continued

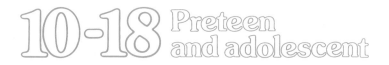

7-9 Early school age

Interested in what's being done, and why. Capable of following directions and problem-solving. Developing a sense of industry, privacy, and independence.

Assessment guidelines
- Ask the child to sit or lie on the examination table, whichever he prefers.
- Ask the child if he wants his parents to leave or stay. (He'll probably want them to stay.)
- Explain what you're going to do and why, using terms the child can understand, and show him the appropriate equipment as you talk. Use play techniques, including riddles and stories. (Remember, this age group has good verbal skills.) Demonstrate procedures on a doll or the parent. For example, before taking the child's blood pressure, demonstrate the procedure on his parent, and allow him to watch the sphygmomanometer. Explain that you want to see how high the needle will go.
- Provide a drape or gown. Although a child this age is developing a sense of modesty, he probably won't mind undressing if he can cover himself.
- Encourage the child to ask questions, and answer them.
- Encourage cooperation with flattery. Since the child probably enjoys being the center of attention, ask him questions and give him directions as you work.
- Follow a head-to-toe format, but assess his genitalia last.

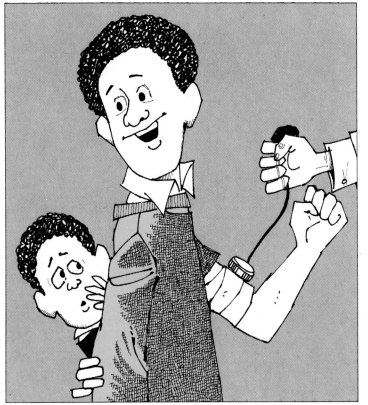

10-18 Preteen and adolescent

Interested in what's being done and why; beginning to take responsibility for own health-care needs. Concerned with body image, changes, and functions.

Assessment guidelines
- Allow the adolescent to sit up, if he prefers.
- Ask him if he'd like his parents to stay or leave. (He'll probably want them to leave.)
- Explain what you're going to do and why, and answer any questions he may have.
- Allow him to undress in private, and to wear a gown during the examination. Talk to him while you're examining him.
- Follow a head-to-toe format. Expose only one part of the body at a time. *Important:* Examine his genitalia last, since he may find this embarrassing.
- If appropriate, reassure the adolescent that everything looks normal.
- Encourage him to ask questions and express concerns. Teach him about his body and health-care needs, as necessary.

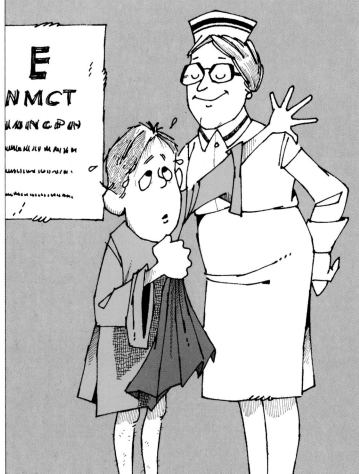

Assessing vital signs and growth

1 *Imagine that you're planning to perform a routine physical assessment of 7-year-old Ginny Lowenstein. The first step's documenting her vital signs and making general observations about her growth and development. For guidelines, read this photostory.*

First, obtain an oral thermometer, sphygmomanometer and pediatric blood pressure cuff, stethoscope, and scale with height measurement bar. If you plan to measure Ginny's head circumference, also obtain a tape measure.

Give Ginny and her mother an explanation of each procedure as you go along—even if Ginny's undergone physical assessments in the past. Remember to use words that Ginny can easily understand. Answer any questions Ginny or her mother asks. Then, wash your hands. *Important:* Try to take all vital signs measurements while the child's quiet. But if she won't settle down, take them anyway, and document the child's behavior during the procedure. (If the child later becomes quiet, repeat the measurements.)

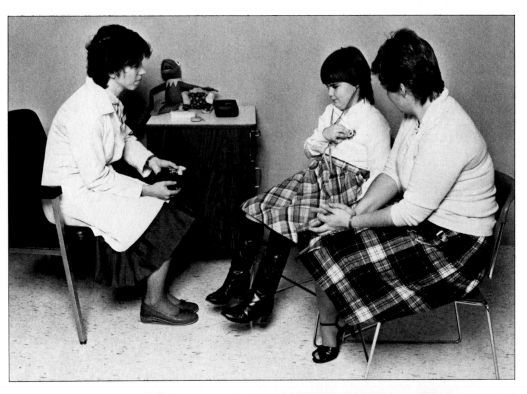

2 First, determine your patient's weight. (Before beginning, make sure that the scale is properly balanced.) Weigh an older child, like Ginny, in her underwear or a light patient gown; weigh a toddler or infant without clothing. (To weigh an infant, of course, you'll need to use an infant platform scale.)

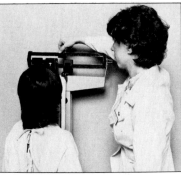

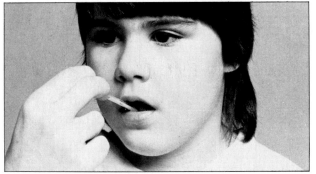

3 Now, determine your patient's height. Measure an older child's standing height, as shown here. But if your patient is less than age 3, place her in a supine position on the examination table and measure her recumbent height. With her legs fully extended, mark the table paper at the vertex of her head and the heels of her feet. Then, measure the distance between the marks. Or, measure the child using a measuring board.

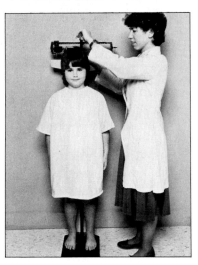

4 Next, prepare to take Ginny's temperature. Since she's older than age 5, use an oral thermometer. *Note:* If Ginny's had anything to drink in the last 20 minutes, wait 15 minutes before beginning.

Place the thermometer tip well under her tongue, as shown. Instruct her to close her mouth and hold the thermometer securely under her tongue, but remind her not to bite down. If you're using a glass thermometer, leave it in place for 7 minutes. (If you're using an electronic thermometer, leave it in place until the machine signals.)

If your patient's less than age 5—or if she's recently had oral surgery or is mouth-breathing—use the rectal route instead. Leave a glass thermometer in place for 3 minutes. Keep in mind that rectal temperature is normally about 1° higher than oral temperature. (An electronic thermometer compensates for this difference.) If the child objects to the rectal route, use the axillary route instead. Leave a glass thermometer in place for about 10 minutes. Axillary temperatures are slightly lower than oral temperatures.

Assessment

Assessing vital signs and growth continued

5 If you're taking an oral temperature with a glass thermometer, you'll have time to assess several other vital signs while you wait. For example, now's a good time to measure Ginny's respiratory rate. Because telling the child what you're doing may make her self-conscious (temporarily raising her respiratory rate), try to unobtrusively observe her respiratory rate for 1 minute. As an alternative, gently place your warm hands on her chest and count her breaths, as the nurse is doing here. Document the rate.

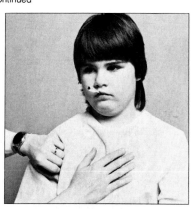

6 Next, take the child's pulse for 1 minute. For an older child, like Ginny, record the radial pulse rate. For a child younger than age 2, record the apical pulse. Document your findings (including which pulse you used). *Note:* A child's pulse rate may fluctuate rapidly.

Are 7 minutes up? Remove the oral thermometer and document Ginny's temperature, as well as the route used.

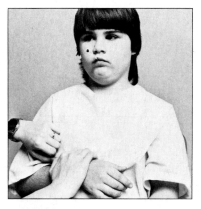

7 Now, take the child's blood pressure. Make sure to use the proper cuff size: the cuff's bladder should be one fifth longer than the circumference of the child's arm. When you apply the cuff, it should cover about two thirds of her upper arm. Document your reading. Keep in mind that her blood pressure will be temporarily higher than normal if she's upset, if she's just eaten, or if she's just urinated or defecated.

Note: The diastolic sound you hear in a child or infant won't be as distinct as an adult's.

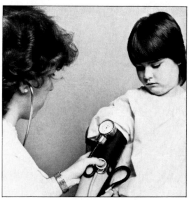

8 Chances are, you won't measure an older child's head circumference. But if your patient's under age 3, or if her head's unusually large or small, a head measurement provides a valuable developmental indicator. To get an accurate one, use a paper tape measure, because a cloth tape may stretch, altering the measurement. Pass it around the most prominent part of the occiput and the supraorbital ridges (the area just above the eyebrows). For accuracy, take three measurements, and record the largest one.

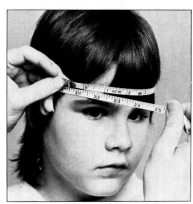

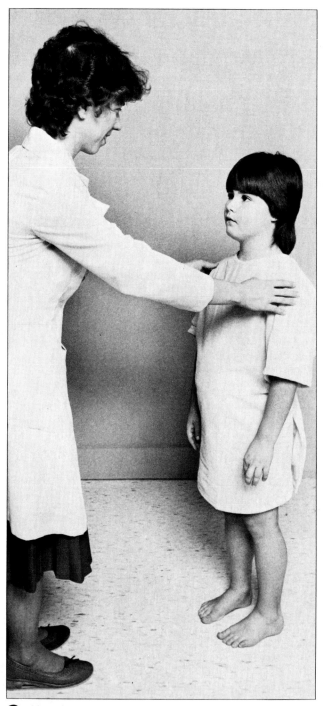

9 Now that you've completed the first part of your assessment, what's your overall impression of the child's health and development? Does she seem well-nourished? Is she in any apparent distress? Document in your nurses' notes your subjective impressions, and continue to observe the child throughout other phases of the assessment.

For guidelines on normal height, weight, and vital signs measurements, consult this book's appendices.

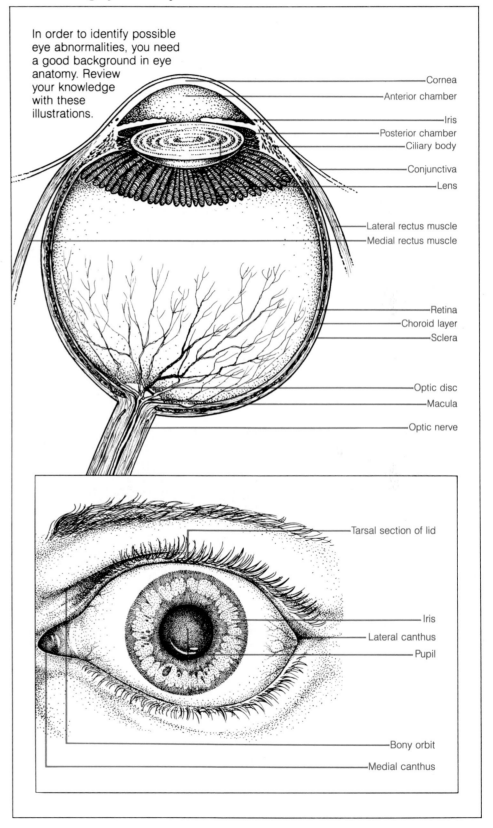

MINI-ASSESSMENT

Using the flush technique

If your patient's less than age 1, you may have difficulty hearing diastolic and systolic sounds when you attempt to measure his blood pressure. To estimate his mean blood pressure, use the flush technique. Elevate the infant's arm or thigh. (Either is okay, since arm and thigh pressures are equal in children under age 1.) Wait until the skin blanches. Now, apply the proper size cuff to the infant's limb and inflate the cuff to about 75 mm Hg. Then, lower the limb and begin deflating the cuff. Note the pressure reading when the entire limb flushes with color. This reading is the infant's approximate mean blood pressure.

Evaluating a child's skin

The condition of a child's skin can tell you a great deal about his general condition. Document it thoroughly, paying particular attention to these assessment variables.

Color: Observe for signs of pallor, cyanosis, and jaundice. Also check the nailbeds for cyanosis and the sclerae for jaundice (especially if the child's black). Note any skin discoloration, including hyper- or hypopigmented spots, erythema or redness, ecchymosis, or bruises.

Turgor: Gently grasp abdominal skin between your thumb and index finger; then, pull it away from the abdomen. Quickly release the skin—it should immediately return to its original position. If it returns slowly, or appears wrinkled, suspect dehydration or poor nutrition.

Texture and temperature: Note the dryness, oiliness, moistness, and smoothness of the skin, as well as any lesions. Check for uniform skin temperature, keeping in mind that exposed skin (such as the skin on the hands) may be slightly cooler than other areas. Although the extremities may be slightly cooler than other parts of the body, expect their temperatures to be equal bilaterally.

Hair: Describe its color, distribution, texture, and location.

Hands: Observe for clubbing of fingertips (a sign of cardiovascular disorders), ragged or bitten nails (a possible sign of chronic anxiety), or a single transverse (simian) crease in each palm (a sign of Down's syndrome).

Important: Never overlook or ignore signs of child abuse; for example, multiple bruising, human bite marks, cigarette burns, or numerous healing lesions. To learn more about child abuse and how to deal with it, see the fourth section of this book.

Understanding eye anatomy

In order to identify possible eye abnormalities, you need a good background in eye anatomy. Review your knowledge with these illustrations.

Cornea
Anterior chamber
Iris
Posterior chamber
Ciliary body
Conjunctiva
Lens
Lateral rectus muscle
Medial rectus muscle
Retina
Choroid layer
Sclera
Optic disc
Macula
Optic nerve

Tarsal section of lid
Iris
Lateral canthus
Pupil
Bony orbit
Medial canthus

Assessment

Inspecting a child's eyes

1 *To assess your patient's eyes, you'll need a penlight and an ophthalmoscope. Here's what to do:*

First, explain the procedure to the child, and show her the ophthalmoscope. Turn on the light for her, and allow her to play with the instrument if she wishes.

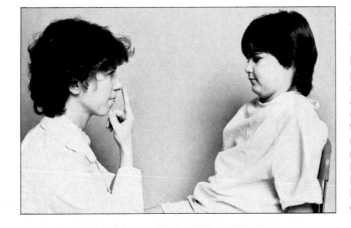

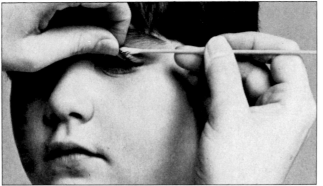

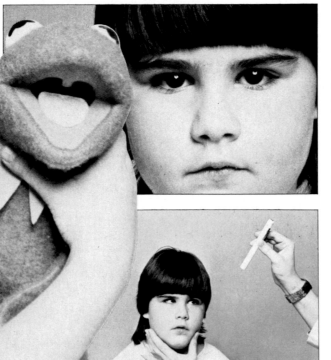

2 Now, inspect the child's eyes for general appearance. To do so, place yourself at the child's eye level, 1' to 2' from her face, and instruct her to look at your nose. Observe eye placement and alignment, color, size, shape, and movement. Possible abnormalities include drooping lids (ptosis), asymmetrical blinking, nystagmus (involuntary rapid eyeball movement, possibly indicating blindness, ear infection or damage, or brain tumor), strabismus (eye malalignment, including cross-eyes and lazy eye), squinting, inflammation, discharge, or excessive tearing.

3 Next, evert the child's upper and lower eyelids and examine the conjunctivae. Expect them to be shiny pink. Inflammation may suggest conjunctivitis, irritation, or eyestrain; pallor suggests anemia.

4 Suppose you suspect strabismus, but you're not sure. (For example, an Oriental child may have epicanthal folds that make her eyes *appear* malaligned, when in fact they're normal.) To investigate further, check the child's corneal light reflex. Stand 14' to 16' (4.2 to 4.8 m) from the child, and shine a flashlight or gooseneck lamp directly into her eyes. The light should reflect from the same spot on each pupil, as shown here. If the light doesn't reflect symmetrically, strabismus is present.

5 To check the child's extraocular movement, hold up your penlight or a toy about 12″ (30 cm) in front of her nose, and ask her to watch it without moving her head. Slowly move the penlight, first to one side, then the other. Next, slowly move the penlight up and down. Watch the child's eyes closely for abnormal eye movement; for example, jerking, oscillation, asymmetry, or lagging. These signs may indicate extraocular muscle problems.

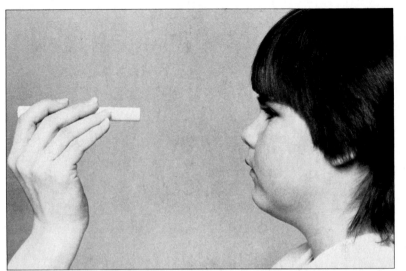

6 Now, test the child's pupils for accommodation and their reactions to light. To test reactions to light, shine your penlight into one of her pupils; it should constrict. When you remove the light, her pupil should dilate. Repeat the test on the other pupil.

To test accommodation (the eyes' ability to focus at different distances), quickly bring your penlight or some other bright object toward the child's eyes. As you do so, her pupils should constrict equally.

Record normal findings as PERRLA (pupils equal, round, reacting to light; and accommodation).

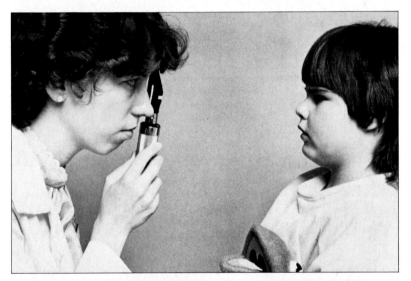

7 If you're skilled at using an ophthalmoscope, prepare to examine the child's cornea and retina. First, darken the room. (Darkness causes the pupils to dilate, exposing more of the retina's periphery.)

Set the ophthalmoscope's lens setting at zero, and turn on the ophthalmoscope's light. Choose the appropriate aperture. (For most patients, the large, clear aperture is best.)

To inspect the child's right eye, as the nurse is doing here, position yourself on the child's right side at her eye level, at a distance of about 12″ (30 cm). Place the ophthalmoscope in front of your right eye and against your forehead, as shown.

Expect to see a red or orange glow, called the red reflex, on her pupil. (If your patient's black, the red reflex may be lighter in color.) Absence of the red reflex may indicate corneal lesions, cataracts, or retinal detachment. Repeat the procedure on the other eye.

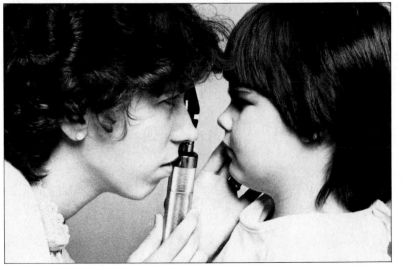

8 Next, prepare to examine the fundus (the eye's deepest portion) by asking the child to focus on a picture on the wall. Tell her to try to keep her eyes as still as possible. Then, positioning yourself as above, move your ophthalmoscope closer to the child's eye. Look into the middle of the fundus to locate the optic disc. (Rotate the ophthalmoscope's lens setting as necessary to focus properly.) The optic disc should appear flat with distinct edges. Examine the blood vessels surrounding the optic disk and spreading over the retina for hemorrhages, aneurysms, or exudate.

Note: Retinal hemorrhage may result from head trauma. Consider the possibility of child abuse. (For other possible signs of abuse, see the fourth section of this book.)

Then, locate the macula (about 3 mm from the optic disc's temporal edge). It should appear to be without blood vessels, and have a bright spot in its center. Repeat the procedure on the other eye.

Document all your observations. If you noted any abnormalities, refer the child to an eye care specialist for further evaluation.

Assessment

Testing vision

1 *Even if your patient has no apparent vision problems, don't neglect to give her a routine vision test. By doing so, you may identify a vision disorder, such as a refraction error, before it makes the child uncomfortable or affects her schoolwork.*

In the following photostory, we'll show you how to test vision, using a handy flip chart. It's designed to test the child's vision at a distance of 10' (3 m), which makes it convenient if your assessment room is small. Although the chart we're featuring displays numbers, you may use a letter chart instead, or (for a preschooler) an E or picture symbol chart. Here's how to proceed.

First, explain the test to the child. Show her the chart, as the nurse is doing here. *Note:* If you're using an E chart, show her a demonstration E card to acquaint her with the symbol. Tell her that during the test, you'll ask her to look at similar Es on the chart and describe which way the legs are pointing. Or, you may ask her to use her first three fingers to imitate the E's position.

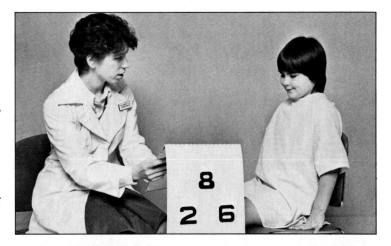

2 Next, give her an eye occluder protected with a disposable cover, or a clean paper cup (as shown here), and show her how to use it. Instruct her to keep both eyes open during the test, even when one's covered. (For infection control, discard the cup or occluder cover after use by one child.)

🖘 *Nursing tip:* If you prefer, use a clean opaque card instead of an eye occluder or cup. Properly dispose of the card after use.

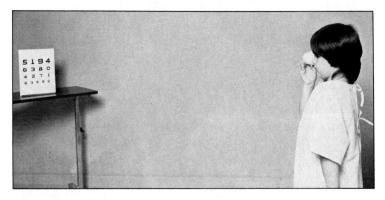

3 Place the flip chart on a table at the child's eye level. Position the child so she's standing 10' (3 m) away from the chart. Ask her to cover her right eye, and look at the chart. Then, ask her to describe the smallest line of numbers she can see clearly. (Many charts contain colored horizontal lines, for easy reference points.) Instruct her to cover her left eye, and repeat the test. Document her visual acuity in each eye. For example, record normal vision as O.D. (right eye) 20/20; O.S. (left eye) 20/20.

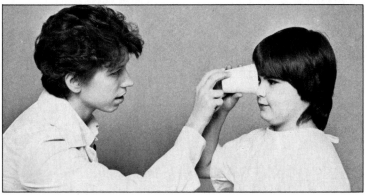

4 What if the child has difficulty seeing even the largest number? Move her closer to the chart, until she can clearly see the largest number with her left eye. Document the distance she's standing from the chart. Then, test and document her right eye's vision.

Refer your patient to an eye care specialist if you identify any of these problems: an obvious disorder, such as cross-eyes (regardless of visual acuity), a one-line difference in acuity between her eyes, or visual acuity of 20/40 or less in either eye. (If your patient's less than age 4, refer her for further evaluation if her vision's less than 20/50 in either eye.)

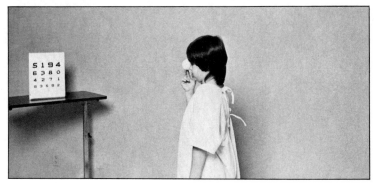

Using a wall chart: Making preparations

In the preceding photostory, you saw how to test a child's vision using a flip chart. But suppose you're using a wall chart instead? For accurate results, follow these guidelines:
• Hang the chart on a light-colored wall. Position it so the 20/20 and 20/30 lines are at the child's eye level. *Note:* Consider whether the child will be standing or sitting for the test.
• Secure the chart at all four corners, so that it's flat.
• Make sure the room's brightly lighted, but eliminate glare from windows or lamps. (If you have a light meter, adjust the lighting until the chart's illumination intensity is 10 to 30 foot-candles.)
• Using a strip of tape, mark a spot exactly 20 feet (6 m) from the chart. During the test, position the child so his heels rest on this mark. Or, if he's sitting, position the chair so its back legs rest on the mark.

Visual acuity: What's normal?

As you probably know, a child doesn't develop 20/20 vision until he's nearly school age. How clearly should a younger child be able to see? Use the following as a guide.

Age	Visual acuity
Newborn	20/300
4 to 5 months	20/200
11 to 12 months	20/100
1½ to 2 years	20/40
3 to 4 years	20/30
5 to 6 years	20/20

Identifying vision impairment

If your patient's between the ages of 6 months and 3 years, identifying impaired vision may take some detective work. The child himself may not realize that anything's wrong—or, if he does, he may be too inarticulate to tell you. These factors also make formal vision testing unreliable. But by piecing together your clinical observations with what the parents have noticed about the child's behavior, you may be able to identify some common disorders. Stay alert for the clues listed at right.

Problem	Signs and symptoms	Behavioral clues
Congenital blindness	• Nystagmus or slow, lateral eye movements • Fixed pupils • Easily-observable strabismus • Possible lack of pupillary response to light	• Can't fix eyes on moving objects • Can't initiate or maintain eye contact • Doesn't respond to visual stimuli
Refraction disorders (myopia, hyperopia, astigmatism)	• Blurred vision • Dizziness • Headache • Nausea • Esotropia or cross-eyes (caused by child's attempt to compensate for hyperopia)	• Writes, reads, or draws with face close to paper • Habitually tilts head, or carries it thrust forward; appears clumsy • Frequently rubs eyes or blinks • Does poorly at school
Strabismus (including amblyopia, or lazy eye)	• Observable malalignment, such as cross-eyes • Diplopia (double vision) or blurred vision • Photophobia • Dizziness and headache *Note:* May accompany Down's syndrome, cerebral palsy, or mental retardation	• Frowns or squints in order to see clearly through one eye • May exhibit poor depth perception • Habitually tilts head to one side
Glaucoma	• Child may see halos around lights • Blurred vision • Loss of peripheral vision • Photophobia • Chronic or acute eye discomfort • Eyeball enlargement • Pupil dilation (acute glaucoma)	• May blink spasmodically • May vomit or complain of nausea during onset of acute glaucoma
Cataract	• Milky-white pupil • Opaque lens • Strabismus • Blurred vision • Child may see halos around lights • Loss of peripheral vision • Photophobia	• May have difficulty reading, writing, or drawing • May exhibit poor vision in bright lighting; better vision in dim lighting
Retinal detachment	• Gray, opaque retina • Painless, progressive vision loss • Child may see spots, shadows, and floating objects, or flashes of light (especially when looking quickly to one side) *Note:* Extreme myopia may predispose a child to retinal detachment.	• May complain of seeing spots or flashing lights

Assessment

Dealing with common eye infections

A child will put his hands almost anywhere—including in his eyes. That's why he's so prone to eye infections. Learn about three of the most common eye infections by studying the following chart.

Problem	Signs and symptoms	Possible causes	Nursing considerations
Conjunctivitis	• Watery to purulent discharge possible • Generalized redness • Itching, pain *Note:* Vision may be normal or slightly blurred.	• Bacterial, chlamydial, viral, or (rarely) fungal infection • Allergy or irritation • Rocky Mountain spotted fever • Parasitic diseases	• Apply antibiotic eyedrops or eye ointment such as chloramphenicol (Chloroptic Ophthalmic*), as ordered, to treat infection. • Tell parents that conjunctivitis is highly contagious. Warn them not to allow family members to share washcloths, towels, or pillows. • Instruct the child not to rub his eyes. Consider covering his hands with mittens or socks to prevent eye scratching. If the child continues to rub his eyes, then consider restraining him, but only as a last resort. • Teach him and his parents proper handwashing technique, to minimize risk of spreading infection. • Teach the parents to correctly instill eyedrops and ointments without touching the child's eyelids or eyelashes.
Keratitis (inflammation of the cornea)	• Opaque cornea • Mild to severe pain • Watery to purulent discharge possible • Prominent redness at corneal-scleral margin • Photophobia • Blurred vision • Interruption of red reflex	• Previous damage to cornea • Infection by herpes simplex type 1 virus, bacteria, or fungus • Inability to protect cornea by blinking and closing eyelids • Congenital syphilis	• Apply anitibiotic eye ointment such as chloramphenicol (Chloroptic Ophthalmic*), as ordered, to treat infection. • If the child can't close his eyes, tape his eyelid closed or provide a protective covering. • Prevent further irritation by applying an eye pad over the affected eye, as needed.
Stye (hordeolum)	• Redness and swelling of eyelid • Abscess at eyelid margin; eyelash may point out from its center • Abscess in conjunctiva (internal stye)	• Staphylococcal infection	• Treat the same as conjunctivitis. • Teach parents how to apply warm compresses, as ordered. Tell them to dispose of the compress after each use, or launder it separately, to avoid spreading infection. • Warn child and parents against squeezing the stye, because this may spread the infection and cause eyelid cellulitis.

*Available in both the United States and in Canada

Examining your patient's ears

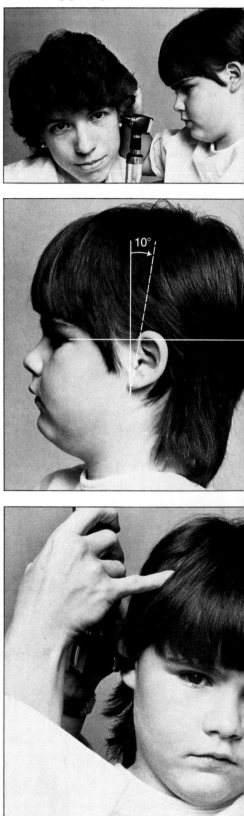

1 As the next step in your assessment, prepare to examine your patient's external ears (auricles or pinnae), external ear canals, and eardrums (tympanic membranes). To do this, you'll need an otoscope with a small speculum attachment. Follow these steps.

First, acquaint the child with the otoscope, and tell her what you're planning to do. If she's curious, let her examine *your* ear, as the nurse is doing here.

2 Then, inspect each of the child's auricles. To determine if it's positioned properly, imagine a line from the outer (lateral) canthus of each eye to the occiput (back of the head). Then, draw an imaginary line that's perpendicular to the horizontal line and that drops directly in front of the auricle, as shown here. The auricle's upper edge should meet this imaginary line, and its frontal plane should lie within 10° of the perpendicular line (see the dotted line). Low-set ears may indicate mental retardation or a renal disorder.

Examine the earlobes for cyanosis, which may indicate polycythemia or heart disease. Also, observe both auricles for size, symmetry, and prominence; flattened ears on an infant may suggest a history of poor positioning. (If necessary, teach the parents how to position their child.) Palpate the auricles, tragi, and mastoid processes for tenderness.

3 Now, get ready to examine the child's ear canal. Ask her to sit as quietly as possible, with her head turned to one side. Try to make the procedure like a game, by telling her that you're looking for an elephant or potato chip. *Note:* If your patient's an uncooperative toddler, ask her parent to hold her in the restraining position shown on page 45.

Hold the otoscope upside down, between your fingers and thumb. For stability, rest a finger on the child's head, as the nurse is doing here. To straighten the external ear canal, use your other hand to gently pull the auricle up and back. *Note:* If your patient's less than age 3, pull her auricle *down* and back.

Pointing the speculum downward and forward, insert it into the ear canal. Since her ear canal is only about 1″ (2.5 cm) long, take care to insert the speculum only ¼″ to ½″ (0.6 to 1.3 cm) into the ear canal. *Note:* As you advance the speculum, take care not to pack cerumen against the eardrum.

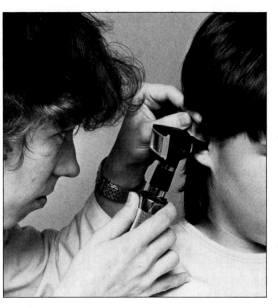

4 Examine the external ear canal, rotating the otoscope as necessary for a complete view. Normally, the external ear canal is pink, with a small amount of brown or orange wax (cerumen). Abnormal observations include redness, swelling, lesions, foreign bodies, scales, or exudate. If a wax plug blocks your view, notify the doctor—he may order an ear irrigation. *Note:* Does the child seem restless or uncomfortable? Keep in mind that inflammation may make an otoscopic exam painful for her.

If the ear canal's free of wax, consider that the child's parent may have cleansed it with a cotton swab. Advise the parent against inserting any object in the child's ear canal, and assure her that some wax accumulation is normal.

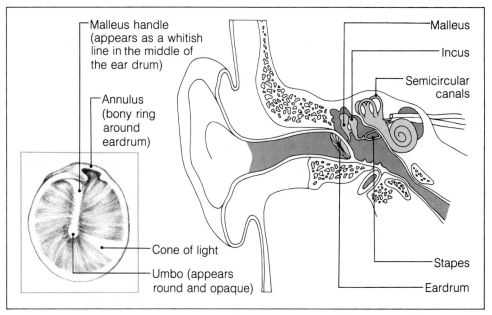

Malleus handle (appears as a whitish line in the middle of the ear drum)

Annulus (bony ring around eardrum)

Cone of light

Umbo (appears round and opaque)

Malleus

Incus

Semicircular canals

Stapes

Eardrum

5 Finally, inspect the patient's eardrum. If everything's okay, it'll look like a shiny, pearl-gray or pale pink disc that's slightly concave. A deep pink or red eardrum may indicate inflammation; a bulging white eardrum may indicate purulent drainage accumulation in the middle ear; a retracted eardrum may indicate scar tissue or a congenital malformation; and a blue eardrum may indicate accumulated blood. *Note:* If the child has recently been crying, the eardrum may be reddish.

Look for the malleus handle, which extends downward behind the center of the eardrum (as shown in the inset illustration).

If you can't see it, the eardrum may be bulging or scarred.

If the eardrum's positioned properly, you'll see a cone of light at the 5 o'clock position in the right ear, and at the 7 o'clock position in the left ear. Normally, the cone points toward the eardrum's center. If it's displaced or absent, your patient's eardrum may be bulging, retracted, or inflamed.

Document all your findings, including the amount, color and consistency of cerumen accumulations. *Note:* If you're not using a disposable cover on your speculum, remove the speculum and clean it with alcohol.

Assessment

Testing hearing ability

1 *Finished examining Ginny's ears? Then you're ready to assess her hearing. For a child older than age 4, like Ginny, use Weber's, Rinne, and whisper tests. To learn how, read on.*

For both Weber's and Rinne tests, you'll need a tuning fork in the C octave, such as the 256-hertz tuning fork featured in these photos. Make it vibrate by gently striking it against your fist, by pinching and releasing the fork's prongs, or by stroking the prongs upward.

Show the fork to the child, let her listen to the sound it makes, and explain the procedure to her in words she can understand. For example, tell her you want to play a game with her, to see how well she can hear the music the fork's making. *Note:* Don't try to assess your patient's hearing unless your own hearing is normal. Any hearing problem you have may compromise test results.

To perform Weber's test, hold the vibrating fork between your thumb and index finger and place the base of the tuning fork in the middle of the child's forehead, as shown here. Then, ask her if she can hear the sound equally well in each ear. If all's well, she'll hear the same volume and quality of sound in each ear.

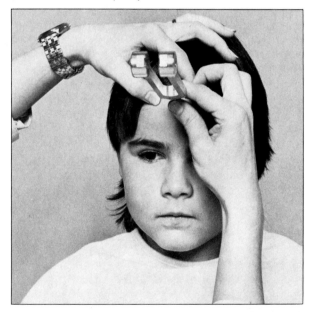

2 Perform the Rinne test to assess both bone and air conduction of sound. Again, vibrate the fork. Then, place the base of the tuning fork against the child's right mastoid process, as shown here. Ask the child to tell you when she hears a sound (she should hear it instantly), and when she no longer hears it. Note the length of time she heard the tone.

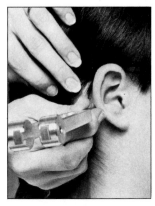

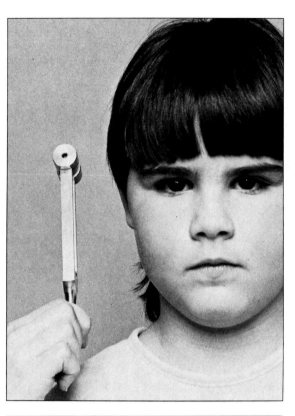

3 As soon as the child reports that she no longer hears the sound, reposition the vibrating tuning fork ½" (1.3 cm) from her right external ear canal, as the nurse is doing here. Make sure the prongs are directly in front of the ear canal, without touching the ear. Again, ask the child to tell you when she no longer hears the sound. If everything's okay, she'll hear this tone twice as long as she heard the previous sound. Why? Because air conduction normally sustains a sound longer than bone conduction.

Repeat steps 2 and 3 on her left ear.

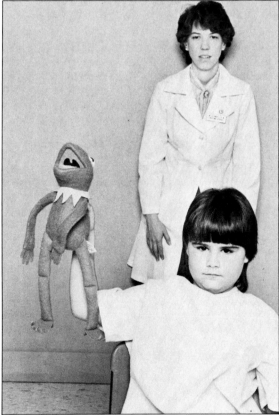

4 Now, to test the child's ability to hear high frequencies, perform the whisper test. Tell her that you're going to stand behind her and talk to her in a whisper. Instruct her not to turn around and look at you. Then, stand 8' to 10' (2.4 to 3 m) behind her and whisper a simple command, such as, "Please hold up your toy."

Document all your observations and the type of tuning fork you used. If the results of any test are questionable, refer the child for an audiogram. *Note*: If the child has cerumen accumulations or a cold, clearly document this. Either condition can affect her hearing ability.

Performing the toy test

1 *Alan Wolfe, your 4-year-old patient, is too young to reliably report how well he hears, so don't try to test him with the Rinne and Weber's tests. Instead, use a simple toy test. Here's what to do:*

First, assemble seven toys. Explain to Alan that you're going to play a game with him.

You'll ask him to pick up a special toy and put it on his lap. Then, to make sure he knows the names of all the toys, ask him to hand them to you as you name them. Eliminate toys he can't identify from the test. Remember, you're testing his hearing ability, not his vocabulary.

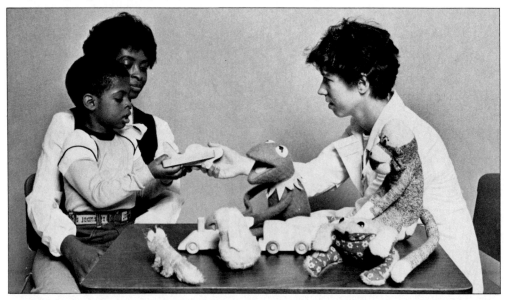

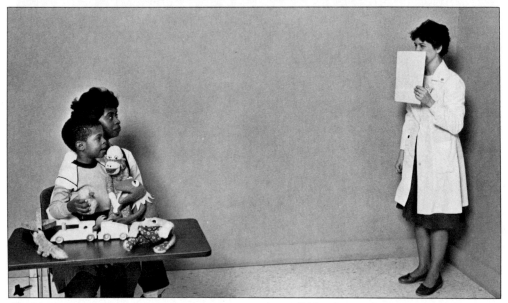

2 Now, stand about 10' (3 m) away from Alan, and hold a piece of paper or file folder in front of your mouth, so he can't lip read. (However, don't hold it so close to your mouth that it muffles the sound.) Using a normal conversational tone, ask him to pick up several toys as you name them, and move them from the table to his lap.

To test Alan's ability to hear high frequen-

cies, tell him that you're going to whisper the name of some toys. Then, repeat the test, using the whisper.

Document your observations. If Alan seemed to have difficulty hearing your commands, refer him for further testing. *Remember:* Head congestion or cerumen accumulation may temporarily impair the child's hearing ability.

MINI-ASSESSMENT

Hearing impairment: Tell-tale signs

Now you know how to use a few simple tests to identify hearing impairment. But what if your patient's too young to cooperate with you, even for the simplest test? Then, your observations (as well as the parents') are especially valuable. By recognizing the clues listed below, you may be able to help the child before his handicap seriously affects his development.

If your patient's an infant, suspect hearing impairment if he:
• fails to show blink or startle reactions to a loud noise.
• sleeps through nearby noisy disturbances.
• responds more readily to loud noises than to a voice.
• doesn't turn his head toward familiar sounds.
• babbles in a monotone.
• fails to babble, coo, or squeal frequently; doesn't babble in response to a human voice.

If your patient's a toddler, suspect hearing impairment if he:
• fails to speak clearly at age 2.
• habitually yells or shrieks when playing or communicating.
• responds to facial expressions rather than spoken words.
• appears shy or withdrawn; prefers playing by himself to socializing.
• seems inattentive, dreamy, or stubborn.
• often looks confused or puzzled.
• lacks interest in hearing stories and nursery rhymes or in playing vocal games, such as riddles.

Assessment

Inspecting the nose, mouth, and throat

	Equipment	Procedure	Abnormal findings
Nose	Penlight, nasoscope with light, ophthalmoscope or otoscope with light, or nasal speculum (for older, cooperative children only)	• Observe the size, shape, placement, and general condition of the child's nose.	• Discharge, inflammation, asymmetrical placement
		• Observe nostrils for symmetry of size and shape.	• Flaring nostrils, which suggest respiratory difficulty
		• Test for nasal obstructions by holding a small mirror under the child's nostrils. Observe the condensation circles that appear as the child breathes.	• Condensation circles of varying sizes, indicating a partial nasal obstruction; or an absent condensation circle, indicating total nasal obstruction
		• Ask the child to tilt his head back; then, gently push up the tip of his nose. Using a penlight, observe the mucous membranes, septum, and inferior turbinate.	• Gray, pale, red, or swollen mucous membranes • Discharge or purulent drainage • Foreign object • Deviated septum (septum which inclines toward one side or the other, giving it an S shape) • Perforated septum (indicated if light shines through the perforation into opposite nostril) • Nasal polyps (pale shiny balls with stalks) attached to turbinate
		• Using a nasal speculum, carefully expand the nostril and observe the inferior and middle turbinates. *Note:* Don't use a nasal speculum when examining a young or uncooperative child; you may injure him.	• Nasal polyps • Purulent drainage • Pallor and engorgement (may indicate allergic rhinitis)
Mouth and throat	Penlight, tongue depressor	• Observe color and condition of lips.	• Lesions, cyanosis, pallor *Note:* Lips normally are slightly darker than surrounding skin.
		• Ask child to open his mouth and say "Ahh." Observe his mucous membranes. If the child's Caucasian or Oriental, they should be smooth and pink; if he's black, they should be a patchy pink color.	• Lesions, bleeding, odor, or tenderness
		• Observe gums and teeth. 📖 *Nursing tip:* Is your patient age 2 or younger? Estimate the number of teeth he should have by subtracting six from the number of months in his age.	• Puffy, tender, or bleeding gums • Discolored, broken, maloccluded teeth; delayed eruption of teeth *Note:* Teach the child and his parents good dental hygiene and refer the child to a dentist, if necessary. Tell his parents that permitting the child to sleep with a bottle promotes tooth decay and malalignment. Also, keep in mind that poor gum condition may indicate malnutrition.
		• Ask child to stick out tongue; observe for velvety-pink appearance.	• Smoothness, cracks, coating, glossitis (tongue inflammation), lesions, lack of mobility
		• Observe palate, uvula, tonsils, and pharynx. *Important:* Use a tongue depressor with caution, and only if the child's cooperative. To avoid stimulating his gag reflex, depress only one side of his tongue at a time.	• Cleft palate and/or uvula • Enlarged, inflamed tonsils *Note:* During childhood, tonsils normally become larger, with a glandular (not smooth) appearance. • Pus, exudate, or follicles on pharynx

Assessing the chest and abdomen

Even during a routine assessment, don't neglect to examine your patient's chest and abdomen. Systematic inspection, auscultation, percussion and palpation may identify a previously unsuspected problem. This chart outlines what to do, and what to watch for. (For accurate auscultation findings, auscultate *before* you percuss and palpate. For a review of auscultation, percussion and palpation techniques, see the detailed information provided in the NURSING PHOTOBOOK ASSESSING YOUR PATIENTS.)

Note: Remember to warm the stethoscope's diaphragm before using it.

Heart

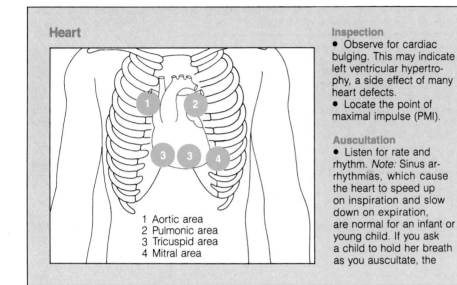

1 Aortic area
2 Pulmonic area
3 Tricuspid area
4 Mitral area

Inspection
• Observe for cardiac bulging. This may indicate left ventricular hypertrophy, a side effect of many heart defects.
• Locate the point of maximal impulse (PMI).

Auscultation
• Listen for rate and rhythm. *Note:* Sinus arrhythmias, which cause the heart to speed up on inspiration and slow down on expiration, are normal for an infant or young child. If you ask a child to hold her breath as you auscultate, the sinus arrhythmia should temporarily disappear.
• Listen for heart sounds S_1 and S_2, using the auscultation areas shown at left. (You may have some difficulty distinguishing them, because your auscultation area's so small.) *Note:* You may also hear S_3 in some children and young adults. Also, although S_4 may be present in normal children, it usually suggests ventricular ejection obstruction.
• Listen for heart murmurs. (For details on murmurs, including innocent murmurs, see this book's third section.)

Percussion
• Identify the size and location of the heart. Its borders should resemble a triangle.

Palpation
• Feel for PMI location. Expect to locate it at the fifth intercostal space, midclavicular line. (In an infant, it's at the third or fourth intercostal space, at left midclavicular line.)
• Note thrills or rubs, and other adventitious sounds.

Lungs

Inspection
• Watch for respiratory rate and symmetry. *Note:* Diaphragmatic breathing is normal for young children and infants.
• Observe for paradoxical breathing (the diaphragm falls, rather than rises, on inspiration), and other signs of respiratory distress.
• Look for developmental abnormalities, such as funnel chest or pigeon chest (either may indicate rickets), or barrel chest, which may indicate chronic respiratory disease.

Auscultation
• Moving from apex to base, auscultate over all lung fields, anteriorly, posteriorly, and laterally.
• Compare sounds from each side of chest.
• Note abnormal breath sounds, such as rales, rhonchi, wheezes, and rubs. *Note:* Coarse sounds may indicate that the child has mucus in her trachea.

Percussion
• Lightly percuss anteriorly and posteriorly, following the sequences shown in the first two diagrams below. Expect to hear resonance over normal, air-filled lungs; dullness over fluid-filled organs (heart and liver), or in plueral effusion; flatness over bone and muscle; and tympany over the stomach. When percussing the back, you should hear only resonance. *Note:* If you hear hyperresonance over the left side of the child's chest, don't automatically suspect a pneumothorax. It may indicate only that she has air bubbles in her stomach.

Palpation
• Feel for symmetrical chest expansion, using the hand position illustrated at left.
• Assess tactile fremitus. Expect to feel fremitus in the upper chest, close to the bronchi; it should be equal bilaterally. Expect to find little or no fremitus in the lower chest.

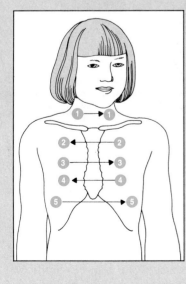

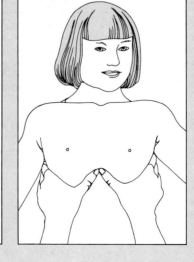

Assessment

Assessing the chest and abdomen continued

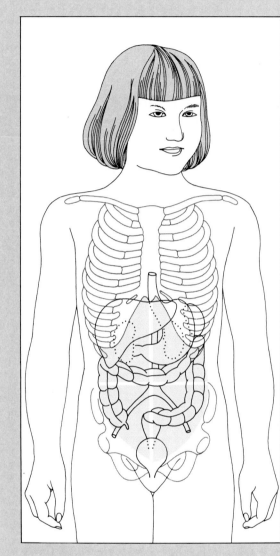

Abdomen

Inspection
• Observe abdominal contour. In a young child, expect it to be cylindrical and prominent.
• Note general appearance and tone. A concave appearance may indicate malnourishment; a flabby appearance suggests obesity. When coupled with thin arms and legs, a distended abdomen suggests malnutrition; in an otherwise-normal child, it may indicate a bowel obstruction.
• Note skin condition. Expect it to be smooth and taut.
• Assess movement; the abdomen should rise and fall synchronously with chest.
• Watch for peristaltic movement. Expect to see a slight wave-like motion (especially in infants and thin children) or no movement at all. Prominent undulating waves (especially when accompanied by a distended abdomen and cramping pain) may indicate a bowel obstruction.

• Look for hernias, including umbilical hernia.
• Note painless inguinal swellings, which normally appear when the child cries, strains, or coughs.
• Observe for aortic pulsations midline, in the epigastric area.

Auscultation
• Beginning at the right upper quadrant (see the illustration at left), auscultate in a clockwise direction.
• Record number of bowel sounds per minute.
• Note the pitch of bowel sounds; document friction rubs, bruits, or venous hums.

Percussion
• Begin at the right upper quadrant and percuss in a clockwise direction. Note the location and size of the liver (dull sound) and the stomach (tympany).
• Listen for extensive dull sounds, which may indicate free abdominal fluid, and for extensive tympany, which indicates free abdominal air.

Palpation
• Palpate from the lower quadrants to the upper quadrants, placing one hand on the child's abdomen, and the other directly behind it, on the child's back.
• Perform superficial palpation to assess skin tension and identify tenderness.
• Perform deep palpation to assess the size and position of blood vessels (especially the aorta) and organs (such as the liver and spleen), and to identify any unusual masses. (The liver and spleen may not be palpable in older children.)
Important: Never palpate the abdomen if you know or suspect that the child has Wilms' tumor.

Assessing genitalia

Do you sometimes feel uncomfortable conducting a genital assessment? Knowing exactly how to proceed and what to look for will put you more at ease. The following information and illustrations will help.

To conduct a genital assessment on either a girl or a boy, you'll use only inspection and palpation techniques. To proceed, you'll need good lighting and a generous measure of tact. Remember, even a young child may find a genital examination embarrassing. To encourage him to relax, provide privacy and don't expose him any longer than necessary. If you must ask him or his parent about possible problems, cover the child while you talk. Whenever appropriate during the examination, reassure him and his parents with a statement like this: "Everything looks fine." Also, take this opportunity to discuss any questions or concerns the child or parent has and to provide patient teaching about hygiene, anatomy, and sexuality.

Always begin with an explanation of what you're going to do and why. Then, wash your hands and proceed in a systematic, matter-of-fact way. After the procedure, thoroughly document all your findings.

Examining a girl
As a rule, you'll perform only an external examination on a girl. If your patient's very young, allow her to lie supine on her parent's lap with her feet on your lap, soles together. Position an older girl flat on her back, with her knees bent, her feet flat on the exam table, and her legs slightly apart. Cover her legs with a sheet or drape.

To begin the procedure, first tell the child what you're going to do, and warm your hands. Then, inspect and palpate her mons pubis, as described below. Next, expose the child's external genitals by placing your index and middle fingers on each side of the labia majora, and gently pulling the sides away from each other. (Or, ask the mother or the child herself to do this.) Inspect and palpate her genitals, following the systematic approach outlined here. Use the first illustration at right as a general guide to appearance, but keep in mind that variations exist among individuals.
Mons pubis: Look for skin discoloration and palpate for masses. In an adolescent, observe for hair distributed in an inverted-triangle shape and extending along the labia majora. Irregular or scanty hair growth may indicate a hormonal imbalance. Also, inspect and observe for pubic lice.
Clitoris: Inspect for size and position. However, because of the clitoris' sensitivity, don't palpate it.

Labia majora: Observe for lesions, such as chancres, warts, and tumors. A localized swelling may suggest a labioinguinal hernia; carefully palpate it to learn whether it communicates with the abdomen. If the labia majora are warm and swollen, possibly indicating vulvitis, suspect an underlying vaginal infection.

Note: Venereal warts or a hematoma may suggest sexual abuse, even in a very young child. For more on dealing with child abuse, see the fourth section of this book.

Bartholin's and Skene's glands: Normally, these glands are neither visible nor palpable. Enlarged, palpable glands may indicate gonorrhea or cysts.

Labia minora: In a newborn, this structure is prominent; it gradually atrophies until it's almost unobservable. At puberty, it again enlarges. Examine this area for adhesion (a transparent membrane that may cover the vaginal opening), which may be present from birth. Also, look for accumulations of thick, sticky smegma, indicating poor hygiene. Remember, even a mother who's otherwise scrupulous about hygiene may neglect to adequately clean the child's genitals. Provide instruction, if necessary.

Urinary meatus (urethral opening): Look for any signs of urethritis, such as inflammation, erythema, and discharge. If you see any such signs, take culture specimens as ordered. If you notice prolapse of the urethral mucosa, ask whether the child has a history of hematuria, dysuria, or any other urinary signs and symptoms.

Vaginal opening: Look for foul-smelling discharge or evidence of irritation, indicating an infection, pinworm infestation, or, possibly, a foreign body in the vagina. Take culture specimens, if ordered. Note whether the hymen is present and intact; however, keep in mind that a perforated or absent hymen is also normal. But, notify the doctor if the hymen is swollen with colorless fluid or blood. (A bloody or mucous discharge may be normal in an infant who's less than 1 month old.) Also be alert for a grapelike, fleshy, malignant growth (sarcoma botryoides) originating beneath the vaginal epithelium. This condition is most common in infants, and requires immediate medical attention.

Examining a boy

When examining a boy, first determine whether his testicles have descended into the scrotum. Normally, the testicles descend shortly before birth, although in some children, they descend later in childhood. Failure of the testicles to descend by late childhood requires surgical intervention.

Note: Although contraction of the cremaster muscle (called the cremasteric reflex) draws descended testicles back into the abdomen, the term *undescended testicles* refers only to testicles that have never descended into the scrotum.

Prepare to palpate the scrotum by soaping your hands or applying lotion. This precaution prevents you from gripping the testicles too firmly, possibly injuring them. Next, warm your hands and explain the procedure to the child. Remember, the touch of cold hands and emotions such as anxiety can stimulate the cremasteric reflex, so do your best to make him comfortable. *Important:* If the child has an erection at any time during the examination, take care to assure him that this is a normal reaction to touch.

Position the child in a squatting position, sitting with his legs crossed in front of him. Or (if he's an infant) position him supine with his legs raised and spread. These positions stretch the cremaster muscle and may prevent it from contracting. As a further precaution, block the inguinal canal by gently pressing upward from behind the scrotum with your thumb and index finger.

Suppose you can't palpate one or both testicles? If your patient's an older boy, seat him in a chair with his knees drawn up against his chest; this position may force the testicles to descend. If your patient's a

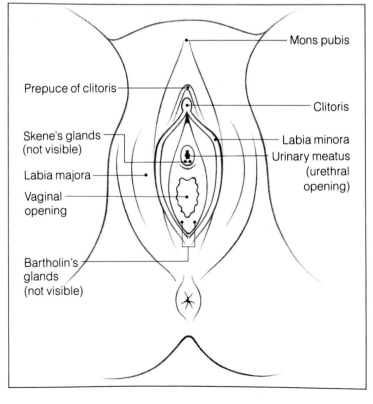

Mons pubis

Prepuce of clitoris

Clitoris

Skene's glands (not visible)

Labia minora

Urinary meatus (urethral opening)

Labia majora

Vaginal opening

Bartholin's glands (not visible)

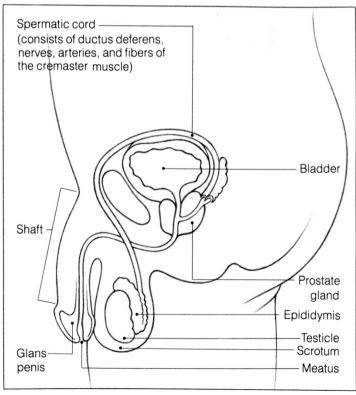

Spermatic cord (consists of ductus deferens, nerves, arteries, and fibers of the cremaster muscle)

Bladder

Shaft

Prostate gland

Epididymis

Testicle

Scrotum

Glans penis

Meatus

Assessment

Assessing genitalia continued

young child, consider seating him in a tub of warm water. The heat may force down the testicles.

Palpate descended testicles for size and symmetry. Normally, they're ⅗" to ⅘" (1.5 to 2 cm) long from birth to about age 11; subsequently, they grow to a length of 1½" to 2" (3.5 to 5 cm).

If you can't palpate both testicles, palpate the femoral, inguinal, perineal, and abdominal areas to locate them. If you find no evidence of testicles, be alert for other signs of sexual ambiguity (see the box at right).

🔖 *Nursing tip:* Well-formed scrotal rugae (wrinkles) usually indicate that the testicles have descended, even if they aren't presently palpable in the scrotum.

After you've determined whether the testicles have descended, follow these guidelines to continue the examination.

Scrotum: Examine the appearance of the scrotum itself, which consists of two sacs covered with loose, wrinkled skin. It should hang freely from the perineum behind the penis. One sac may hang lower than the other. Assess the scrotum for edema, inflammation, or lesions. (Sebaceous cysts are considered normal.) Red, shiny scrotal skin may indicate orchitis (inflammation of a testicle). Also,

palpate the spermatic cord within the scrotal sac. Simultaneously compare each side, and note any thickening or nodules. A boggy mass may indicate hematoma caused by trauma to the cord.

In addition, palpate the inguinal area for hernias.

Glans penis: If the child's uncircumcised and older than 4 months, gently retract the foreskin. (Don't disturb the foreskin of a younger child, because it may tear.) If it doesn't pull back easily, ask the parents if the child's had any difficulty urinating. Also, observe the glans for edema, which often accompanies a tight foreskin. If the child's experiencing urinary difficulty or edema of the glans, the doctor may advise circumcision.

Genitourinary meatus: Note its position and size. It should be centered at the top of the penile shaft. Notify the doctor of any deviation in position, or of an unusually small, pinprick-sized opening. Either condition may require surgical repair. Also, check the meatus for ulcerations (more common in circumcised children) and any other lesions.

Penile shaft: Inspect and palpate the shaft of the penis for size, swelling, or palpable long cords, which may indicate urethritis.

Recognizing sexual ambiguity

Because of the child's embarrassment (or his parents'), you may be tempted to skip genital assessment. But don't. In addition to the possible problems described in the preceding pages, you may discover evidence of sexual ambiguity: hermaphroditism (presence of both male and female gonads), or pseudohermaphroditism (presence of one set of gonads, along with some external genitalia of the opposite sex). As you know, early recognition and treatment of sexual ambiguity is essential for the child's normal development. Make sure you know what to look for by reviewing the following information. If you observe signs of sexual ambiguity, refer the child for appropriate treatment.

If your patient's a girl, check for these abnormal signs:
• an enlarged clitoris, which may be a small penis (especially if it contains a urethral opening)
• prominent, fused labia, which may be a small scrotum; palpable masses within them may be testicles
• absence of a vaginal opening.

If your patient's a boy, check for these abnormal signs:
• a small penis (in a newborn, shorter than 1" or 2.5 cm, which may be an enlarged clitoris
• a small, smooth-skinned scrotum with midline separation and without any palpable testicles, which may be an enlarged labia.

Assessing the musculoskeletal system

Throughout the assessment procedure, you've had a chance to observe your patient as he moves and plays. Have you noticed anything unusual about his posture, gait, or coordination? If so, he may have a musculoskeletal problem. Use these specific tests to help identify abnormalities:
• Test the child's range of motion (ROM) by having him do ROM exercises. If your patient's a toddler, encourage him to do these exercises by playing a game, such as Simon Says.
• Ask the child to undress from the waist up (if he hasn't already done so), and to stand up straight. While standing behind him, observe for asymmetrical hips and shoulders, which may indicate scoliosis (C- or S-shaped lateral deviations of the spine).
• Ask the child to bend at the waist, so his back's parallel to the floor. Instruct him to let his arms hang straight down, and to bring his hands together. While standing to his side, look for

asymmetry or unusual prominence of the rib cage.
• Now, instruct the child to slowly straighten up, until he's standing straight again. While continuing to stand to one side of him, observe his spine's mobility. Then, when he's standing straight, note any sign of lordosis (a swaybacked appearance of his lumbar and cervical spines), or kyphosis (a hunchbacked appearance of his thoracic spine).
• Observe and palpate his major joints (ankles, knees, hips, elbows, and wrists) for tenderness, edema, or deformity.
• While the child stands and walks, look for bowlegs, knock-knees, clubfoot, toeing-in, and toeing-out. (Keep in mind, however, that a toddler naturally has a broader stance than an older child.)
• Document your findings. If you observed any abnormalities, refer the child for further evaluation and treatment.

Procedures

After completing an assessment on your pediatric patient, you've determined that he has a health problem. To investigate further, the doctor's ordered blood and urine tests. Do you know how to proceed, no matter how old the child is?

Read the following section for guidance. You'll learn how to:
* help a child collect a urine specimen, with a parent's help.
* collect a urine specimen from an infant, using a U bag.
* assist with a suprapubic tap on an infant.
* choose a venipuncture site.
* perform femoral vein and capillary puncture.

Of course, an essential preliminary to any pediatric procedure is preparing the child *and* his parents. So, in the following pages, we'll also provide valuable information about patient/parent preparation.

Pediatric procedures: Preparing the child

When Mrs. Margolis brings 2-year-old Johnny into your outpatient clinic for blood tests, she pulls you aside. "I haven't told Johnny a thing about these tests today," she whispers to you. "He's really too young to understand much about it. And anyway, he'd just be scared."

How often has a parent told you something like this? Right away, you know you have a totally unprepared child on your hands—one who may quickly become frightened and uncooperative when he realizes what's in store for him.

Through overprotectiveness or their own lack of information, many parents simply fail to tell their child about medical and nursing procedures. Consider teaching the child—and his parents—to be your responsibility. Sure, it takes some time. But think about the consequences of *not* taking the time: a frightened, untrusting child whose confidence in adults—especially nurses—has been seriously shaken.

What's the first step? Enlisting the parents' cooperation. Explain to them that informing the child will make him more cooperative in the long run. Take care to emphasize the importance of their support and comfort to the child.

Also, do your best to relieve their own anxieties. Remember, parents can't bear to see their children hurt. If they communicate their anxiety to the child, they'll feed the child's own fears. Tell the parents exactly what you'll do, and how long the child's pain (if any) will last. Encourage them to ask questions. Then, if they're calm and supportive, encourage them to stay with the child during the procedure and to comfort him afterwards.

Now, let's consider how to approach the child himself. Follow these basic guidelines:
* Explain all procedures to the child, in words he can understand. And don't neglect to explain a procedure just because he's experienced it before. Give him another explanation that's appropriate for his older age.
* Always be honest with a child. If a procedure will hurt, tell him so. But, to avoid terrifying him, temper the bad news with a positive statement. For example, you might say something like this: "This will hurt. But the hurt will go away very soon. Then, if you like, you can pick out a colorful bandage to put on."
* Consider every nursing procedure a teaching opportunity. Whenever you use a stethoscope, blood pressure cuff, and other equipment, explain their function, and let the child play with them, if possible. (But don't let him handle equipment he could break, such as a glass thermometer.)
* When teaching, involve as many of his senses as possible. For example, don't just show him a stethoscope. Let him handle it, and show him how to hear his heartbeat.
* After you've explained the procedure to the child, ask him to tell you what's going to happen. His answer may reveal a startling misconception that you can set straight.
* Assure the child that it's okay to cry during painful procedures. Then, if he does cry, take care to remain supportive.

Obtaining a urine specimen

Tracy DuBois, your 4-year-old patient, is scheduled for a myringotomy. The doctor wants a urine specimen for routine preoperative testing. How do you proceed when your patient's this age?

Since Tracy's toilet trained, plan to obtain a clean-catch specimen. Of course, because she's so young, she'll need help to correctly perform the procedure. Teach one of her parents how to assist; the child will probably feel more comfortable with one of them than with you.

On the following pages, you'll find a self-care aid you can copy and give to the child's parent as a guide. But remember, no aid's a substitute for face-to-face patient teaching. To adequately prepare the child and parent, take them to a private, quiet room, and explain the procedure to them. Of course, the child won't absorb as many details as her parent will. But take care to include her anyway.

Keep these particular points in mind:
* Explain why the specimen's necessary.
* When speaking to the child, use words she knows. For example, use *pee, tinkle,* or *go to the bathroom,* instead of *urinate.*
* Give her a clean specimen container to play with.
* Speak to the parent in simple, nonmedical terms. If you use a technical term, such as *urethral opening,* take care to explain it, if necessary.
* Stress the importance of keeping all equipment as clean as possible.
* Tell the parent why a midstream specimen's best. But can a child Tracy's age urinate a small amount, stop, and then resume urination? Probably not; in fact, she may consider such a request upsetting. As a compromise, direct the parent to position the specimen container under the stream just moments after the child begins urinating.
* Ask when the child last urinated. If she urinated within the past hour, wait at least 30 minutes before attempting the procedure. In the meantime, offer her something to drink (unless contraindicated), to increase urine production.
* Provide the parent with disposable wipes and a specimen container. Then, take the parent and child to a private bathroom. Assure them that they may take as much time as they need to complete the procedure.

Note: An older child may prefer to perform the procedure by himself, privately.

Procedures

Self-care

Helping your child collect a urine specimen

1 Dear Parent:
The doctor wants to test your child's urine for this reason: _____
_____

The nurse will give you a kit containing the equipment you need. Before you begin, read this entire teaching aid carefully. Then, to make sure the test results are as accurate as possible, follow these steps:

First, help the child wash his hands. Wash your hands, too. Using simple words, explain this procedure to your child and answer his questions.

Next, spread a fresh paper towel on a clean, dry surface. Open the kit and remove the disposable wipes and other contents. Without touching the wipes themselves, open their wrappers. Place the opened wrappers on the paper towel, as shown here. By leaving the wipes on their wrappers, you can keep the wipes perfectly clean until you're ready to use them.

2 Without touching the inside of the plastic specimen cup or the lid, remove the lid from the cup. Place the cup on the paper towel. Lay the lid next to it, flat side down.

3 If your child's a girl, skip ahead to steps 5 and 6. But if he's a boy, here's how to cleanse his penis and collect the specimen:

First, gently grasp his penis, and pull back his foreskin (if he's uncircumcised). Pick up one of the wipes and make a stroke from the urethral opening toward his abdomen, as shown here. Discard the wipe; don't use it again. Repeat this procedure with each of the remaining wipes, discarding each after one use.

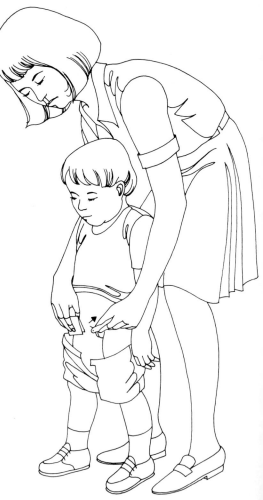

4 Now, pick up the specimen cup and have it ready. Position the child in front of the toilet, and ask him to urinate. (If he has difficulty, try turning on the water faucet.) As soon as he's urinated a small amount into the toilet, position the cup under the stream. Try to hold it close enough so the urine doesn't splash, but not so close that the child's penis touches the cup. Take the cup away when it's about two-thirds full (don't let it overflow); then, let the child finish urinating. Place the lid on the container. Remember not to touch the inside of the cup or the lid with your fingers. Wash your hands, and encourage the child to wash his, too. Praise him for his effort.

Write your child's name on the cup's label, and return the cup to the nurse.

5 If your child's a girl, follow these steps: First, help her undress from the waist down, and sit her on the toilet or potty seat. Using the fingers of your left hand (if you're right-handed), gently separate her labia (the folds of skin around her urethral opening). Keep the labia separated for the rest of the procedure.

Use a wipe to cleanse one side of the labia, using just one front-to-back stroke. Discard the wipe. Then, cleanse the other side with a clean wipe. Still moving from front to back, use the third wipe to cleanse the urethral opening (located in the center of the labia). Discard the wipe and pick up the specimen cup.

6 While still holding her labia apart, ask her to urinate into the toilet. (If she has difficulty, try turning on the water faucet.) After she's urinated a small amount, position the cup under the stream. Try not to touch the cup's rim to her skin. Take the cup away when it's about two-thirds full (don't let it overflow), and let her finish urinating. Now put the lid on the container. Remember not to touch the inside of the cup or the lid with your fingers. Set the cup down in a safe place, and help the child dress and wash her hands. Wash your own hands, too. Praise the child for her effort.

Finally, write her name on the cup's label, and return the filled cup to the nurse.

Procedures

Using a U bag

1 *Debra Lister, your 8-month-old patient, has the signs and symptoms of a urinary infection. To confirm his diagnosis, the doctor's ordered a urine culture. But how can you collect a specimen from a child who's not yet toilet trained?*

Chances are, you'll collect a specimen with a U bag (urine collection bag). This noninvasive plastic device fits temporarily over the child's perineal area, capturing urine as she excretes it. Some models have a nonreflux flap to prevent urine from escaping. To learn how to collect a specimen using a U bag, read on.

First, collect the equipment shown here: a U bag, nine 4"x4" sterile gauze pads (or cotton balls), antimicrobial solution, sterile normal saline solution or water, and a sterile specimen container with lid. To help secure the bag, also obtain 1" (2.5 cm) nonallergenic tape.

✆ *Nursing tip:* Unless contraindicated, give the child something to drink 30 minutes before performing the procedure. This helps insure adequate urine production.

Thoroughly wash your hands. Open all of the sterile gauze pads. Moisten three of them with antimicrobial solution, and three with sterile saline solution. Let the other three remain dry. Make sure all your equipment's within easy reach.

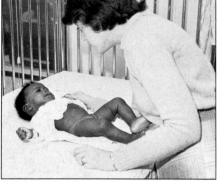

2 Place the child in a supine position, and remove her diaper. Even though she's too young to understand an explanation of the procedure, remember to speak soothingly to her, as the nurse is doing here.

Important: If Debra's parents are present, tell them why the specimen's needed, and describe the cleansing and collection procedures. Assure them that the procedure's not painful, but that the child may find the bag uncomfortable or annoying. Tell them that you'll remove the bag as soon as enough urine has accumulated (usually within 20 minutes).

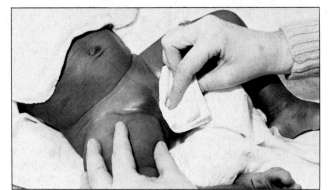

3 Now, prepare to cleanse Debra's perineal area. First, position Debra with her legs apart, as shown here, and separate her labia. Using one of the pads moistened with antimicrobial solution, gently cleanse one side of the labia, as the nurse is doing in this photo. Cleanse from front to back, to avoid fecal contamination. Discard the gauze pad and repeat the procedure on the other side of the labia, using another pad moistened in antimicrobial solution. Finally, take the last of these pads, and cleanse the urethral opening. To prevent irritation, rinse her perineal area with the gauze pads soaked in sterile saline solution. Follow the same procedure as for cleansing.

Then, use the dry gauze pads to dry the perineum. This step reduces the risk of skin chapping and allows the adhesive strip to stick securely to her skin.

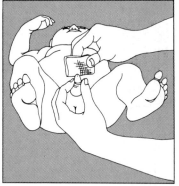

4 If the child's an uncircumcised male, pull back his foreskin. Then, take a wipe moistened with antimicrobial solution, and begin cleansing the head of the penis, working from the urethral opening toward his abdomen. Discard the wipe after one stroke. Repeat the cleansing procedure with each of the remaining two wipes, discarding each wipe after one use. Rinse the penis, following the same procedure as for cleansing, and dry the area.

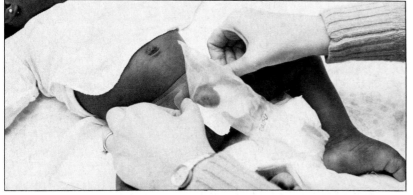

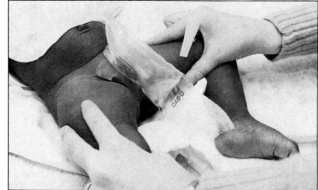

5 Remove the paper backing from the U bag's top adhesive strip. Then, center the bag's opening over the child's labia, and press the adhesive firmly in place. When the bag's properly centered, remove the U bag's bottom adhesive strip, and firmly press this adhesive in place, too. Smooth out any loose edges or bubbles in the adhesive strips. For added security, consider reinforcing them with a strip of 1" (2.5 cm) nonallergenic tape.

If your patient's a boy, place his penis inside the bag, and firmly press the backing against his skin. Reinforce the adhesive with nonallergenic tape, if necessary.

Unless contraindicated, place the child in semi-Fowler's position, to facilitate drainage into the bag. Give her a toy to play with, or ask her parents to distract her, if she's active.

Nursing tip: If you apply a diaper over the bag, allow the bottom of the bag to protrude from the diaper, so you can check urine accumulation.

6 Check the bag at least every 15 minutes, to assess urine production. As soon as about 20 ml of urine accumulates, remove the bag. By removing the bag as soon as possible, you reduce the risk that it'll loosen, which may spill or contaminate the specimen.

Note: If the infant doesn't urinate within 30 minutes, remove the bag, prep her perineal area again, and apply a new bag. This precaution minimizes the risk of specimen contamination.

Pour the urine specimen into the sterile specimen container, and cover it securely with the lid. Label the container, and send it to the lab at once. Properly dispose of the U bag and other soiled equipment. Wash your hands, and document the procedure.

Assisting with a suprapubic tap

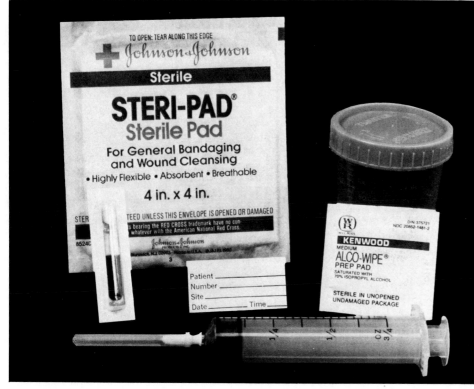

1 You've been trying to collect a urine specimen from 13-month-old Kevin Borelli. But because he has diaper rash, the bag's adhesive strip won't stick firmly to his skin. What's more, Kevin's becoming increasingly upset as the bag irritates his already-inflamed skin. To spare Kevin prolonged discomfort, the doctor's ordered a suprapubic tap.

As you probably know, a suprapubic tap allows the doctor to obtain a sterile urine specimen. Although it's an invasive procedure, a suprapubic tap carries fewer risks of infection or trauma than does catheterization. What's your role? To find out, read the following photostory.

First, gather the sterile equipment you'll need: 20 ml syringe, 20G or 21G 1½" needle, specimen container, and 4"x4" gauze pad. In addition, obtain a patient label for the specimen container, a povidone-iodine prep and an alcohol wipe.

Unless contraindicated, offer Kevin fluids before the procedure, to help ensure adequate urine production. Inform the doctor if Kevin's urinated within the past hour. The doctor will probably postpone the procedure until the bladder has time to fill again.

Procedures

Assisting with a suprapubic tap   continued

2 Before the doctor begins the procedure, speak soothingly to Kevin so he's as quiet as possible. But if your patient's an older child, provide a simple explanation of the procedure. For example, tell him that the doctor will prick his tummy, and that it will hurt. But emphasize that the discomfort will last only a very short time, and tell the child that he can help you and the doctor by holding as still as possible.

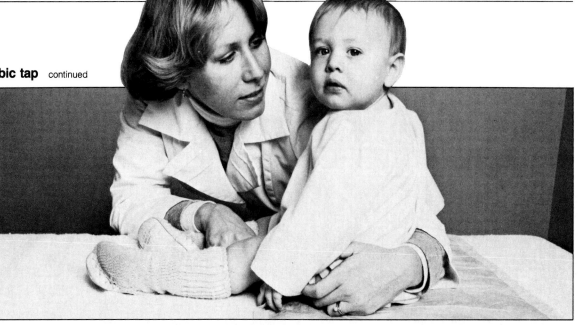

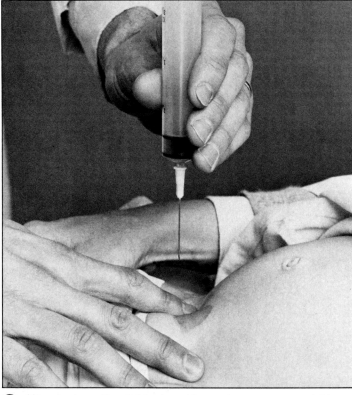

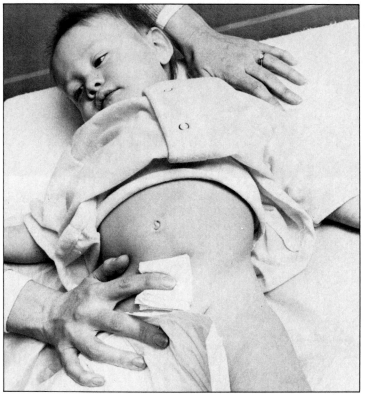

3 Now, undress the child, place him supine on an exam table, and restrain him in the frog-like position shown on page 39. Or, grasp both his feet in one hand, and draw them toward his body. Speak reassuringly to the child throughout the procedure.

While the child's restrained, the doctor will palpate his bladder and cleanse the puncture site.

Before the doctor aspirates the specimen, he may ask you to apply pressure to the child's urethra. If necessary, ask a co-worker to restrain the child. Then, gently squeeze the penis, to occlude the urethra. (If your patient's a girl, apply direct pressure on her urethra; or, apply upward pressure through her rectum.) Then, the doctor will insert the needle into the bladder, as shown, and aspirate a urine specimen.

4 As soon as the doctor removes the needle, apply gentle pressure over the puncture site with the sterile gauze pad. As you do, comfort and praise your patient. After bleeding stops, dress him and make him as comfortable as possible. An older child may want you to put a colorful adhesive bandage strip over the puncture site.

Eject the urine specimen from the syringe into the sterile container, label the container, and send it to the lab at once. Document the procedure in your nurses' notes.

Important: Following the procedure, observe the child for hematuria (bloody urine). Document any blood traces you see, and notify the doctor immediately if bleeding is prolonged or seems excessive.

Performing capillary puncture

1 *Does your laboratory use micromethods to perform routine blood analyses? If so, you'll need to obtain only 0.1 to 1 ml of blood from your patient (depending on the specific tests ordered). To spare her the trauma of venipuncture, use the capillary puncture technique. Here's how:*

First, obtain the equipment you'll need: a sterile lancet, capillary collection tubes (or micropipettes, depending on the size of the specimens you need), sealing putty, alcohol swabs, a sterile gauze pad or cotton ball, and adhesive bandage strips or dots. (To determine the number and type of collection tubes you need, consult your lab manual.)

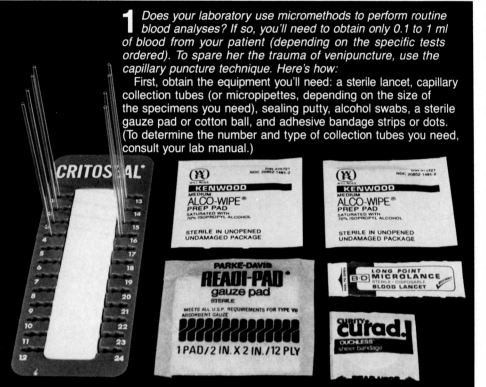

2 Now, prepare the child and her parent for the procedure. (See the guidelines on pages 29 and 37.) If the child seems calm and cooperative, allow her to sit on her parent's lap during the procedure, if she wishes. Or, she may prefer sitting next to her parent. If she's not cooperative, despite your best efforts to prepare her, ask an assistant to help you hold her during the procedure. (Remember, never ask the parent to restrain a struggling child for a painful procedure; this will further upset both the child and her parent.)

What puncture site's best? For a child older than age 2, choose a fingertip (unless contraindicated because of burns or other injury). To minimize risk of postprocedure trauma to the puncture site, make the middle finger of her nondominant hand your first choice. If using a fingertip is contraindicated, choose a site on her great toe instead. And if the child's less than age 2, use the lower outer aspects of either of her heels, as shown in the inset illustration. (Take care to avoid calluses.) By using one of the outer aspects, you avoid puncturing the lateral or medial plantar arteries. Dilate the heel vessels by applying warm, wet compresses to the heel for about 10 minutes before performing the puncture.

3 Let's say you've chosen a fingertip. To prepare the site, first make sure the child's hands are as clean and warm as possible by helping her wash them. Then, wash your own hands.

Place your equipment on a nearby clean surface, so it's easily accessible. If your lancet is in a sterile wrapper, leave it on the open wrapper until you're ready to use it.

Next, tell the child that you're going to cleanse her fingertip with a cold, wet pad. Assure her that the pad won't hurt her. Then, cleanse the puncture site with the alcohol swab, using a circular motion.

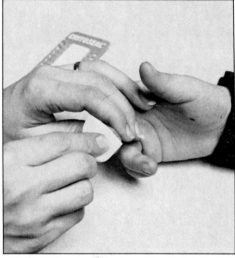

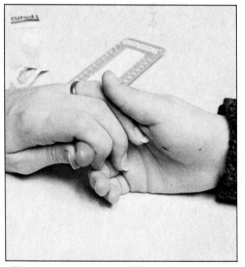

4 To engorge the capillaries, firmly grasp the child's finger near its tip. Take care not to contaminate the puncture site with your fingers. If necessary, use a stroking motion to milk her fingertip toward the tip. When the fingertip's flushed, you're ready to do the puncture.

Procedures

Performing capillary puncture continued

5 Tell the child that you're ready to prick her finger. Reassure her that it'll hurt only a short time, and encourage her to stay as still as possible.

Now, work quickly to minimize the child's anxiety. Grasp the lancet between the thumb and forefinger of your dominant hand, and stabilize her fingertip with your nondominant hand. (Continue to apply firm pressure, to maintain flushing.) Position the lancet about 2″ (5.1 cm) from the side of her fingertip, as shown here.

[Inset] Then, with one quick, firm motion, move the lancet in a short arc, so it penetrates the fingertip at a 90° angle. Immediately withdraw the lancet.

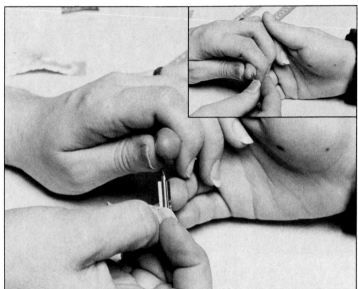

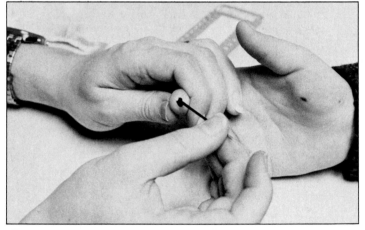

6 When a large drop of blood accumulates, place the tip of a capillary tube against the drop. To allow capillary action to pull blood into the tube, make sure you don't obstruct the top of the tube with your finger. When the tube's full, firmly place your fingertip over the top of the tube. Then, press the open end in the sealing putty. By occluding one end of the tube with putty, you prevent blood from spilling when you remove your finger. If your sealing putty container provides slots to hold the tubes, securely place the tube in one.

Repeat this step until you've filled all the tubes required.

7 Suppose bleeding stops before you've collected all the blood you need? First, try positioning her finger below her heart level, and firmly squeezing the fingertip several times, until more blood collects. Pause briefly between each squeeze, to allow the capillaries to refill. Also, try rewiping her finger with a clean alcohol pad.

If blood flow continues to be inadequate, you'll see air bubbles in the capillary tube. Since air bubbles can alter test results, repeat the capillary puncture procedure on another finger to insure adequate blood flow.

Important: Carefully explain to the child why you must prick her again, so she won't think you're punishing her. Provide additional support and encouragement.

You may also secure adequate blood flow by performing an X incision. With a sterile lancet, make a second puncture nearly perpendicular to the original puncture to make an X-shaped incision.

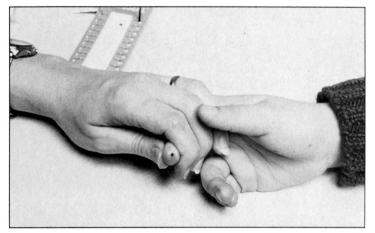

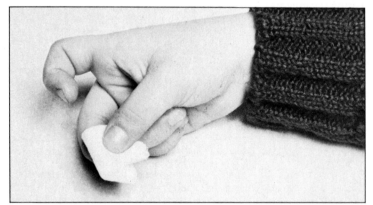

8 Finished filling the tubes? Then press a dry sterile gauze pad over the puncture site, until the bleeding stops. If possible, ask the child to hold it for you. This responsibility may take her mind off the pain. Also, take care to assure her that the bleeding will stop soon. *Note:* If you used a heel site, apply additional pressure, as necessary, to prevent hematoma formation.

Praise the child for her cooperation, and comfort her if necessary. When the bleeding's stopped, place a brightly colored adhesive bandage strip or dot over the puncture site. Caution the child not to put her finger in her mouth.

Finally, fill out the lab slip and send the blood specimens to the lab at once. Document the procedure in your nurses' notes.

Choosing a venipuncture site

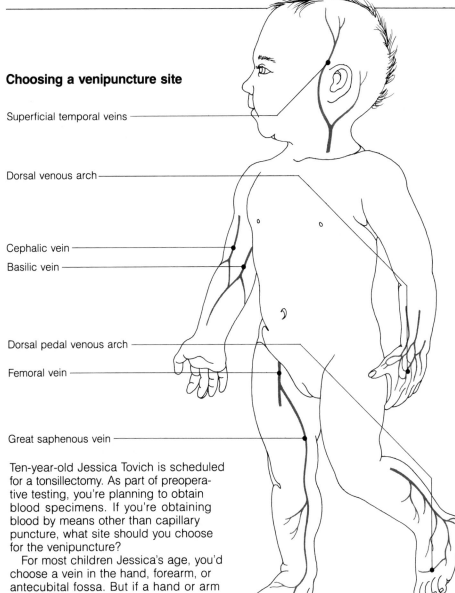

Superficial temporal veins

Dorsal venous arch

Cephalic vein

Basilic vein

Dorsal pedal venous arch

Femoral vein

Great saphenous vein

Ten-year-old Jessica Tovich is scheduled for a tonsillectomy. As part of preoperative testing, you're planning to obtain blood specimens. If you're obtaining blood by means other than capillary puncture, what site should you choose for the venipuncture?

For most children Jessica's age, you'd choose a vein in the hand, forearm, or antecubital fossa. But if a hand or arm site is undesirable for any reason, you may also consider the femoral vein, or a vein in her lower leg or foot. To learn the location of veins commonly chosen for venipuncture, examine the illustration above. *Note:* Under some circumstances, the doctor may perform venipuncture on the external jugular vein.

Although you may use a scalp vein for long-term I.V. therapy on an infant, this vein is a poor choice for simply withdrawing blood samples. Chances are, the child and her parents will find venipuncture at this site upsetting, especially since you'll have to shave off some of her hair.

Before making a decision on what vein to choose, ask yourself these questions:
• Is the child small or debilitated? A hand or arm vein may be difficult to find. Consider using another site; for example, the large, easily located femoral vein. *Important:* Before proceeding, make

sure venipuncture of the femoral vein is a nursing responsibility at your hospital.
• Does she have a condition, such as burns or an infection, that affects a possible venipuncture site? To avoid complications, choose a vein away from the affected area.
• Is the child bedridden? If so, avoid using a lower extremity vein, because of the risk of thrombophlebitis or embolism. However, a one-time venipuncture on an ambulatory child's lower extremity usually does no harm.
• Does the child have an I.V. in place? Choose a site in another extremity. *Important:* Never attempt to withdraw blood through an I.V. needle or catheter that's been used to infuse medication or I.V. fluid.

Preparing the child for venipuncture

Suppose, as part of patient assessment, you need to obtain blood specimens from a child. What's your immediate reaction? If you usually find performing venipuncture on a child frustrating and unpleasant, you may not be preparing him properly. Although nothing *guarantees* success, careful patient preparation is likely to produce a cooperative child. Try the following tips. You may be pleasantly surprised by the results. (Use these same techniques to prepare a child who needs I.V. therapy. For more information, see the section beginning on page 70.)
• Plan enough preparation time so you're not rushed. But don't prepare the child too far in advance of the procedure, since waiting will make him anxious.
• Project a positive attitude. Approach the child in a matter-of-fact way, as if you expect his cooperation. If he perceives that you expect trouble, his anxiety will grow.
• Don't mislead or deceive the child. You'll destroy your rapport with him if you tell him needle insertion won't hurt at all, or that it feels "like a mosquito bite." With a child, as with any patient, honesty's the best policy. Tell him the procedure will hurt, but assure him that the hurt will last only a short time.
• Don't use words like *shot* or *needle*—they're likely to frighten a child. Instead, teach an older child the words *injection* or *venipuncture.* A toddler may like a playful but descriptive word like *ouchie.*
• Use a toy, such as a teddy bear, to demonstrate venipuncture (using a syringe without a needle, of course). Then, let the child try. By pretending to do the procedure himself, he regains a sense of control, and may release many of his fears and frustrations.
• Give the child a chance to make choices, if possible. For example, you might allow an older one to choose the venipuncture site. After the procedure, allow him to select an adhesive bandage strip to place over the site. Once again, this gives him a sense of control.
• Be sensitive to any fears or misconceptions the child may have. For example, he may view the painful procedure as punishment. Assure him that other children need a blood test from time to time, so the doctor can see what's going on inside their bodies.

Also remember that a child probably has no understanding of hematopoiesis. He may consider any blood loss a deadly threat. Take care to assure him that you're taking only a very small amount, and that his body will quickly make more.

Procedures

Preparing the child
for venipuncture continued

A child may also fear that his insides will leak out the puncture hole. Assure him that they won't. Applying an adhesive bandage strip to the puncture site may relieve this fear.

Encourage the child to ask questions or comment on your explanation. He may reveal other misconceptions or fears.
• Tell him that he's allowed to cry. If he does, remain supportive.
• After the procedure, comfort and praise the child. Try to find something encouraging to say, even if he wasn't very cooperative. For example, say, "It was hard to hold still, wasn't it? But I could tell you tried."

Include the parents

When your patient's a child, preparing his parents is as important as preparing the child himself. Remember, his attitudes often mirror his parents'. Provide a complete explanation of the procedure to the parents, and encourage them to ask questions. In addition, emphasize the importance of their emotional support for the child. Even an infant will tolerate a painful procedure better when he's being held and soothed by a parent. Encourage the parents to hold or sit with the child during venipuncture, and to comfort and praise him afterward. But *don't* ask them to restrain the child.

Other nursing considerations

• Never attempt venipuncture on a child before you've become experienced at doing the procedure on adults. Remember, a child's small veins are even more difficult to find than an adult's. And if, for any reason, you aren't successful after two tries, ask someone else who's experienced at venipuncture to take over.
• Learn to perform the procedure with one hand, so you can stabilize the child's arm throughout the procedure.
• Set up all your equipment before you explain the procedure to the child. If he's already apprehensive, waiting and watching while you prepare may frighten him further.
• Help control the child's pain by teaching him rhythmic deep breathing, and encourage his parents to coach him. In addition to helping him control his anxiety, this technique keeps his veins dilated, making needle insertion easier. To reduce the pain of venipuncture, insert the needle when the child exhales.
• Continue to reassure him during the procedure. Remember, like many adults, a child may become concerned or upset at the sight of his own blood. Compliment him on its nice red color, so he'll know that everything looks normal.

Selecting equipment
to draw blood specimens

When preparing to withdraw blood specimens from a child, take care to select appropriate equipment. Suppose, for example, your patient's older than age 12. To perform venipuncture on any site except the femoral vein, you'll probably use the following equipment: pediatric Vacutainer® collection tube, a 21-gauge Vacutainer needle, and a Vacutainer sleeve. (Smaller-gauge needles are also available. Check with your lab.)

To proceed, you'll screw the needle into the sleeve and perform venipuncture. After puncturing the vein, you'll insert a collection tube into the sleeve, so the needle's free end punctures the tube stopper. The vacuum inside the collection tube then draws blood through the needle into the collection tube. While holding the needle and barrel as still as possible, you'll replace each collection tube with a new one until you've obtained as many specimens as you need, according to the doctor's order.

On a younger or debilitated child, however, you'll probably choose to use a butterfly needle and syringe. Why? Because a Vacutainer tube's powerful vacuum can cause this child's small vein to collapse. To use a butterfly needle and syringe, perform venipuncture with the butterfly needle and attach the syringe to the needle's tubing. Then, slowly aspirate the blood you need. By controlling the suction yourself, you may avoid collapsing the vein. And by grasping the butterfly needle's wings, you can easily stabilize the needle.

Now, suppose you're using a femoral vein for venipuncture. You'll need a needle and large syringe. You'll puncture a large vein, like the femoral, at a steep angle; a needle and syringe gives you the greatest control.

To learn how to obtain a blood specimen from the femoral vein, read the photostory beginning at right.

For details on obtaining blood specimens using Vacutainer equipment, consult the NURSING PHOTO-BOOK CARING FOR SURGICAL PATIENTS.

Performing femoral venipuncture

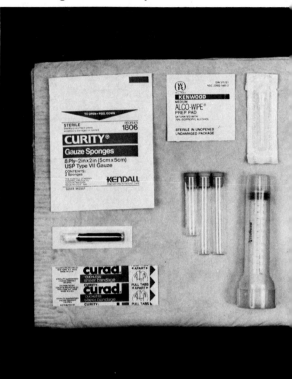

1 *Femoral venipuncture may be a nursing responsibility in your hospital, at least in the pediatric intensive care unit. If it is, you'll use the procedure to obtain blood specimens from very young or debilitated children. Make sure you know the proper procedure by reviewing this photostory.*

First, determine what lab tests the doctor's ordered, and how many collection tubes you'll need. As an example, let's say you'll need to fill three collection tubes, one containing an anticoagulant. Obtain the Vacutainer collection tubes you'll need. (Consult your lab manual for guidelines.)

Because you're puncturing the femoral vein, you'll use a needle and syringe to withdraw blood. Obtain a sterile 21-gauge 1½" needle, and a syringe that can hold the amount of blood required. This permits you to withdraw all the blood you need with one aspiration, eliminating the risk of traumatizing the large femoral vein during repeated aspirations. At the end of the procedure, you'll transfer the blood to the collection tubes.

Finally, you'll need to gather a povidone-iodine prep, sterile 2"x2" gauze pad, bed-saver pad, and adhesive bandage strip. Because the femoral vein's large and easy to locate, you won't need a tourniquet.

Important: Find out if the child's sensitive to iodine. If he is, cleanse the site with alcohol instead of povidone iodine.

2 Now, speak soothingly to the child and give his parent an explanation of the procedure. Place the bed-saver pad on a firm surface, such as an examination table, and lay the child on his back on the bed-saver pad. Ask a co-worker to stay with him while you thoroughly wash your hands; you'll also need her help to restrain him during the procedure. *Note:* If necessary, wash the child's upper leg before you begin the skin prep. Remember, because his upper leg is difficult to keep clean, you must take some special precautions to avoid contaminating the venipuncture site—especially if he still wears diapers.

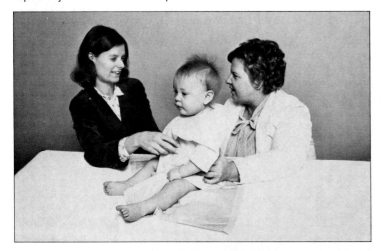

3 Open your equipment, leaving sterile equipment on the sterile wrappers, and assemble the needle and syringe. Place all equipment within reach.

Now, after your co-worker's warmed her hands, ask her to restrain the child in the frog-like position shown here. As you see, she's using her forearms to pin down his arms. In addition to holding the child still, this position provides easy access to the femoral vein.

If necessary, ask your co-worker to hold the child's diaper out of the way. But don't remove the diaper—it'll protect the venipuncture site from contamination if the child urinates.

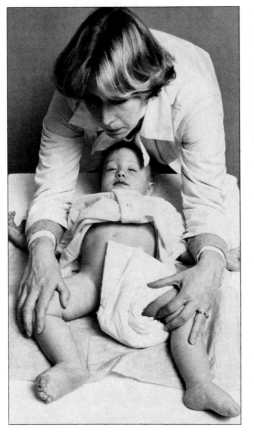

4 Now, palpate to find the femoral vein. To do so, first locate the femoral artery. You'll recognize the artery by its strong pulsation. The femoral vein is located slightly medial to the artery, as shown in the illustration on page 40.

When you've located the vein, mark the puncture site by straddling the vein with your index and middle fingers or your thumb and index finger, as the nurse is doing here. In addition to marking the site, your fingers will stabilize the vein.

Using a brisk circular motion, cleanse the site with the povidone-iodine prep. Continue cleansing for at least 1 minute. Wait about 30 seconds for the povidone iodine to dry. (If you're using an alcohol wipe, cleanse for 3 minutes.)

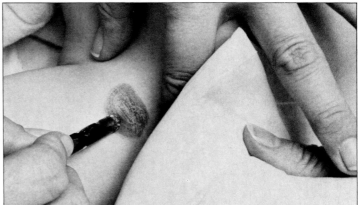

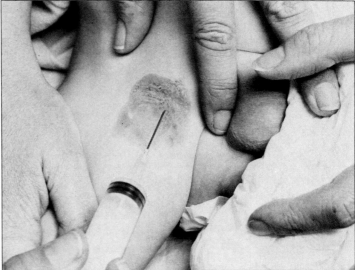

5 To puncture the vein, hold the syringe like a dart, grasping it near the needle hub. Position the needle at an angle between 45° and 90°. (You may rest it just slightly on the skin surface to stabilize its position.) Then, with one firm, quick motion, insert the needle through the skin and into the vein. When the needle punctures the vein's muscular wall, you'll feel a popping sensation.

To affirm that you're properly in the vein, gently pull back on the plunger and look for blood backflow in the syringe. If you don't see backflow, remove the needle, apply direct pressure to the puncture site until any bleeding stops, and prepare to repeat the procedure on the child's other femoral vein.

Procedures

Performing femoral venipuncture continued

6 As this illustration shows, the femoral vein lies very close to the femoral artery. If you mistakenly puncture the artery instead of the vein, how will you know? First, you'll probably feel arterial pulsation through the needle. Second, arterial blood pressure may force up the syringe plunger. And finally, arterial blood is a brighter red than venous blood.

Suppose you *have* entered the artery—what now? For most blood tests, arterial blood is just as informative as venous blood, so go ahead and withdraw the specimen you need. But take care to clearly document on the lab slip that you obtained an arterial specimen, so the lab technician can take this into account. *Note:* You must obtain *venous* blood if the doctor's ordered a test of lactic acid levels.

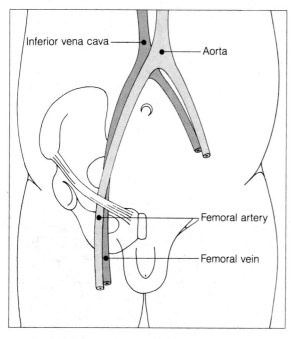

Inferior vena cava

Aorta

Femoral artery

Femoral vein

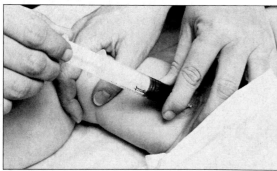

7 To aspirate the blood you need from the femoral vein, *gently* pull back on the syringe plunger. Fast aspiration may cause the vein to collapse, stopping blood flow.

Nursing tip: If blood flow stops, try releasing the plunger for several seconds, to allow the vein to refill with blood. Then, slowly resume aspiration.

8 When the syringe is as full as necessary, quickly withdraw the needle from the vein, maintaining exactly the same angle at which you inserted it. Then, using the sterile gauze pad, apply direct pressure to the puncture site for at least 1 minute, or until the bleeding stops. If you punctured the artery, apply pressure for at least 5 minutes.

When the bleeding's stopped, apply an adhesive bandage strip to the puncture site, and release the child from the restraining position. Reassure him and make him as comfortable as possible. *Note:* If the child's very active, or if you punctured the artery, consider folding a sterile 2"x2" gauze pad in half and taping it securely over the puncture site.

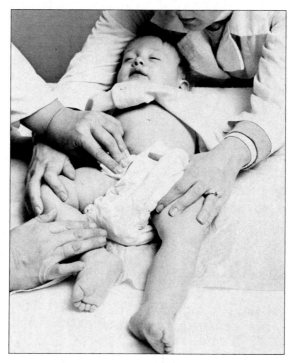

9 Now, transfer the blood into the three collection tubes, following the sequence outlined in the text at right. Simply insert the needle into the stopper of a tube; the tube's vacuum will pull blood into the tube until the tube's nearly full. Repeat the procedure until all three tubes are filled. Gently invert the tube containing anticoagulant five or six times. (*Don't* vigorously shake it.)

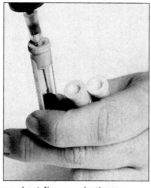

Label the tubes and fill out the necessary lab slips. Send the specimens to the lab at once.

Document the procedure. Continue to monitor the child closely for bleeding or hematoma formation.

Filling collection tubes in proper sequence

Before transferring blood from a syringe to Vacutainer collection tubes, make sure you know what sequence to follow. Avoid jeopardizing test results, by learning these guidelines:
* Fill sterile blood culture tubes first, to minimize the risk of contaminating the specimen. These collection tubes contain a culture medium.
* Next, fill tubes that contain anticoagulant additives, such as oxalates or heparin. These additives appear as white powder or clear liquid. By transferring blood into anticoagulant containers as quickly as possible, you minimize the clotting that occurs after venipuncture. (Remember to gently invert these containers five or six times, to thoroughly mix the blood and additives.)
* Fill any empty tubes last.

Hospitalization

We've already discussed many methods and techniques for preparing a child for nursing and medical procedures. And of course, you'll use these techniques for all aspects of pediatric care, whether you work in a doctor's office, a clinic, or a hospital.

Now, let's focus on preparing a child for hospitalization, because it poses special challenges. Think of it from the child's point of view. Suddenly, he's taken from his safe, familiar home, and thrust into a world of strangers and possibly painful procedures. He's separated from his parents—perhaps for the first time ever. In addition to being frightened and confused, he may actually feel guilty, subconsciously believing that he's being punished for some misbehavior.

But careful planning by you, other members of the hospital staff, and the child's family can relieve much of the understandable emotional stress your patient feels. In the following pages, you'll see how.

Helping parents prepare the child

Mrs. Foreman, mother of 3-year-old Robbie, asks to speak to you in private. "The doctor wants to take out Robbie's tonsils," she tells you, looking worried. "Robbie's never been away from home overnight. I think his father and I will miss him as much as he will miss us!"

Sound familiar? As a pediatric nurse, you know that preparing the parents for a child's hospitalization is as important as preparing the child himself. Otherwise, they may communicate their own anxieties to the child.

Parents have a strong desire to protect their child from fear and pain. To them, hospitalization may represent a threat to their ability to care for him. They may even feel somehow guilty about his illness.

Understanding the parents' concerns will help you prepare them for temporary separation from their child. To help satisfy their natural desire to care for him, include them as part of the health-care team. Such action, of course, has another advantage: These days, a child may be admitted to the hospital the day of surgery—or only the day before. More and more, health-care professionals *must* rely on parents for preparation.

If you work in a hospital pediatric unit, you'll probably have little contact with the parents before the child's admitted. But if you work in a doctor's office or in an outpatient clinic, you have an opportunity to help the child and parents prepare. Consider using the following suggestions.

Informing the parents

The first step is encouraging the parents to find out as much as possible about the child's illness and about the hospital routines he'll experience. If you're familiar with the hospital, tell them about visiting hours and other policies yourself. If you're not, or if the parents have questions you can't answer, encourage them to call the hospital for more information. Also, if the hospital provides a preadmission brochure, see that they get a copy.

Urge them to question you or the doctor about anything they don't understand. Being well-informed serves two purposes for parents: It helps relieve their own anxieties, and it permits them to answer the child's questions with confidence.

When you talk to the parents, you'll probably hear some of the questions listed below. To help you answer them, we've supplied some sample replies. But remember, always offer any advice with tact. Never imply that just because you're a nurse, you know what's best for the child. After all, no one knows him better than his parents. But as a nurse, you *do* know more about hospitalization. Chances are, the parents will be grateful for your insights.

When should I tell my child about his hospitalization? This depends on your child's age and maturity. But as a rule, if he's age 7 or older, you should inform him a week or two before admission, or as soon as possible. He needs this time to get used to the idea of hospitalization and to think of questions. Let him participate in planning for the event; this gives him a feeling of control that'll reassure him.

Hospitalization

Helping parents prepare the child continued

A younger child needs preparation only a few days to a week before admission. Young children, especially toddlers, have a very limited ability to imagine future events.
How much should I tell him about the hospital experience? I don't want to frighten him.
Many parents believe that a child's better off not knowing what's going to happen. But I've discovered that a child will be less afraid and more cooperative if he knows what to expect. After all, what a child imagines may be far worse than what he really faces.

Try to describe the hospital environment, personnel, and routines to the child, in words he'll understand. Concentrate on the aspects that most concern him. A younger child, for example, will wonder: What will my room look like? Who'll take care of me? What will I eat? When can I see you?

Keep in mind that you can't anticipate *everything* that'll happen to your child. Try to avoid giving him too many details, or you may inadvertently mislead him.
I know that surgery causes pain. What do I say when he asks if it'll hurt?
Be honest, but stress the positive. For example, you might say that his throat will hurt for a while after he wakes up, but it'll feel better each day. Encourage him to tell the nurses if he feels uncomfortable; make sure he understands that the nurses will help him get well as soon as possible.
What if he's upset, or starts crying?
It's perfectly normal for a child to be frightened, or even angry, at the thought of separation from you and his home. Don't scold him if he cries; that's a normal reponse. Instead, try to discuss his fears with him. In addition, help him express his feelings through play. By drawing, writing, or acting out his feelings, a child's better able to cope with them.
Can he bring anything from home to the hospital?
Certainly. Help him pick out a favorite toy to bring with him. This familiar object will provide a sense of security. And re-

member, no matter how tattered it may be, an old toy's likely to provide more reassurance than a new one. Label the toy with your child's name, so it won't get lost.
What else can I do?
Some hospitals provide orientation tours or programs for pediatric patients. Such a tour helps prepare the child by familiarizing him with hospital equipment, personnel, and routines beforehand. Consider participating. Also, if the hospital provides coloring books or brochures geared toward young patients, read through them with the child.
Suppose I think of other questions later?
Jot them down on a piece of paper, so you don't forget them. Then, don't hesitate to call me, the doctor, or the hospital for answers.

What not to say

Parents may unintentionally upset a child by saying the wrong thing. Help them avoid some common pitfalls by giving this special advice:
• Don't bribe the child, or lie to him about his destination. He'll probably feel betrayed and may be angry with you. Keep in mind that your careful preparation will make such measures unnecessary.
• Don't mislead the child about the hospital experience. To reassure him, you may be tempted to tell him that the hospital will be fun, like a party. Do, of course, stress the positive aspects of hospitalization,

but don't give him the wrong impression. Discuss both the pleasant and unpleasant aspects of hospitalization in a matter-of-fact manner.
• Don't try to insure the child's good behavior by telling him the nurse or doctor will give him an injection if he's bad. Teach the child that nurses and doctors want to help him, not punish him.
• Don't give the child false reassurances. For example, don't tell him that you'll sleep in the same room or next door, if you're unable to do so. Instead, find out what hospital policy allows, and tell the child exactly where you'll be.
• Don't overwhelm the child with more details than he can absorb at one time. Give information in small doses, using his own curiosity and questions as a guide.
Note: For suggested reading for pediatric patients, see page 157 of this book.

Getting to know your patient

When a child's admitted to the pediatric unit, you have a lot to remember. In addition to introducing him and his parents to his new roommate, orienting them to the facilities, and applying an identification band, you'll take an admission history. But no matter how busy you are, don't neglect to collect personal information about the child as well as recording his health history. The more you know about the child, the better able you'll be to support and comfort him in his new environment.

Explain to the parents that you want to know as much as possible about the child so you can make him comfortable in the unit. Then, ask them to give you background information in a few key areas.

To save time, your hospital may provide a form for you (or the parents) to fill out. If not,

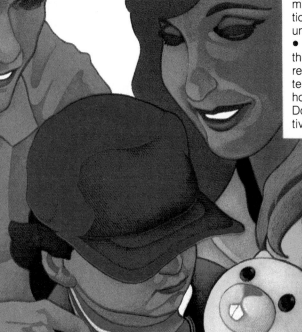

consider making your own, using the following topics as a guide.

General information: Record the child's full name and nickname, his sex, and his age. Find out why he's being admitted, and how much he knows about his illness and treatment. Also, find out about anything the parents may not want him to know, and ask them to explain why they feel this way. Ask if the child has any particular fears or expectations about being hospitalized.

Previous hospitalizations: Has the child been hospitalized before? If so, where and why? How did the child react to the experience?

Home life: Who spends the most time caring for him at home? Record the names of his immediate family members, and the ages of brothers and sisters. Note the names of family pets. Also, document any major recent changes in the family, such as a divorce, death, birth, or a parent's job loss. How is the child coping with such a change?

Visitation plans: How often can family members visit? Does anyone plan to stay with the child, or be present at meals? Ask if family members would like to participate in the child's care, and if so, to what extent.

Toilet habits: What words does the child use for urination and bowel movement? Is he fully toilet trained, or does he need diapers or training pants? Does he use a potty seat? Does he use the bathroom at night? Record when he had his last bowel movement, and how frequently they normally occur. Also, note any difficulties he has eliminating, and any particular routines or rituals associated with elimination.

Eating habits: Does the child

feed himself, or does he need help? Is he accustomed to a morning, afternoon, or evening snack? Is he allergic to any foods (or anything else)? What foods does he particularly like or dislike? Note any special aids or rituals the parents use to encourage the child to eat.

Sleep habits: Does the child usually have a morning or afternoon nap? What's his bedtime? When does he normally arise? Does he sleepwalk, wet his bed, or have nightmares? (If he has one of these problems, ask how the parents deal with it.) Does he sleep with a toy? Also note whether the child sleeps in a crib or a bed when he's at home.

Hygiene: How often does he bathe and brush his teeth? Does he object to either?

Play habits: Document whether the child prefers to play with others, or alone. What are his favorite games and toys? What toys has he brought with him to the hospital?

Fears: Does the child have any special fears? For example, is he afraid of being alone? Of the dark? Certain animals or places? Doctors or nurses? Injections? (If necessary, reassure the parents that many children have fears like these.)

School and religion: If the child's school age, ask how well he likes school, and whether he'll continue with school work while in the hospital. Also, document the child's religion, and note whether he will continue any religious practices (including bedtime prayers) in the hospital.

Discipline: Ask parents how they discipline the child when he misbehaves. Who in the family usually disciplines the child? How does the child respond? Is the discipline usually effective?

Other: Note whether the child has any difficulty communicating, or if he has any physical disabilities that limit his mobility.

Parents' comments: Finally, give the parents a chance to volunteer any additional information that will help you make the child feel at home. Encourage them to describe the child's temperament, and to tell you how he expresses anxiety, annoyance, and anger.

Helping a child cope

Early this morning, 6-year-old Colin Frawley was struck by a car outside his home. When Colin arrived at the hospital with his distraught parents, he was conscious and alert. Subsequent examination revealed no broken bones. But, because Colin suffered a head injury and possible internal injuries, the doctor admitted him to your unit for observation and further testing.

A child like Colin presents a special challenge. Because he's unprepared for hospitalization, he may cope poorly with the stress of a new environment and even suffer some long-term emotional effects as a result.

Consider how Colin may feel. In addition to his understandable pain, fright, and confusion, he may feel guilty about the accident. "I was bad to play in the street," he may tell you. "I hope Mommy's not mad." And if his hospitalization's prolonged, or he must undergo surgery to repair a ruptured spleen, he's likely to become even more upset.

Fortunately, your sensitive nursing care can make a difference. Most children, when treated with kindness and respect, cope with the stress of hospitalization remarkably well. And you're in the perfect position to help them do so.

Although a child who enters your unit with little or no preparation may need extra attention and support, you'll use the same basic techniques to help *all* your patients cope with the stress of hospitalization. Make the following guidelines part of your nursing routine.

• Provide one-to-one nursing care, if possible. You or another nurse, a nurse's aid, or any other staff member can serve as the child's special friend throughout his hospital stay. In addition to playing with him, this staff member should be available for support during any stressful procedure, especially if the parents aren't present.

• Assess the child's under-

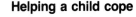

Hospitalization

Helping a child cope continued

standing of his illness and treatment by asking him why he thinks he's in the hospital. Use his responses to plan patient teaching and assess his need for special emotional support.
• Plan teaching sessions when the child's rested and alert. Don't prolong them beyond the child's attention span.
• Foster the child's trust with consistency and honesty. Tell him that you'll warn him before you do anything that'll hurt; then, keep your promise. This way, he won't feel he must be on guard all the time.
• Prepare him for treatments, including surgery, by describing the events and sensations he'll experience. But avoid being *too* specific, because he may become upset if events don't happen exactly as you predicted. To help the child cope with any unexpected threat, ask him to remember anything that happens to him that's different from what he expected. Then, you can discuss it with him later.
Important: Tell him about painful or unpleasant aspects of treatment last. Otherwise, he may become too anxious to

listen to the rest of your explanation.
• Choose your words carefully, especially if your patient's a preschooler. Remember, a child this age thinks in literal terms, and in terms of his own experience. For example, if you tell him that he'll be "put to sleep" for surgery, he may think of the old family dog who never returned from the veterinarian's. Likewise, if you tell him that surgery will occur when he's asleep, he may be reluctant to fall asleep at night, fearing that something awful will happen if he does so. Emphasize that anesthesia's a *special* sleep he'll experience when the doctor gives him a special medicine, and that the doctor will wake him up when surgery's all over.
• Question the child about his conception of treatments and procedures. Suppose, for example, he asks you, "How does the doctor take out my tonsils?" Reply by saying, "How do *you* think he does it?" Listen carefully to his explanation. In addition to revealing his misconceptions, it can help you understand his unique fears and fantasies.
• Use group-teaching techniques, when possible. In addition to saving you time, group teaching provides peer group support for each child.

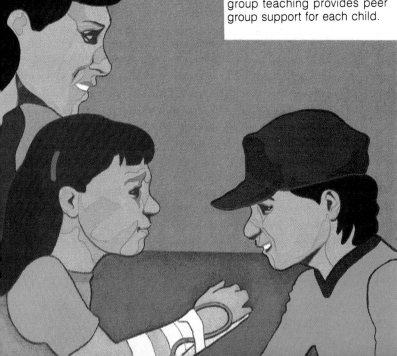

• Perform all painful or upsetting procedures in the treatment room—not the child's bedroom. Let his bedroom be a safe haven, where he needn't worry about being hurt.
• Give him a sense of control by offering realistic choices. For example, you can't allow him to choose whether or not to have an injection. But you *can* ask him if he'd like another minute to get ready.
• Ask another child to help you prepare a newcomer for an unpleasant procedure. For example, if the new patient's afraid of an injection, a more experienced child may be able to reassure him that it's not so bad.
• Build playtime into your daily routine. This encourages the child to associate you with comfort and fun, not just pain. And it gives you a chance to learn more about the child.
• Use play therapy to explain procedures to the child, and to help him work through his emotions. For example, if he's scheduled for a tonsillectomy, you might bandage the throat of his teddy bear or other toy, to show him where the pain will be. Assure him that the pain will occur *only* at this spot. Also tell him that he'll still be able to swallow and talk, although his throat will hurt at first. After surgery, he can care for his toy as you care for him.
Play also provides clues to how well the child's adjusting to his illness and treatment. Violent or destructive play suggests anger or fear; drawings that distort body parts suggest poor self-image and fear of mutilation. Encouraging a child to express himself through play helps him work through his feelings. But if the child seems unusually disturbed, consult with a child psychologist or specially-trained social worker.
• Tell the child that no one will be mad if he cries. Remain supportive of the child, no matter how negatively he behaves.

The child's parents: Part of the team

How do you feel about your patient's parents? Do you regard them as an important part of the team?
If not, you're missing a valuable opportunity to make the child's hospital stay as pleasant as possible. Never underestimate the importance of parents' presence to a child. When parents are treated as allies rather than nuisances, everyone benefits.
Of course, not all parents are willing or able to fully participate in their child's care. For example, they may have jobs, and other children at home to care for. But regardless of the extent of their participation, accept them as part of your team. Here's what you can do.
• Ask them to give you as much personal information about the child as possible, using the suggestions on pages 42 and 43. This way, you can try to make the child feel at home, even when the parents aren't present.
• Encourage them to help care for the child. For example, they can support and entertain him simply by reading or playing with him. Also, they can help with simple responsibilities, such as feeding, bathing, and ambulating him.
• When appropriate, congratulate the parents on the good job they did preparing the child. This reinforces the idea that you're all working together as a team.
• Ask the parents to inform you of any problems or behavioral changes they notice. Remember, because they know the child best, they're likely to be the first to notice any developing problems. Then, discuss with them possible ways to help the child.
• Encourage parents to support the child during especially frightening periods; for example, the day of surgery. The child's separation anxiety will decrease his ability to cooperate, and increase any pain or discomfort he feels.

Restraints

"No!" Anyone who's worked as a pediatric nurse dreads hearing a child utter this word with all the determination he can muster. As we've already discussed, you'll always do your best to elicit a child's cooperation before beginning a procedure. But let's face it—sometimes your best efforts will fail. Or, your patient may be just too young or ill to reason with. What then?

For the child's safety and comfort, you may have to restrain him. If you're obtaining a blood sample or giving an injection, you'll restrain the child for only a short time. To do so, you probably won't need an artifical restraint. Instead, you (or an assistant) may be able to safely and effectively restrain the child by holding him in a restraining position. In the following pages, you'll see how.

But suppose your patient needs long-term restraining; for example, after surgery. Then, you'll need to apply an artifical restraint, as ordered. In this section, we'll acquaint you with several different types.

Although you'll use artificial restraints only as a last resort, they're basic to pediatric care. Consider using them to:
• protect an I.V. or surgical site.
• prevent a child from rubbing inflamed eyes, scratching skin eruptions, or irritating any other medical condition.
• maintain proper body alignment during prolonged immobilization; for example, while a child's in traction.
• prevent an active child from climbing out of bed, or a disoriented child from injuring himself.

How to restrain a child

1 *Let's say you're examining 4-year-old Alan Wolfe, who has a foreign object in his ear. Because he's upset, you do your best to relax him before beginning your otoscopic exam. For example, you show him the otoscope, allow him to touch it, and explain that its light will let you see into his ear. But when you begin the exam, Alan squirms continuously, preventing you from completing the procedure. Although Alan's not really afraid, he simply doesn't understand why he must hold still. How would you solve this problem?*

Ask Mrs. Wolfe to hold Alan, as shown here. Seat the child sideways on Mrs. Wolfe's lap, with his legs between her legs. Ask him to hug his mother, using the arm nearest to her. Then, ask Mrs. Wolfe to gently grasp Alan's free arm with one hand, and hold his head against her chest with the other. To avoid frightening the child, remind Mrs. Wolfe not to block his view with her hand. With the child held securely in this position, you can quickly examine his ear. To examine his other ear, just reposition him facing in the opposite direction.

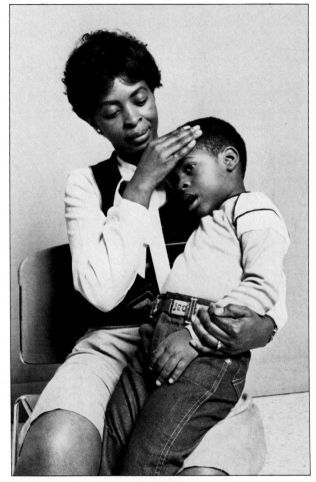

2 Suppose the doctor's ordered a diphtheria, tetanus toxoids, and pertussis (DTP) vaccine. If you're giving the injection at an upper leg site, how can you restrain Alan long enough to prevent injury while you give the injection? Try the position shown here. If the child's quiet and calm, you can hold him securely between your arm and side.

Note: Use this position to hold a younger child while you give an injection at a ventrogluteal or dorsogluteal site. However, never use the dorsogluteal site in a child under age 3, since these muscles aren't developed well enough to protect the child from injury.

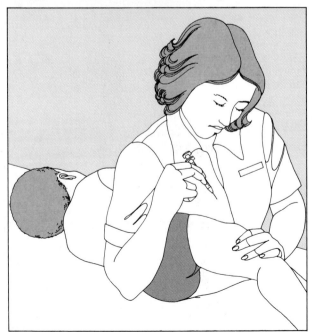

Restraints

How to restrain a child continued

3 As an alternative, ask an assistant to hold the child in this position. (Take care to introduce the assistant to the child first.) Keep in mind that, because this position is more restrictive, the child may find it more frightening.

Don't use it unless the position shown in step 2 is inadequate.

Important: Never ask a parent to restrain a child during a painful procedure. Instead, ask another health-care professional to help you.

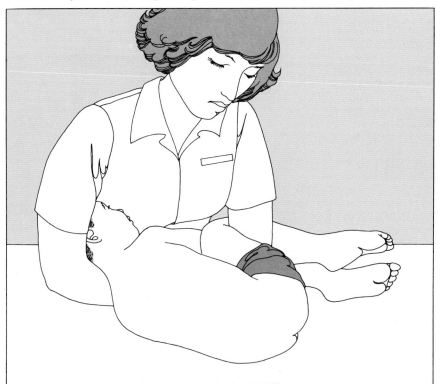

4 What if you're giving Alan an injection in his arm? Ask an assistant to hold the child in his lap, like this, crossing his arms over the child's chest.

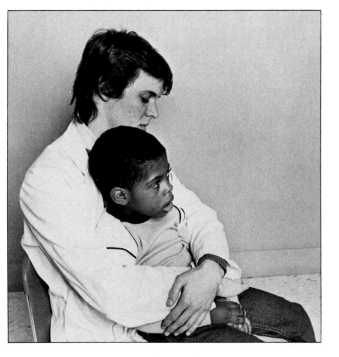

Using restraints: Some guidelines

Now you know how to hold a child in a restraining position. But what if the child needs long-term restraining—after eye surgery, for example? Then, you'll probably use an artificial restraint.

As a rule, you need a doctor's order before you can apply (or remove) any of these restraints. However, in an emergency, you may apply a restraint first, then obtain an order immediately afterwards. *Note:* Many hospitals also have specific procedures for checking and removing restraints. Learn your hospital's policy.

No matter what type of restraint the doctor orders, follow these guidelines:

DO tell the child and his parents that a restraint is necessary to protect the child from possible injury. Never make the child feel that you're punishing him for misbehavior.

DO position a young child on his side or abdomen, if possible. This reduces the risk of aspiration if he vomits.

DO position him so his body and restrained limbs are well-aligned and in natural positions. Help him change position every 2 hours.

DO check the patient every 1 to 2 hours for signs of abrasions, bruises, or developing pressure sores under the restraint. Also, check his peripheral pulses, skin color, and temperature distal to the restraint. If necessary, loosen or reposition the restraint, or apply additional padding.

DO remove the restraint at least once every 2 hours, and massage the affected limb or body area. Help the child perform range-of-motion exercises. Massage his heels, hips, elbows, and other pressure points.

DO give an older child a bedpan, or help him to the bathroom every 2 hours. Check an infant or toddler every 30 minutes, and change his diaper as needed.

DO use restraints decorated with bright colors or designs, if possible.

DO let the parents remove the restraint, if you feel they can prevent the child from injuring himself. But tell them to call you before they leave the child, so you can reapply the restraint.

Avoiding pitfalls

To use restraints properly, keep these additional points in mind:

DON'T use a restraint as a substitute for observation and personal attention.

DON'T tie the restraint to the side rails. Tie it to the bed or crib frame, out of the child's reach.

DON'T position a tongue depressor or tube restraint so it presses into the child's skin.

DON'T restrain the child any longer than absolutely necessary.

DON'T threaten to restrain a child if he doesn't cooperate.

Making a mummy restraint

1 *Your 5-month-old patient may have an eye infection. To immobilize him while the doctor examines his eyes, make a mummy restraint. Here's how:*

First, place a drawsheet (or blanket) flat on the bed or examination table. Then, lay the infant in the middle of the sheet. Make sure the sheet's top is at his shoulder level, as shown here, and its bottom extends about 12″ (30 cm) beyond his feet.

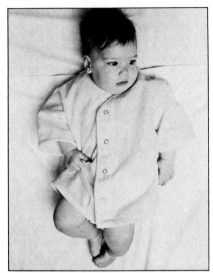

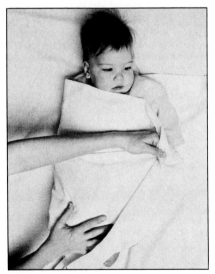

2 Next, position one of the infant's arms at his side, in a natural position. Grasp the top corner of the sheet on the same side. Then, fold the edge of the sheet downward over his arm and across his torso, as shown. Tuck it under the opposite side of his body.

3 Put his other arm at his side, in a natural position, and repeat the procedure.

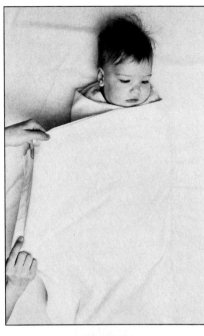

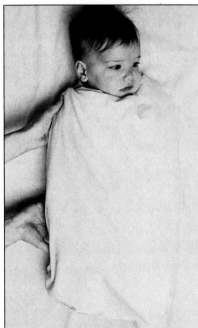

4 Finally, grasp each corner of the sheet's bottom, and bring the bottom edge up to his shoulder level. Tuck both corners of the sheet under his shoulders. Secure the restraint by crossing one side of the sheet over the other, underneath the infant. Finally, tuck in any excess.

Making an arm restraint

1 *Need to restrain an infant's arms? The doctor may order one of the restraints shown below.*

Suppose your hospital supplies ready-made elbow restraints. This type of restraint consists of tongue depressors presewn into a piece of fabric (see inset). Wrap the restraint around one arm, and secure it with tape or gauze ties, as shown. If necessary, tie the restraint to the bed frame with gauze ties, or pin the restraint to the bed linen.

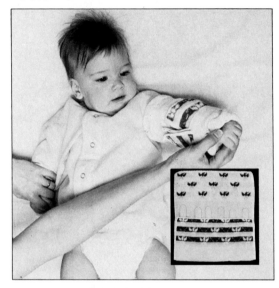

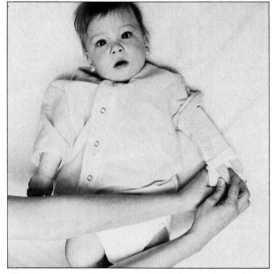

2 If your hospital doesn't supply ready-made elbow restraints, you can easily make your own. Obtain a piece of stockinette that's twice the length of the child's arm. Pull it inside out to half its length, and slip it on his arm. Then, place two to four tongue depressors (depending on the size of his arm) in the folded stockinette, as the nurse is doing here. Secure the restraint as described above.

Restraints

Making an arm restraint continued

3 If your patient's an infant or toddler, consider applying stockinette without tongue depressors to his arms. Pin the stockinette to the bed linen.

Or, roll a washcloth into a long band, and fold it over the child's forearm. Then, pin the washcloth to the bed linens, as shown here. Place the pin close to his wrist, so he can't pull his hand through the washcloth.

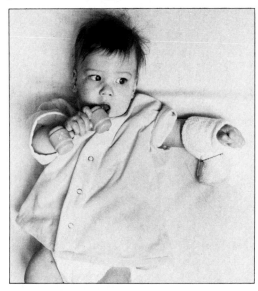

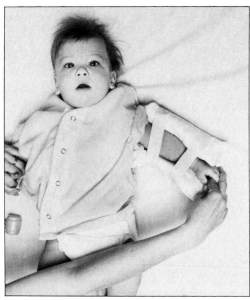

4 As an alternative, try this arm restraint made from a diaper. Fold the diaper in thirds or in half (depending on the child's size), and lay his arm in its middle. Roll the edges of the diaper toward his arm, until the rolls form splints beside his arm. Secure the restraint with two pieces of double-backed tape, as shown.

Making a wrist restraint

1 *To restrain an older child's arms, consider making one of the wrist restraints shown here. These restraints work equally well on the child's ankles, if you must restrain his legs.*

A clove-hitch restraint won't tighten when the child pulls against it. To make one, use a gauze tie that's long enough to loop twice around the child's wrist and then tie to the bed frame. With this gauze, fashion two loops, as shown in the inset illustration. The arrow indicates where you'll insert the child's hand.

Next, pad the child's wrist with cotton, a dry surgical dressing (Surgipad™), or a gauze pad (depending on the child's size). Place his hand through the loops, and adjust the loops so they fit snugly (but not tightly). Tie the ends of the gauze loops to the bed frame, as shown.

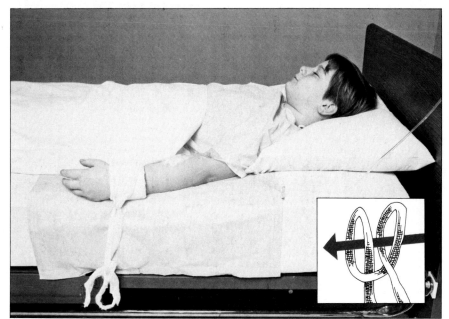

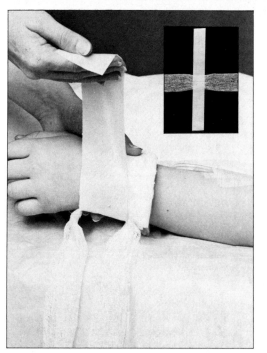

2 As an alternative, cut a strip of regular adhesive tape long enough to wrap 1½ times around the child's wrist, and lay it sticky-side up on a flat surface. Then, cut a cotton or gauze tie that's long enough to run double between the child's wrist and the bed frame. Lay the tie across the middle of the tape, so that equal parts of the tie rest on each side of the tape (see inset).

Then, wrap padding around the child's wrist, and secure it firmly (but not tightly) with the strip of tape. Position the tape so the ties hang down from the underside of the child's wrist, as shown. Tie the ends of the restraint to the bed frame. *Note:* Don't use paper tape or nonallergenic tape to make this restraint, because they tear easily.

Using ready-made restraints

On the preceding pages, you saw how to make several types of restraints. This chart will acquaint you with some of the ready-made restraints available.

Crib net

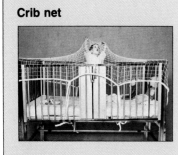

A net stretched over the top and sides of an infant's crib or playpen. The flexible net permits the child to stand, but prevents him from climbing out.

Indications
For any active child capable of climbing out of his crib or playpen

Nursing considerations
• Tie the net to the bed frame, not the side rails. This way, you can raise and lower the side rails without removing the net.

Mitten

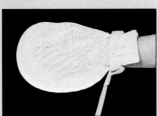

A translucent mitt with extra strap for tying to bed frame. May be used without the strap.

Indications
To prevent a child from scratching his skin, or from disturbing a surgical or I.V. site

Nursing considerations
• Don't allow the restraint to bind or bend the child's fingers. Maintain the natural position of partial hand flexion by placing a small roll of gauze in the child's hand before applying the mitten.
• Frequently observe the child's hand for changes in skin color.
• When using the strap, tie it to the bed frame.
• If the restraint immobilizes the child's elbow (or any other joint), remove the restraint at least once every 2 hours and help the child perform range-of-motion (ROM) exercises.

Crib cage

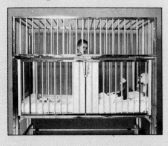

An enclosed metal cage attached to the crib and extending above it, to permit the child to stand

Indications
For any active child capable of climbing out of his crib or playpen

Nursing considerations
• Supervise the child closely, to make sure he doesn't climb up the cage and fall.
• Provide additional emotional support, since the child may feel like he's imprisoned.

Sandbag

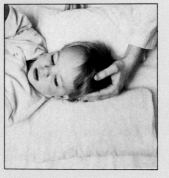

Sand encased in water-impervious oilcloth. Available in varying sizes.

Indications
To immobilize a child's head, to separate his legs, or (when placed on each side of a young child) to maintain proper body alignment

Nursing considerations
• Cover sandbag with a pillowcase before use.
• Supervise the child carefully, and perform ROM exercises on immobilized joints every 2 hours.
• Maintain proper body alignment.

Jacket

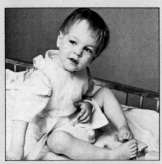

A vest with long restraining tapes at waist level; some types also restrain at the shoulders. Fastens with cloth ties.

Indications
Use as an alternative to the crib net or crib cage restraints, or to secure a child in a high chair or wheelchair

Nursing considerations
• Apply jacket with the ties at the child's back, so he can't undo them.
• Secure the jacket's tapes to the bed or chair frame, never the side rails.
• Frequently observe the child, to ensure that he doesn't entangle himself in the restraint's tapes.
• If the child's positioned flat, frequently check him for proper body alignment.

Restraining board

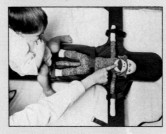

A hard-plastic, cross-shaped board padded with vinyl-covered cushions. Includes Velcro® straps for securing arms, legs, head, and torso.

Indications
For complete, short-term immobilization during procedures or transport

Nursing considerations
• Provide emotional support while the child's restrained, since being restrained this way may frighten him.
• Release the child immediately after the procedure.
• Don't attempt to use this restraint for a child who's too big to comfortably fit on it.

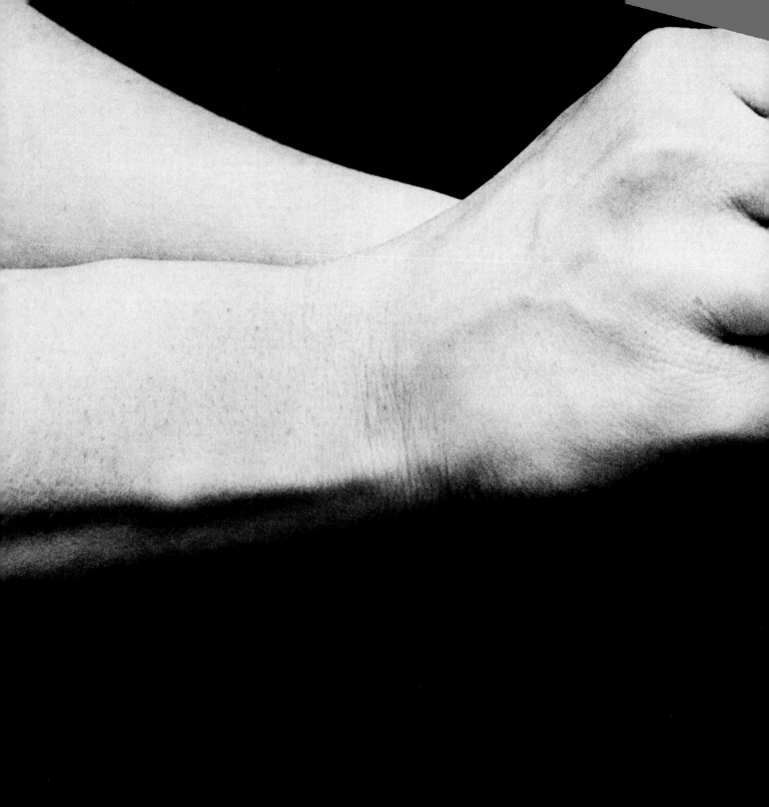

Administering Medications

Precautions
Oral
Dermatomucosal
Parenteral
Rectal

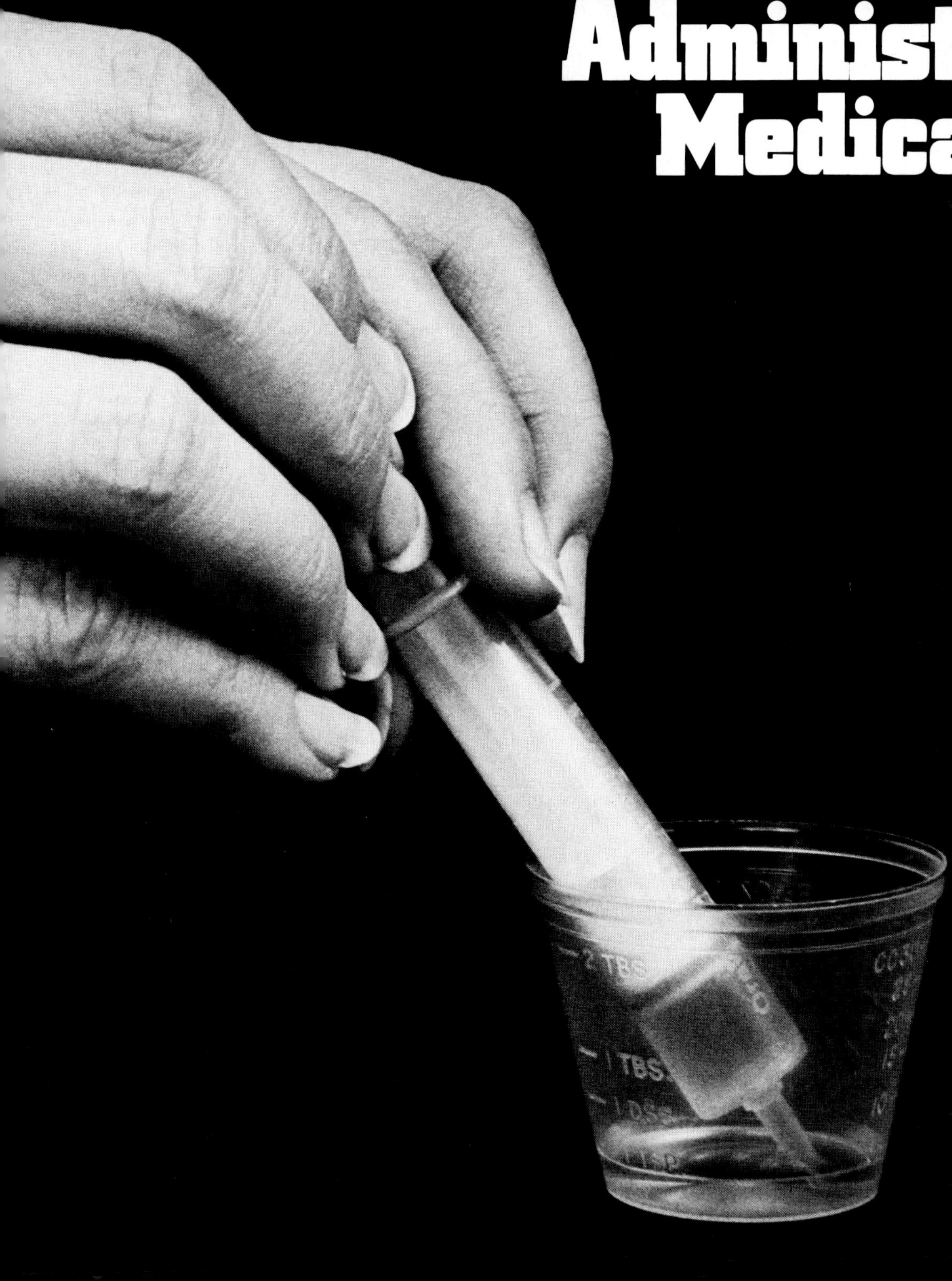

Precautions

As you know, before you give a child (or any patient) his medication, you have to take certain precautions. These include checking and confirming the doctor's order, making sure the dose and dosage are appropriate for your patient, and knowing what foods and other medications affect absorption. Afterward, you must clearly and accurately document medication administration, according to your hospital's policy.

For more information on these and other points to remember when administering medications, read the next few pages.

Observing the Five Rights

When administering any drug, make sure you confirm the patient's identity and compare the doctor's order with the order written on your patient's medication card or Kardex. To do so, use the system known as the Five Rights; it will help you prevent errors and ensure safe drug administration.

Ask yourself:
• **Right patient name:** Are the names on the order, Kardex and identification band identical?
• **Right drug:** Is the ordered drug the same?
• **Right dose:** Does the dose you're administering match the ordered dose on your patient's Kardex? Is the dose appropriate for the patient's age and size?
• **Right route:** Is the ordered route the same? Is the route correct for the prescribed drug? Is the route correct for the dose?
• **Right time and frequency:** Are the time and frequency of administration the same, and appropriate for the patient's age and size?

If you find any discrepancy, withhold the drug until you can check with the doctor or pharmacist.

Important: Except in an extreme emergency, avoid accepting verbal drug orders (unless your hospital policy dictates otherwise). During an emergency, immediately write the verbal order on your patient's chart so you can easily refer to it. If possible, have another nurse listen to the order on a phone extension. Then, have the doctor countersign the order as soon as possible.

$$\frac{300\,mg \times 85.8}{150} = 171.6\,mg$$

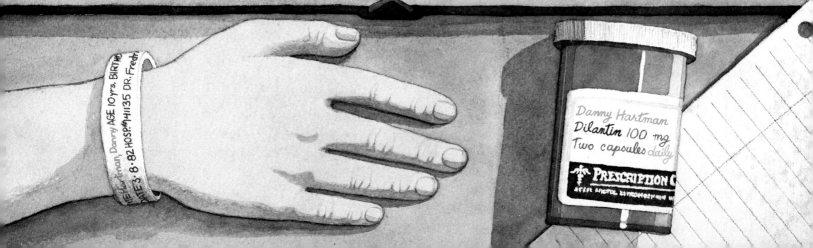

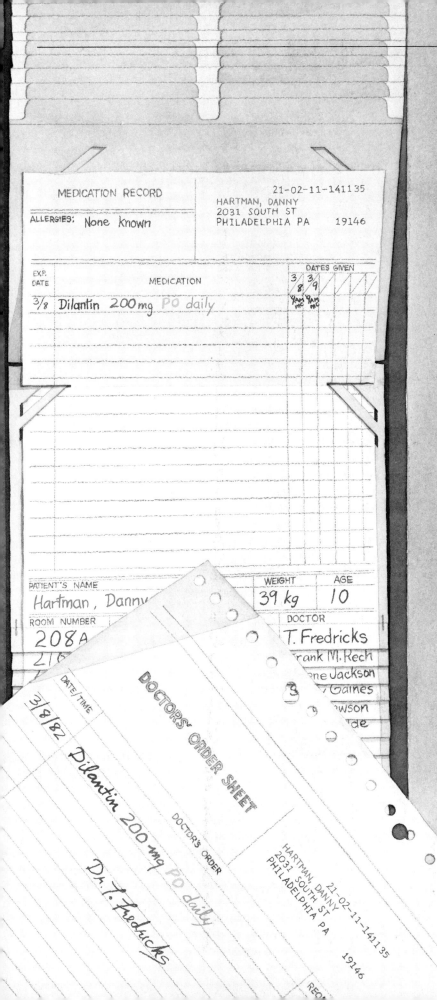

MEDICATION RECORD   21-02-11-141135
                                     HARTMAN, DANNY
ALLERGIES: None known   2031 SOUTH ST
                                     PHILADELPHIA PA   19146

EXP. DATE	MEDICATION	DATES GIVEN
		3/8	3/9
3/8	Dilantin 200 mg PO daily	9am mc	9am mc

PATIENT'S NAME   WEIGHT   AGE
Hartman, Danny   39 kg   10
ROOM NUMBER   DOCTOR
208A   T. Fredricks
                        Frank M. Rech
                        ene Jackson
                        Gaines
                        wson
                        de

DOCTORS' ORDER SHEET
DOCTORS' ORDER
DATE/TIME
3/8/82   Dilantin 200 mg PO daily
         Dr. T. Fredricks

HARTMAN, DANNY
2031 SOUTH ST
PHILADELPHIA PA
21-02-11-141135
19146

Checking dose and dosage

Suppose the doctor's ordered 200 mg phenytoin sodium (Dilantin) orally once a day for your 10-year-old patient, Danny Hartman. Do you know if such a dosage is appropriate for seizure control in a child Danny's age and size?

Before giving any drug, you're responsible for determining whether or not the dose and dosage are safe for your patient. If you're unsure, follow these guidelines.

To check the prescribed *dose* (the amount of drug given at one time), use one of the formulas below. If the result of your calculation differs significantly from the prescribed dose, withhold the drug and check with the doctor or pharmacist.

Young's rule:
$$\frac{\text{adult dose} \times \text{child's age (in years)}}{\text{child's age} + 12} = \text{dose}$$

Clarks' rule:
$$\frac{\text{adult dose} \times \text{child's weight (in pounds)}}{150} = \text{dose}$$

Fried's rule (for a child less than age 1):
$$\frac{\text{adult dose} \times \text{child's age (in months)}}{150} = \text{dose}$$

Surface area rule:
$$\frac{\text{adult dose} \times \text{surface area of child (in square meters)}}{1.7} = \text{dose}$$

Note: Use a body surface area nomogram to determine surface area. (See the appendices to this book.)

Now, suppose you question the prescribed *dosage*. As you know, dosage includes the prescribed dose, the frequency of administration, and the number of doses to be given. To check dosage, you must consult a drug reference book or the pharmacist. Always double-check the dose and dosage for a potent drug with another nurse.

Know your medications

When caring for a patient—whether he's a child or an adult—make sure you know as much as possible about the medication you're administering. To determine what effect the medication will have on your patient, remember these important points:
• If you believe the prescribed medication's inappropriate for your patient's condition, consult the doctor.
• If you're not sure the prescribed dose and dosage are safe, calculate the dose again (see above). Then, call the pharmacy, or consult a drug text to confirm dosage. If a problem exists, withhold the medication, and contact the doctor.
• Make sure the ordered route is compatible with your patient's condition. For example, if the ordered route is oral and your patient's been vomiting, notify the doctor.
• Make sure the medication's compatible with other medications your patient's taking. Notify the doctor of any medication incompatibility.
• Know what foods or other medications will affect the absorption of the medication you're administering. Doing so allows you to gauge your patient's response to the medication and helps you determine the cause of any adverse reactions.
• Find out the anticipated effect of the medication, and any possible side effects, so you can recognize complications.
*Available in both the United States and in Canada

Precautions

Protecting a child from an allergic reaction

As you know, if you give your patient a drug to which he's allergic, you can endanger his life. And if your patient's a child, the risk of inadvertently doing so increases. Because a young child hasn't been exposed to as many substances as an adult has, he may have an allergy that hasn't yet been discovered.

You're responsible for doing everything you possibly can to determine if your pediatric patient's allergic to a particular drug. So remember to be thorough in your determination.

First, never assume that your patient has no allergies, even if the allergy information space on his Kardex is blank. Make sure you question his family. Is his father or mother allergic to a particular drug, such as penicillin? If so, the child may be allergic to it, too.

In addition, your patient may be allergic to various foods or animals. If so, he may have an allergic reaction to some serums or vaccines; for example, Attenuvax*, a measles (rubeola) virus vaccine cultured in eggs, or Dryvax, a smallpox vaccine cultured in cows. Check for these kinds of allergies as well.

Never leave a blank space on the allergy information section of your patient's Kardex. If he has any allergy (including a food allergy), docu-ment this in red on his Kardex, medication administration record, and chart. If your hospital provides color-coded identification bands for patients with allergies, see that he gets one.

Suppose, after a thorough check, you find that your patient has no known allergies. Write on the Kardex, "No allergies known."

If the doctor orders a drug that you suspect the patient's allergic to, obtain an order for a substitute. Or, obtain an order for a skin test before giving the suspicious drug. (For detailed information on giving an intradermal skin test, turn to page 70.)

When performing a skin test (or administering any suspicious drug), always keep a syringe of epinephrine hydrochloride (Adrenalin Chloride) available to counteract the effects of anaphylactic shock. Watch your patient closely for 24 hours if you're administering the drug orally; watch him for 30 minutes when giving the drug subcutaneously or intramuscularly; and stay with him for at least 5 minutes when using the I.V. route.

Anytime you receive a new drug order for your patient, familiarize yourself with the drug's properties and components. If you're unsure of them, check a reference book before administering the drug.

Documenting medication administration

As you know, you must keep an accurate record of all medications you administer. Since record-keeping systems vary from hospital to hospital, you'll have to learn your hospital's system. For example, you may use medication cards, medication Kardexes, or a combination of both. But no matter what system you use, you'll need the following information: your patient's name and room number; the date; the medication; dose, route, frequency, and time of administration; and your name and title.

To help remember other important documentation points, keep these questions in mind:
• Have you recorded the injection site for the parenteral medication you're administering? Doing so will make proper site rotation easier, and will prove helpful if problems arise with a specific site. You may use letters, numbers, or abbreviations to identify the body parts used as administration sites. (You may also use different colored ink to distinguish a change in shifts.) Check your hospital policy.
• Are your abbreviations and numbers written clearly on your patient's Kardex? If they're not, they may confuse other health-care professionals who are caring for your patient. For example, never abbreviate the word UNIT. Someone may misread the letter U for a poorly-written zero, and administer the wrong dose.

Also, place a zero before the decimal point when writing a fractional dose; for example, 0.4 ml epinephrine hydrochloride. Then, the dose won't be mistaken for 4 ml epinephrine hydrochloride.
• Do you document the medication's administration as soon as possible? You should, so you won't forget. In addition, if a drug's ordered for your patient, but not given for some reason, indicate this on the medication form. Then record the reason in your nurses' notes.

When giving a medication that's to be administered when needed, such as an analgesic, document why it was given, whether or not it was effective, and if it caused an adverse reaction.
• Does state law regulate dosage of the ordered medication? Remember, orders for some medications (for example, narcotics, antibiotics, sedatives, and anticoagulants) must be periodically renewed by the doctor. Check your hospital policy for guidelines.
• Has your patient's medication regimen been discontinued because of surgery? If so, make sure you indicate the change on the appropriate medication forms.

*Available in both the United States and in Canada

Oral

As a nurse, you probably administer oral medications every day. But, are you aware of all the information you need to properly perform that function—particularly if your patient's a child? For example:
• Can you safely administer a tablet to a child?
• Are you familiar with special equipment you can use to administer liquid oral medication?
• Do you know how to persuade a child to take an unpleasant-tasting liquid medication?

You'll find answers to these questions and others in the following pages.

Do's and don'ts of administering oral medications

You're trying to give Jason Byerly, your 6-year-old patient, the oral medication his doctor's ordered for him. But Jason tells you he doesn't want to take it. He says that the tablet's "too big for me," and that he can't swallow it. What can you do?

You'll probably encounter patients like Jason in your hospital's pediatric unit. They can present special challenges to even basic nursing skills, such as administering medications. Because of their different physical and mental makeup, children require special care. So, when giving them medication, keep these guidelines in mind:
• DO get acquainted with your patient before approaching him with the medication. Use a matter-of-fact but friendly manner to put him at ease. Act as though you expect his cooperation.
• DO check the patient's identification band, and observe the Five Rights of medication administration (see page 52).
• DO find out if he has a nickname and use it, if it makes him feel more comfortable.
• DO check any medication that's unfamiliar to you, and any dose or dosage that seems inappropriate for your patient. Have a second nurse check dose and dosage for potent medications, such as insulin, anticoagulants, and digitalis preparations. Call the pharmacist if you have any questions.
• DON'T try to trick a child into taking his medication. Doing so may make him less cooperative the next time he has to take it, and will make him distrust nurses.
• DO encourage your patient's cooperation by acting as if you expect it. Praise him for cooperating, if he does.
• DO give an older child choices, if possible, to give him some feeling of control over his care. For example, offer him a choice of beverage to take with (or after) his medication.
• DON'T threaten, insult, or embarrass your patient.
• DO taste an oral medication before giving it to your patient. Doing so provides some idea of how the medication will taste to the child, and whether you'll have to mask the taste with flavoring. Don't promise that the medication will taste good if you've never tasted it yourself. (Of course, you won't taste a medication if you think you may be sensitive to it.)
• DON'T tell the child the medication's candy, because he may try to take more than the prescribed dosage. Or, he may not trust you.
• DON'T leave any unattended medications at your patient's bedside.
• DON'T let the medication cart or tray out of your sight while administering medications. Your patient may try to take something from it while you're not looking.
• DO allow the child to become familiar with the oral administration device. For example, if you administer the medication in a souffle cup, give him a chance to play with one.
• DON'T give the child a chewable tablet if he has loose teeth.
• DO explain the relationship between illness and treatment to an older child. He may be more cooperative if he realizes the medication will help him.
• DON'T insist that your patient swallow his medication, or attempt to hold his nose or mouth shut to force him to swallow it. Doing so may cause him to choke.
• DO administer medications to an infant in a manner similar to the feeding activity. By giving medications through a nipple, for example, you take advantage of the infant's natural sucking reflex.
• DO try to comfort an infant while administering the medication, to calm him.
• DO place a tablet or capsule near the back of your patient's tongue, and give him plenty of water or flavored drink to help him swallow it.
• DO encourage the child to tip his head slightly forward, not back, when swallowing a tablet or capsule. Throwing his head back increases the risk of aspiration. Make sure he swallows the medication.
• DO try allowing parents to administer the oral medication to a difficult patient. But check your hospital's policy first.
• DO observe the child closely to see if the medication has the intended effect or any adverse effects on him.
• DO note any special considerations on your patient's Kardex; for example, "Jason will take his tablet only if it's crushed and mixed with a flavoring syrup."
• DO document carefully on the medication record all medications that you administer. Document problems you encountered during the administration in your nurses' notes.

Understanding tablets and capsules

Nearly everyone's taken medicated tablets or capsules at one time or another. But as a pediatric nurse, you need to know much more about these oral medications than most people. Review your basic knowledge by reading the following information. Let's first consider tablets.

Learning about tablets
In addition to the medication itself, tablets normally contain diluents to ensure the proper size and consistency, and disintegrants to speed the disintegration process. Many tablets are also covered with a coating, which may serve one or more of these purposes:
• to add color or a pleasant taste
• to protect the gastric mucosa from irritation
• to protect the tablet from premature disintegration in the stomach and allow it to dissolve in the small intestine (this is called an enteric coating)
• to protect the tablet from light, air, and moisture.

Chewable tablets are flavored and usually pleasant-tasting. Chewing aids the disintegration and digestion of the medication. But, don't tell your patient the pleasant-tasting tablet is candy—he may try to eat more than

Oral

Understanding tablets and capsules   continued

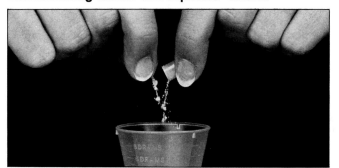

the proper dose. And don't confuse the child by administering chewable and nonchewable tablets at the same time.

If you're administering an uncoated tablet with an unpleasant taste, or if the child has difficulty swallowing a tablet, you can crush it and mix the medication with a flavoring syrup or nonessential food, such as applesauce. Since the medication may change the food's taste, tell the child what you've done. Avoid mixing medication with favorite or essential foods, such as milk, because the child may develop an aversion to those foods. Afterward, offer the child a choice of beverage to help him get rid of any unpleasant aftertaste.

Remember: Before giving any medication with food or a beverage, make sure the food or beverage won't adversely affect how the medication's absorbed. For example, some penicillins decompose prematurely when given with fruit juice.

Some uncoated tablets are scored; if your patient requires only a portion of a scored tablet, you can easily divide it into halves or quarters. But never divide a tablet that's not scored, because you can't be sure the dosage will be accurate. In such a case, ask your hospital's pharmacy to supply the drug in a smaller dose, or in a liquid form, if available.

Don't crush enteric-coated

tablets, because the medication won't be absorbed properly. The coating on the tablet must remain intact, so the tablet will pass through your patient's stomach and dissolve in his small intestine.

Learning about capsules
The medication inside a capsule may be in powder, granule, or liquid form. In addition, one or more diluents, solvents, or other pharmacologically inert substances are usually included. Solid medication particles may be coated with substances that permit sustained release of small amounts of medication over a long period of time.

The medication and inert substances are encased in a hard or soft gelatin shell. Because gelatin dissolves quickly in gastric fluids, medication in capsule form tends to be absorbed more quickly than medication in tablet form. However, some capsules are coated with sustained release or enteric coatings, to delay absorption. *Note:* Check with the pharmacist before opening a capsule.

Storage tips
When storing tablets or capsules, remember these points:
• Protect them from humidity, light, and air.
• Watch for signs of deterioration, such as discoloration and unusual odor. Discard any medication that looks or smells strange.
• Check the medication's expiration date to see if it's outdated. If so, discard it.

Giving a tablet to a child

1 *Let's say you're about to give 7-year-old Paul Clark a tablet. Before you begin, use the Five Rights system to compare the doctor's order with the order written on Paul's Kardex. If the dose looks inappropriate for a child, calculate it yourself (see page 53). Don't administer the medication if you have any questions or doubts about the order. But if all's well, follow the steps shown in this photostory.*

Wash your hands. Make sure the medication cart contains the equipment you'll need: a bottle or blister pack (a single, prepackaged dose) of the ordered medication, a souffle or medicine cup, and a glass of water or other beverage. If you plan to crush the tablet, you'll need a mortar and pestle or a commercially-made tablet crusher; you'll also need a small amount of flavoring syrup or nonessential food, such as applesauce, and a spoon. If you plan to divide a scored tablet, you may also need a knife or a serrated blade.

Now, approach your patient in a calm, reassuring manner. Confirm Paul's identity by checking his identification band, and ask him to tell you his name. Check the Kardex to see if he has a nickname; using it may put him more at ease. Explain the procedure in terms he can understand.

Nursing tip: If appropriate, offer him a choice of beverage to take with his medication. By giving him some control over the procedure, you encourage his cooperation.

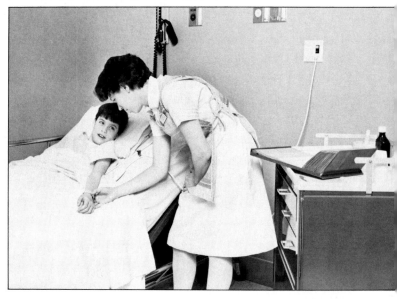

2 If Paul's medication isn't packaged in a blister pack, pour the correct number of tablets or capsules from the bottle into the bottle cap. If you pour out too many, put the excess back.

Important: Never touch the excess medication, because you may contaminate the entire bottle. For the same reason, don't return the unused portion of a divided tablet to the bottle. Instead, discard it.

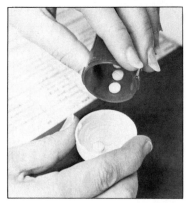

3 Next, pour the tablet or capsule into the souffle cup or medicine cup, and recap the medication bottle. Then, give the cup to the patient, or tap the medication into his hand.

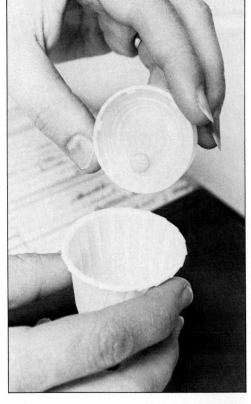

4 If you're crushing the tablet, place the tablet inside a souffle cup and cover that cup with another. Then, place the two cups inside the mortar, and crush the tablet with the pestle, as shown. This procedure keeps the medication from sticking to the mortar and pestle, and insures a more accurate dose. Mix the crushed tablet with the flavoring syrup, or sprinkle it over a small amount of nonessential food.

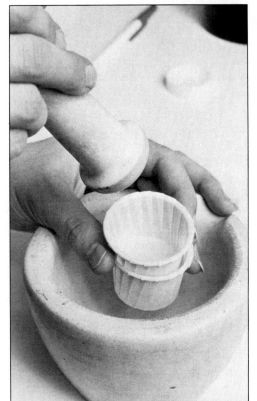

5 Ask Paul to drink some water or other beverage before taking his tablet; doing so should make it easier for him to swallow the medication. Then, tell him to put the tablet or capsule on the back of his tongue. (Help him do so, if necessary.) Avoid touching his mouth or the rim of the medicine cup after he's used it. If you do, wash your hands immediately, to avoid transferring bacteria to your next patient.

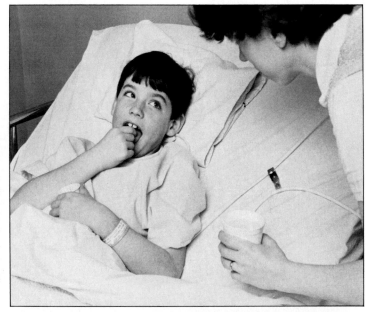

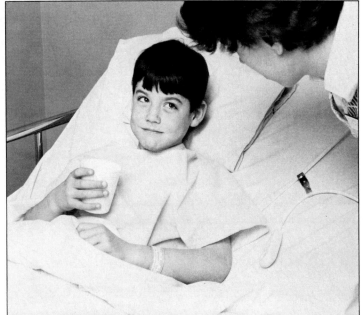

6 Give Paul the cup of water. Ask him to take a mouthful of water, and swallow the tablet. Remember to tell him to tip his head slightly forward when swallowing the tablet, to avoid aspiration.

Finally, discard the used souffle cup or medicine cup. Document any problems in your nurses' notes, and document the medication administration on the appropriate form.

Oral

Learning about liquid medications

If your patient's younger than age 5, you'll probably administer medications in liquid form, rather than as a tablet or capsule. Although a young child may be unable or unwilling to swallow a tablet or capsule, he may be willing to take a pleasant-tasting liquid. To learn about liquid medications, read the following chart.

Type	Description	Nursing considerations
Syrup	• A medication and preservative in a viscous, sugar/water solution; usually flavored	• When giving a syrup for a demulcent (soothing) effect, or for cough relief, don't follow it with water. Tell the child to sip the syrup slowly. • When giving a syrup for a systemic effect, you may dilute it. However, dilute only the dose being given. If you dilute the entire bottle, you may destroy the preservative and hasten contamination or decomposition. Also, subsequent doses taken from the bottle won't be accurate. • Use caution when administering syrups to diabetic children. Check with the pharmacist to see if a sugar-free syrup is available. • When giving syrups with other medications, administer syrups *last.* • Don't tell a child that the syrup is candy, because he may try to take more than the prescribed dose. Keep syrups (and all other medications) out of his reach.
Suspension	• *Magma:* a thick, milky suspension of an insoluble (or partly soluble) inorganic medication, suspended in water • *Gel:* the same as magma but with smaller medication particles • *Emulsion:* droplets of fatty or oily medication, suspended in water	• Always vigorously shake a suspension before giving it. • If desired, you may dilute most suspensions with water before administration. (Dilute only the dose you're giving.) However, don't dilute an *antacid* suspension, or it won't effectively coat the stomach. • Find out what the medication tastes like before giving it, so you can inform the child. You may want to add flavoring.
Alcoholic solution	• *Elixir:* a mixture of medication, alcohol, water, and sugar. Elixirs are less sweet and less viscous than syrups. • *Spirits:* a solution of volatile substances; for example, liquids, solids, or gases. The alcohol in the solution acts as a preservative and solvent. • *Tincture:* a solution of alcohol, or alcohol and water, with a medication • *Fluidextract:* a bitter solution of vegetable medications, usually sweetened with a syrup or flavoring. Fluidextracts are rarely prescribed, because they are unusually potent and unpleasant tasting.	• Check the solution carefully. Never administer an alcoholic solution that has precipitate at the bottom of the bottle. • If you want to dilute the solution, use only a small amount of water. Too much water could cause the drug to precipitate. • Consult the pharmacist before you mix alcoholic solutions with liquids other than water. Mixing with other liquids may counteract the medication. • Follow administration with water, unless you're giving the solution for cough relief. • Store solution in an airtight container. Protect from temperature extremes. Protect fluidextracts from light. • Because a child may not like the alcohol taste, avoid administering this type of solution, if possible. • Use these solutions cautiously if you suspect that your patient abuses alcohol. Never give these solutions to a patient who's receiving disulfiram (Antabuse*).
Reconstituted powders and tablets	• Solid medication reconstituted with water (or another suitable liquid) and given to the patient in suspension or solution form	• Read the directions carefully before reconstituting powders and tablets. Don't use too much water with effervescent tablets, or they'll boil out of the glass. • Some powders become gelatinous very quickly after you mix them. Administer them immediately after reconstitution. • Let effervescent tablets dissolve completely before you give them to the patient. Give without further dilution.

*Available in both the United States and in Canada

Giving liquid medication: Equipment selection

You may use any of the equipment shown below to give a child liquid medication. Which is most appropriate for your patient? What special points should you keep in mind when using each type of equipment? Read this chart for tips.

Note: Thoroughly wash reusable equipment after each use, and store it in the patient's medication box.

Oral dropper

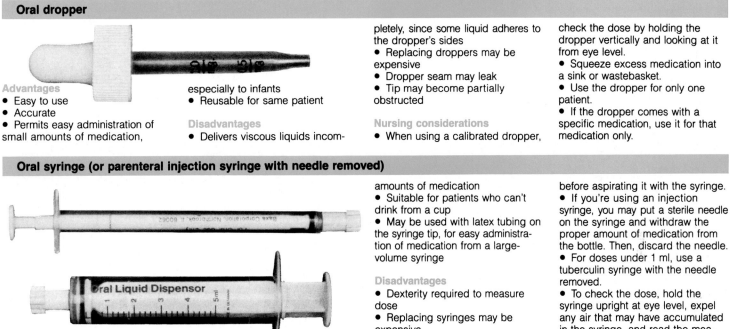

Advantages
• Easy to use
• Accurate
• Permits easy administration of small amounts of medication, especially to infants
• Reusable for same patient

Disadvantages
• Delivers viscous liquids incompletely, since some liquid adheres to the dropper's sides
• Replacing droppers may be expensive
• Dropper seam may leak
• Tip may become partially obstructed

Nursing considerations
• When using a calibrated dropper, check the dose by holding the dropper vertically and looking at it from eye level.
• Squeeze excess medication into a sink or wastebasket.
• Use the dropper for only one patient.
• If the dropper comes with a specific medication, use it for that medication only.

Oral syringe (or parenteral injection syringe with needle removed)

Advantages
• Marked in teaspoons (tsp), cubic centimeters (cc), and milliliters (ml) for accurate measurement
• Delivers complete dose
• Provides low risk of spillage
• Provides precise control over placement and administration speed; as a result, a syringe is especially suitable for young children and infants
• Accurately delivers even small amounts of medication
• Suitable for patients who can't drink from a cup
• May be used with latex tubing on the syringe tip, for easy administration of medication from a large-volume syringe

Disadvantages
• Dexterity required to measure dose
• Replacing syringes may be expensive

Nursing considerations
• Obtain a syringe that has the precise marking you need; don't estimate.
• To avoid contaminating the medication bottle with the syringe, pour the medication into a medicine cup before aspirating it with the syringe.
• If you're using an injection syringe, you may put a sterile needle on the syringe and withdraw the proper amount of medication from the bottle. Then, discard the needle.
• For doses under 1 ml, use a tuberculin syringe with the needle removed.
• To check the dose, hold the syringe upright at eye level, expel any air that may have accumulated in the syringe, and read the measurement from the rubber stopper's top edge.
• To administer the medication, place the syringe's tip in the pocket between your patient's cheek mucosa and second molar. Administer slowly and steadily, to reduce the risk of aspiration.

Oral cylindrical spoon

Advantages
• Easy to use
• Reusable for same patient
• Widely available

Disadvantages
• Risks spillage
• Delivers viscous fluids incompletely

Nursing considerations
• Because a cylindrical spoon is more accurate than a regular household spoon, encourage parents to use it when administering liquid oral medications to their children. If your hospital's policy allows it, give the parents one of these spoons to use at home.

Medicine cup

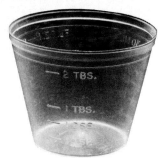

Advantages
• Accurate for larger volumes of medication
• Easy to use
• Inexpensive
• May be reusable for same patient

Disadvantages
• Inaccurate for small doses
• Inaccurate for milileter doses not divisible by 5 (because cups are marked in 5 ml increments)
• High risk of spillage, especially when used for a young child
• Doesn't completely deliver viscous liquids

Nursing considerations
• Choose a disposable medicine cup that has the markings you'll need to measure the dose. Don't estimate measurements between markings.
• Place your thumbnail at the proper mark, and hold the cup at eye level when pouring the medication, to insure an accurate dose.
• To recheck the dose you've poured, place the cup on a level surface and read the base of the meniscus at eye level.
• Discard any excess medication. Don't return it to the bottle.
• Use a straw to administer medication that may stain your patient's teeth.
• If cup is disposable, wash it out well and give to a younger child for a toy.

Oral

Administering liquid medications to an infant

1 *Any oral medication you administer to an infant will probably be liquid, and prescribed in very small doses. Use a dropper to ensure that you give the right amount of medication. This photostory shows you how:*

First, place a bib under the infant's chin and a towel over your shoulder. Position the infant in the crook of your arm, as the nurse is doing here. Hold him so his head's elevated at a 45° angle. If necessary, use one of your hands to restrain his arms.

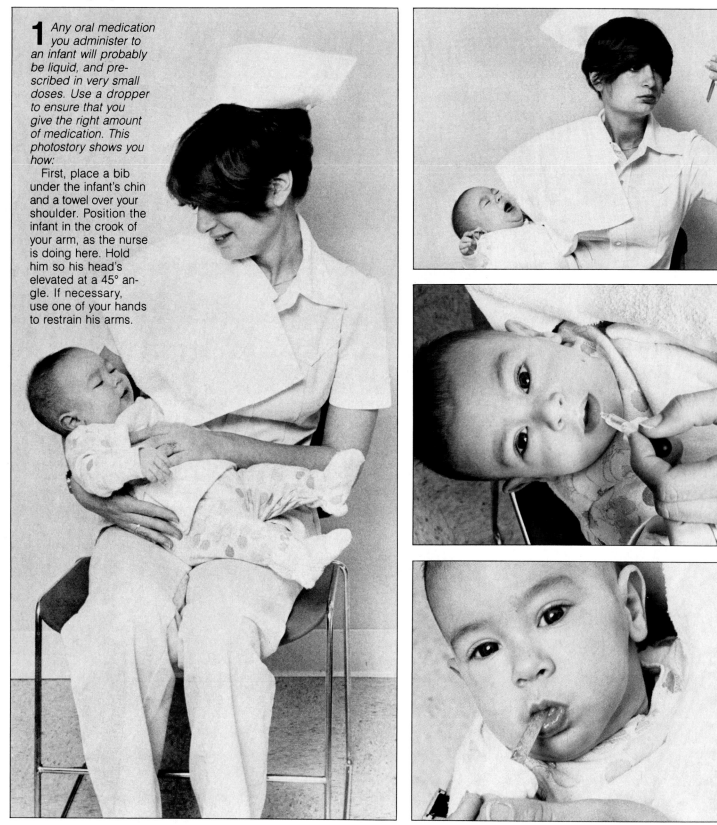

2 Now, using your free hand, withdraw the correct amount of medication from the bottle by squeezing the bulb on the dropper.

Check the dose in a calibrated dropper by holding it vertically at eye level and looking at it. Squeeze excess medication into a sink or wastebasket. Don't return it to the bottle.

3 Next, instill the drops. If the infant won't turn toward you, gently stroke the side of his cheek closest to you. If he won't open his mouth, pinch his cheek gently. Or, get another nurse to gently squeeze his cheeks together or pull down on his chin.

If the dropper's not calibrated, hold it vertically over the infant's open mouth, and instill the prescribed number of drops.

4 If you're using a calibrated dropper, place it between the infant's cheek and gum to instill the medication. Doing so will keep him from spitting out the medication, and reduces the risk of aspiration.

📠 *Nursing tip:* You can also place the medication in a small nipple and give it to the infant. This takes advantage of his sucking reflex. But make sure that he receives all of the medication.

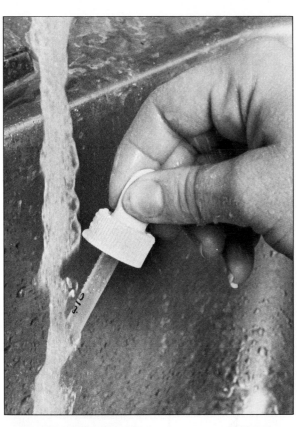

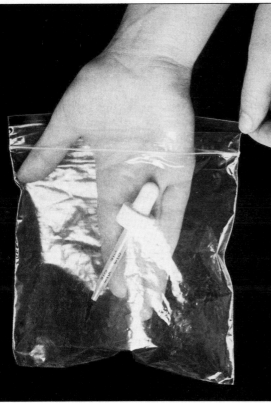

5 If the dropper touches the inside of the infant's mouth, consider it contaminated. Wash the dropper thoroughly with soap and water; then, rinse and dry it.

6 If the dropper's not contaminated, and it's attached to the bottle cap, simply return it to the bottle and tightly screw on the cap. But if the dropper's unattached, rinse out the medication with warm water, dry it, put it in a clear plastic bag, and store it with the infant's medication bottle. Document what you've done.

Important: Never use the same dropper for more than one patient. Keep each infant's dropper separate and labeled with his name. Dispose of the dropper when the medication's finished.

Making liquid medications palatable

How can you encourage your pediatric patient to take a liquid medication that has an unpleasant taste? We've already discussed disguising an unpleasant taste with nonessential food or flavored syrup. Here are some other methods you may try:

• Use a syringe without a needle to bypass your patient's taste buds. Instill the medication into the pocket between his cheek and his second molar.

• Give an older child ice chips to suck on; they'll help numb his taste buds before you give him the medication.

• To dilute the taste, pour the medication over ice and give it through a straw. But don't use this method if you're only giving a small dose, because the accuracy of the dose may be affected.

• If the medication's oily, chill it before administration to improve the taste. Store oily medications in a refrigerator, unless contraindicated.

• To minimize a bitter aftertaste, offer an older patient sugar-free hard candy or chewing gum after administering his medication. Or, ask him to gargle or rinse out his mouth with mouthwash or water.

📠 *Nursing tip:* If you're giving your patient several medications at one time, always administer the best-tasting medication last. This minimizes the unpleasant aftertaste your patient may experience.

Dermatomucosal

Administering eyedrops continued

3 Rest the hand that's holding the dropper or dropper bottle on your patient's forehead. This way, if he moves his head, your hand moves with it.

Note: If your patient's uncooperative, you may have to restrain him. Have a co-worker help hold him.

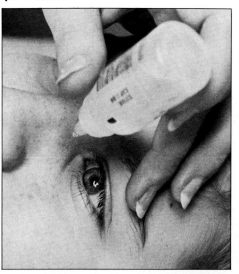

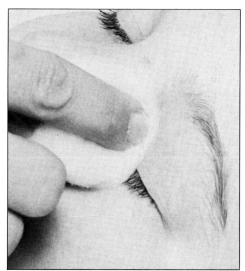

5 After instilling the eyedrops, place gentle pressure on Roger's inner canthus with a clean cotton ball, to minimize the amount of solution entering his tear duct.

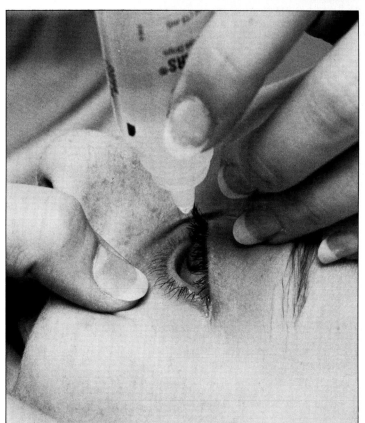

4 Place your thumb on his cheekbone, and gently pull down the skin, exposing the lower conjunctival sac. Take care not to press on his eyeball. Ask the patient to look up. This way, he won't see the drop coming and try to blink his eye.

Now, with your other hand, hold the eyedropper or dropper bottle near the outer canthus of his eye. But don't let the tip touch his eyeball or eyelashes. Squeeze the prescribed number of drops into the conjunctival sac. To prevent possible injury, never place drops directly on your patient's cornea.

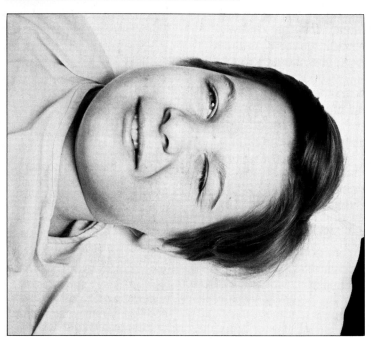

6 Remove the cotton ball, and let him blink to distribute the medication over his eye and inner lids. Use a clean cotton ball to remove excess fluid, working from the inner canthus outward.

Repeat the entire procedure on the other eye, if ordered. Remember, always use fresh cotton balls to cleanse the other eye. Caution your patient not to rub his eyes. Observe him closely for any medication side effects.

Finally, if the eyedropper came with the medication bottle, and you didn't contaminate it during the procedure, return it to the bottle. Store an unattached dropper in a clean plastic bag. If the eyedropper was contaminated during the procedure, discard it and obtain a new one. *Note:* If you contaminated a dropper bottle's tip, dispose of the bottle. Obtain a new one for the next medication administration, if necessary.

Document the procedure in the medication administration record. Note any problems in your nurses' notes.

Administering eye ointments

1 *Let's say you're going to administer an eye ointment to a preteen patient. Before you do, make sure you have the proper medication, and that it's not outdated. Make sure it's labeled for ophthalmic use.*

In addition to the medication, you'll need clean cotton balls or tissue, and an alcohol swab.

Now prepare your patient in the same manner you would for administering eyedrops. Tell him that the ointment will temporarily blur his vision. Reassure him that blurring is normal, and will soon disappear.

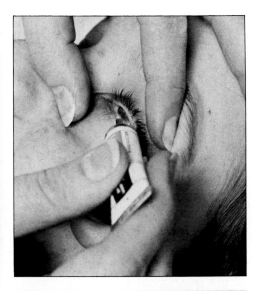

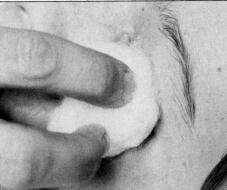

2 After you've prepared your patient, thoroughly wash your hands. Then, remove the cap from the tube of medication. Lay the cap down on its side on a clean surface. Ask your patient to look up and focus on a specific object. With one hand, place your index finger on his upper eyelid to help keep his eye open. Then, place your thumb on his cheekbone and gently pull down on his skin to expose the conjunctival sac.

Next, take the tube of medication in your other hand. Starting at the inner canthus, squeeze a thin ribbon of ointment along your patient's lower conjunctival sac. As you approach the eye's outer canthus, rotate the tube to detach the ointment. Make sure you don't touch his eye with the tube. And use this tube for only one patient.

3 Ask your patient to close his eyes for 2 minutes so the medication can spread and be absorbed. Then, using a cotton ball or tissue, wipe away any excess medication.

Wipe the tip of the tube with the alcohol swab, and replace the cap. Then, store the medication properly.

Document the procedure in your patient's medication administration record. Include any observations in your nurses' notes.

Restraining a child

How can you help a parent easily administer eyedrops or eye ointment to her struggling 2-year-old son? Try teaching her the restraining position shown here.

First, tell her to place a pad on the floor and sit on it, or to sit in the middle of a bed. Then, tell her to place the child between her legs, and put her thighs over the child's arms, as shown. By doing so, the child's head and body is secured between her thighs, and he can't use his arms to struggle. Now the parent can freely administer the medication without help.

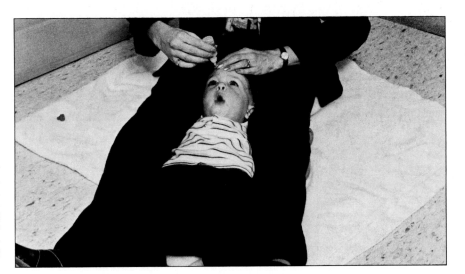

Dermatomucosal

Administering eardrops

1 *Mrs. Clark brings her son Paul into the doctor's office where you work, saying that Paul was awake all night with a painful earache. After examining Paul, the doctor determines that the 7-year-old boy has a severe ear infection. To treat the condition, he orders Cortisporin* otic suspension (polymyxin B-neomycin-hydrocortisone) eardrops. If you're not sure how to administer them, read this photostory.*

First, gather the medication and some clean cotton balls. Check the medication label against the doctor's order. Warm the solution to body temperature by holding the bottle in your hand for 2 minutes. *Important:* Never administer eardrops that aren't near body temperature, because cold solution may cause pain or vertigo when it strikes the eardrum. Also, don't administer eardrops if you suspect your patient has a perforated eardrum. Instead, check with the doctor.

As you warm the eardrops, explain the procedure to your patient, and tell him why it's necessary. Talk to him in a calm, reassuring tone of voice, and answer his questions. Explain that he'll feel and hear something in his ear, but that it won't hurt.

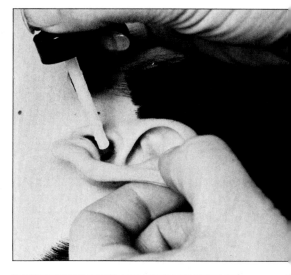

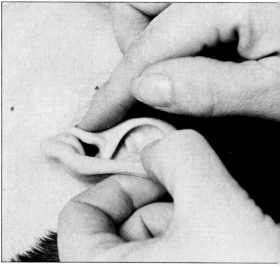

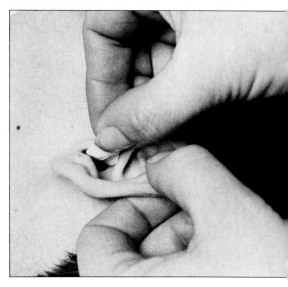

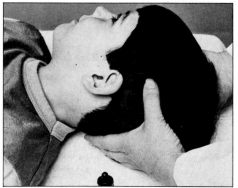

2 Thoroughly shake the bottle, as the label directs, and loosen the cap, so you can easily remove the dropper. Then, wash your hands, and turn your patient's head to one side, so the affected ear is accessible.

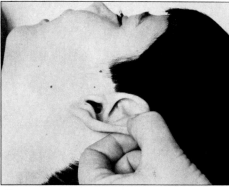

3 Gently cleanse the external ear with a clean cotton ball. Then, straighten the ear canal by pulling the auricle *up* and back. If your patient's age 3 or younger, pull the auricle *down* and back. (An infected ear's painful, so be gentle.)

*Available in both the United States and in Canada

4 With your free hand, remove the dropper from the medication bottle. (Or if you're using a dropper bottle, remove the cap.) Instill the prescribed number of drops into your patient's ear canal. Taking care not to touch the ear with the dropper, direct the drops onto the wall of the external ear canal, as shown in this photo.

5 Continue holding your patient's ear until the medication disappears down the canal. To help the medication progress down the canal, massage the area directly in front of your patient's ear. Ask him to tell you when he no longer feels the drops moving in his ear; that's a sign that they've reached his eardrum. When that happens, release his ear.

6 Tell your patient to remain on his side and to avoid touching his ear for 10 minutes. If your patient's active, place a medication-soaked cotton ball in his ear to help keep the medication in his ear canal. Don't use a dry cotton ball because it may absorb the medication.

If both ears require medication, repeat the procedure in his other ear. Finally, return the dropper to the medication bottle (or recap the dropper bottle). Document the procedure.

Administering nose drops

1 *Imagine that your patient, who's an infant, has nasal congestion. Because he usually breathes through his nose, nasal congestion impairs his sucking reflex. To provide relief, the doctor orders nose drops administered 20 to 30 minutes before each feeding. Read this photostory to learn how to proceed.*

First, wash your hands. Obtain the prescribed medication and check it against the doctor's order. Also, obtain a plastic medication dropper, and tissues.

Hold the bottle of medication up to the light, and check it for discoloration or sediment. If it looks okay, warm the medication by running warm water over the bottle for several minutes, holding it between your hands for 2 minutes, or carrying it in your pocket for 30 minutes prior to administration. Remember to wash your hands thoroughly before beginning the procedure.

Now, position the infant in your arm so his head is slightly tilted back over it, as shown in the photo. You can also use your hand to restrain the infant's arms.

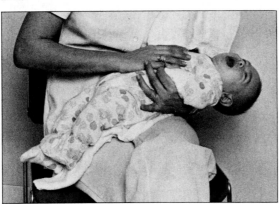

2 If your patient's too large to hold, place her on her back with a pillow under her shoulders. Make sure her head extends over the pillow's edge. Gently tilt back her head, supporting it between your forearm and body, and use one of your hands to restrain her arms and hands. *Note:* Ask an older child to breathe through her mouth as you administer the drops. This discourages her from sniffing, which may propel the drops into her sinuses. Also, warn her that she'll taste the drops.

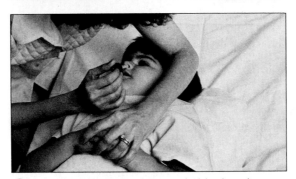

3 Draw enough medication into the dropper to instill the prescribed number of drops into your patient's nostrils. If you don't, you increase the risk of contaminating the medication by reinserting the dropper into the bottle.

If necessary, open your patient's nostrils by gently pushing up the tip of his nose, and get ready to instill the drops.

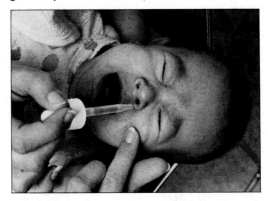

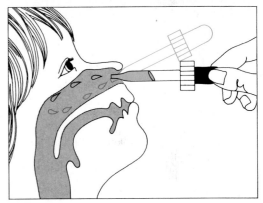

4 Direct the tip of the dropper toward the midline of the superior turbinate, as shown in this illustration. This position permits the drops to flow down the back of the patient's nose, not directly into his throat. Squeeze the dropper bulb to instill the prescribed number of drops. Avoid touching the nostril with the dropper. Repeat the procedure in the other nostril, if ordered.

After instilling the drops, keep your patient's head tilted back for at least 1 minute to allow the drops to reach his superior turbinate.

Watch for signs of aspiration. If he begins to cough, sit him up and pat his back until he's cleared his lungs.

Finally, rinse out the dropper and store it in a plastic bag. Or, if the dropper came with the bottle, reinsert it, provided it's not contaminated. (If it's contaminated, rinse it with warm water before reinserting it into the bottle.) Remember, use the bottle of medication and the dropper for only one patient.

Document the procedure.

Dermatomucosal

Applying a stockinette

1 *Suppose your patient has a severe case of eczema* on his face, and he continues to scratch it. You must find a way to keep the prescribed medication in contact with his skin, and prevent him from irritating the condition. How can you do it, short of restraining him? By applying a cotton stockinette. If you're unsure about the procedure, read the following photostory:

First, gather the equipment you'll need: a roll of stockinette 8″ (20.3 cm) wide, scissors, a marking pen, and a tube of the prescribed medication; for example, betamethasone valerate (Valisone) cream. Then, prepare your patient for the procedure. Since a young child probably can't understand the need for the stockinette, he may resist your efforts to apply it. Try telling him that you're playing a game with him, and that the stockinette is a mask he has to wear.

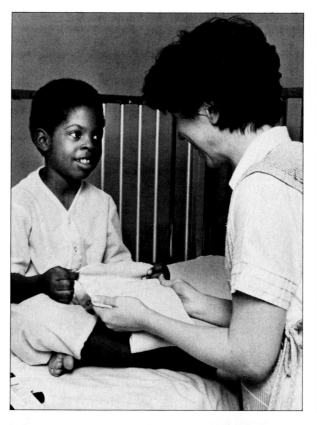

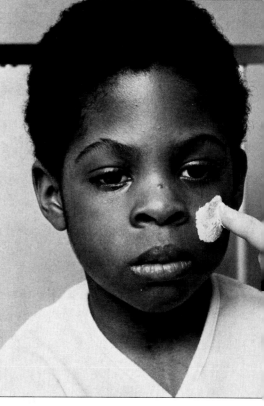

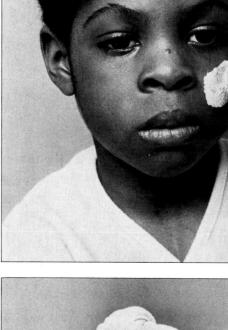

2 Next, prepare the stockinette. Take the scissors and cut a piece of stockinette that's about 16″ (41 cm) long (depending on the child's size). Tie a knot in one end of the piece that you've cut, and place the stockinette over the child's head. Use the marking pen to mark the spots where you'll have to make holes for his eyes, nose, and mouth. Remove the stockinette, and cut holes where you've made the marks.

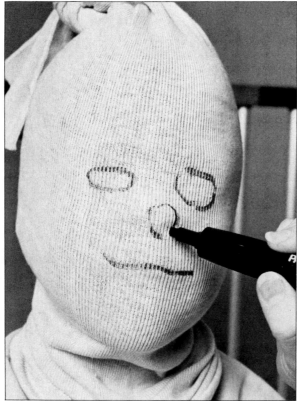

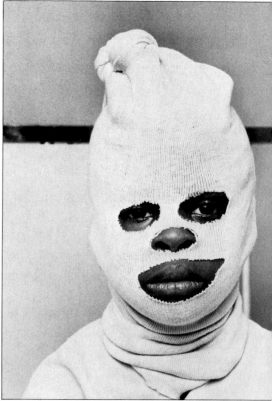

3 Remove the cap from the tube of prescribed cream and apply the cream to your patient's face. If you're applying a large amount of the cream, wear a glove. Take care to avoid getting cream in your patient's eyes, nose, or mouth.

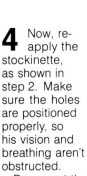

4 Now, reapply the stockinette, as shown in step 2. Make sure the holes are positioned properly, so his vision and breathing aren't obstructed.

Document the procedure in your nurses' notes.

Note: If your patient's uncooperative and keeps trying to pull off the stockinette, you may have to restrain him. See the section that begins on page 45 for more information on restraints.

Teaching parents to apply skin medications

Your pediatric patient's going home. After he leaves the hospital, his parents will have to apply the skin medication the doctor's ordered for him. Make sure they know how to properly apply it by giving them these instructions:
• Wash your hands thoroughly before and after the procedure.
• Use warm water and a mild soap to cleanse your child's skin of old medication. Thoroughly dry the skin.
• To prevent contamination, place the container's cap hollow side up after removing it.
• Apply the medication as directed. If necessary, use an applicator stick or cotton-tipped swab.
• Wear disposable gloves to apply a medication (such as a steroid ointment) that may adversely affect you. Avoid prolonged contact with such a medication.
• To protect your child's clothing, cover the area where you apply the medication with a thin gauze dressing. Don't apply a thick dressing, because it may absorb the medication. (You won't apply a dressing or allow your child to wear clothing over the affected area if the doctor warns against it, of course.)
• Never use medication that's prescribed for one child on another. Also, don't substitute another medication for the one your doctor prescribed.
• Notify the doctor if you notice any of the following: increased swelling or redness at the affected site; increased itching or pain; or a change in the amount, color, consistency, or odor of any drainage that appears.

Learning about head lice

Ever wonder why children seem so prone to head lice (pediculosis capitis) infestation? The reason's simple: Crowded buildings, such as schools, provide ideal conditions for lice to migrate. Once present, these persistent parasites spread rapidly through direct contact, or through contact with clothing and toilet articles, such as combs, hair brushes, towels, hats, scarves, coats, and sweaters.

Adult lice, which are silverish-white, flat, wingless creatures, are 1 to 2 mm long (see illustration). Because they're so small, they're hard to see. But if you look closely, they resemble dandruff that moves.

Female lice lay eggs—or nits—on hair shafts, close to the scalp. When the nits hatch, the young lice pierce the scalp to suck blood. As they do so, they inject a toxin that causes itching.

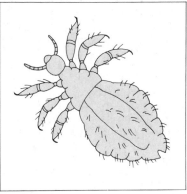

If you suspect that your patient has head lice, part his hair to expose his scalp. Make sure the room's well-lighted. Then, examine the skin on the back of his head or behind his ears, where lice bites are easy to detect. Also examine his eyebrows and eyelashes. Look for these signs and symptoms:
• small, white nits attached to individual hairs near the skin. Unlike seborrheic scales or hair casts, nits can't be moved along the hair shaft and flicked off with your fingers. *Note:* The closer the nits are to the end of the hair shaft, the longer lice have been present.
• a persistent scalp itch, possibly accompanied by infected scratch marks or a rash.

Combating head lice
To treat head lice, the doctor will order lindane (Kwell®) shampoo. To apply it, follow these guidelines:
• First, check the child's scalp for rawness or inflammation. Don't apply the shampoo if you see these signs; instead, notify the doctor.
• If the child's scalp isn't raw, pour 1 ounce (30 ml) of Kwell shampoo onto the affected area and adjacent hair. Vigorously rub the shampoo into the hair for about 4 minutes. Take care to keep the shampoo out of the child's eyes. Then, wet the area thoroughly with warm water, and work the shampoo into a lather. Rinse the hair, and dry it with a clean towel.
• After you're finished shampooing your patient's hair, use a fine-tooth comb dipped in vinegar to remove the nits and nit shells that have been loosened from the hair shafts.
• Change your patient's clothing and bed linen, and have them laundered. (If hospitalized, isolate the clothing and linen, and mark them *lice infested.*)
• If your patient is severely infested, consider wearing protective garb.
• Make sure you avoid touching your own hair after you've cared for a patient with head lice. Wash your hands thoroughly.
• Instruct the parents in home care. Tell them to stop using the shampoo and notify the doctor if the child develops any signs of scalp irritation.

Preventing infestation
Take this opportunity to teach your patient and his parents how to minimize the risk of repeated infestation.
• Stress how contagious head lice are. Recommend laundering all towels and bedding in hot water, and ironing them.
• Urge family members and close contacts of the infested person to be checked for infestation.
• Instruct parents to frequently inspect the child's head for lice—especially if a lice outbreak occurs at his school. *Important:* Warn parents not to use Kwell shampoo more than once a week without the doctor's permission. Repeated or prolonged use of Kwell shampoo may cause skin irritation or systemic toxicosis.
• Warn patients (especially teenagers) that borrowed clothing, such as sweaters and scarves, can be a source of infestation. Tell them to make sure borrowed clothing is clean and to return it freshly laundered.

Parenteral

When it comes to administering parenteral medication, are you sure of your knowledge and skills? For instance, can you confidently select equipment and injection sites appropriate for both a child's size and the ordered parenteral route? Are you certain that your injection techniques are correct and up-to-date?

If you need to brush up on parenteral administration, review the following pages. In addition to covering the basics, we'll show you how to:
● assess an intradermal test reaction.
● evaluate a child's self-injection technique.
● prepare a child for I.V. therapy.
● avoid intramuscular injection complications.

Learning about intradermal injections

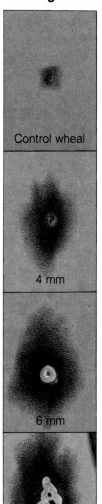

Control wheal

4 mm

6 mm

10 mm

Does your pediatric patient have a possible allergy? If so, the doctor may order an intradermal skin test. If you're not sure about proper testing techniques, review the following photostory. You may also use these techniques to test for some diseases, such as tuberculosis.

To give an intradermal skin test, you'll inject a small amount of diluted antigen solution between the epidermis and dermis tissue layers. Until absorbed, the injected solution causes a small white bump to form under the patient's skin.

The best injection sites on a child are his ventral forearm or upper back. The skin in these areas is lightly pigmented and thinly keratinized, so you can easily observe the reaction.

Important: Since intradermal injections require inserting the needle in your patient's skin at a precise angle, you may need a co-worker's assistance to keep a child still for the injection.

After giving the injection, observe for signs of anaphylactic shock. Be prepared to administer epinephrine hydrochloride (Adrenalin Chloride) 1:1,000, if necessary.

Normally, induration (hardening and possible enlargement of the wheal) occurs within 30 minutes after allergy testing. But, reaction times vary according to the test given and the sensitivity of the child.

The extent of induration tells you whether a specific allergy (or disease) is present. To interpret the results, hold the skin around the injection site taut. Record induration in millimeters and measure any erythema that's present. Then, consult the antigen solution's package insert for a scale to help you interpret the test results.

Tuberculosis testing

If you're testing for tuberculosis, expect induration to occur within 48 and 72 hours. To assess test results, you'll use a scale like the one at left. Measure the area of induration. If the area is:
● less than 5 mm in diameter, consider the test result negative.
● between 5 mm and 9 mm, consider the result questionable and perform another test.
● 10 mm or more, consider the test result positive; your patient may have tuberculosis. After further testing to confirm the diagnosis, the doctor will order treatment.

How to inject intradermally

1 *Twelve-year-old Roger Simms arrives at the clinic where you work to be tested for an allergy to cats. You'll have to administer the test ordered by the doctor. Do you know the proper technique? This photostory will show you.*

First, gather the following equipment: the dilute antigen solution, sterile normal saline solution, two 1 ml tuberculin syringes, two 26G ⅝" needles, acetone wipes, 4"x4" sterile gauze pads, and alcohol wipes. (If your patient's very small, obtain ⅜" needles.) With this equipment, you'll make both a test wheal and a control wheal. Also, obtain a syringe of epinephrine hydrochloride (Adrenalin Chloride) 1:1,000 in case of anaphylactic shock.

Before beginning, thoroughly wash your hands. Then, attach the needles to the syringes. Check the antigen to make sure it's not outdated or contaminated. If the antigen's okay, draw the ordered amount into one of the syringes. Then, cap the syringe and bring all the equipment close to your patient, within easy reach.

To help relax your patient, carefully explain what you're going to do. Let him choose whether to sit or lie down. Ask Roger to hold his arm as still as possible, even though the needle will hurt.

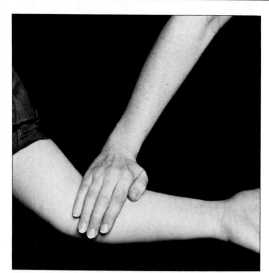

2 Position him with his ventral forearm exposed and supported on a flat surface, and his elbow flexed. *Note:* If your patient's very young, ask a co-worker to help hold him.

Now, measure about a handbreath away from his antecubital fossa, toward his wrist. Use this area for your test. *Note:* Avoid using an area covered with blemishes; they can make the test results difficult to read.

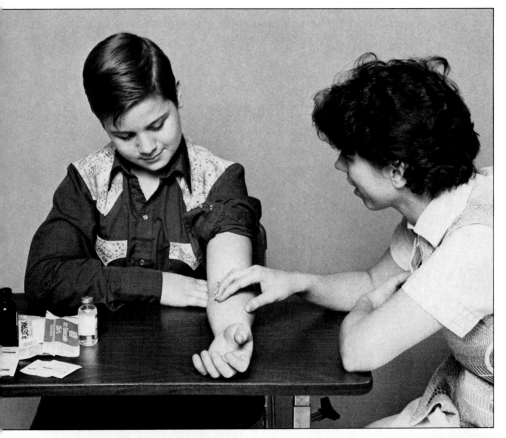

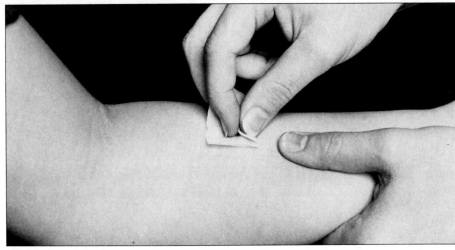

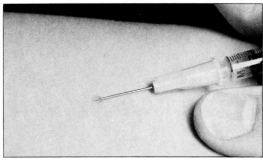

4 Position the syringe so the needle is almost flat against Roger's skin. Make sure the needle's bevel is up.

Slowly insert the needle into his skin. Advance the needle through the epidermis. (You should be able to see the needle's point through his skin.) Stop when the point's resting ⅛" (3 mm) below the skin surface, between the epidermis and dermis layers.

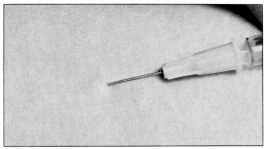

5 Inject the antigen slowly and gently. Expect to feel some resistance, which tells you the needle's properly placed. If the plunger moves freely, you've inserted the needle too deeply. Slightly withdraw the needle, reangle it, and try again.

Watch for a small, white wheal, about 6 mm in diameter, to form as you inject the antigen. When it appears, withdraw the needle, and apply gentle pressure to the site with a gauze pad for about 30 seconds. But, don't massage the site, because doing so may interfere with test results.

Make a control wheal by drawing up 0.1 ml sterile normal saline solution (or antigen solution base) into the other syringe, and injecting the saline solution into the same site on the opposite arm. Use the procedure already described.

Finally, circle the injection sites with indelible ink so you can locate them to read the results. Observe Roger for at least 30 minutes, for signs of anaphylactoid allergic reaction.

Note: If the control wheal shows induration, consider the result a false positive. If ordered, repeat the test later, at different sites.

Tell the child and his parents to avoid washing the sites, and instruct the child not to scratch or rub them. Document the procedure in your nurses' notes.

3 Defat the skin with an acetone wipe. Begin at the center of the injection site you've selected and move outward in a circular motion. Then, prep the skin with an alcohol wipe, using the same motion. Never use an antimicrobial solution that discolors the skin. And don't rub so hard that you cause irritation. Either action could hinder interpretation of test results.

Allow your patient's skin to dry thoroughly. If you inject the antigen while the patient's skin is wet, you may accidentally introduce alcohol solution into his skin tissue, causing burning.

With one hand, hold the syringe upright and expel any air in the needle. Then, hold his forearm in your other hand. Grasp underneath his forearm, and pull the skin tight with your thumb.

Parenteral

Learning about I.V. therapy

If your patient needs a large amount of fluid or special medication, you'll probably administer it intravenously. By using the intravenous (I.V.) route, you deliver fluid and medication directly to the bloodstream, so it has almost immediate effect. This route also eliminates the risk of damaging muscles and other tissue with irritating medication, and delays biotransformation by the liver.

But, like any percutaneous procedure, I.V. therapy has some risks. So, if the medication comes in oral form and the child can safely swallow, the doctor may prefer the oral route.

Choosing a site

Because a child's veins are so small, he has fewer available I.V. sites than an adult has. That's why you must choose a site wisely, and take special care to preserve the vein. (On the following page, you'll learn some special tips for protecting an I.V. site.)

To select a site, consider the child's age. If he's an infant or small child, a scalp vein or superficial hand or arm vein is easiest to locate. If he's an older child, use any accessible arm or hand vein. But avoid using foot and leg veins, because of the high risk of thrombophlebitis and embolism. And, of course, using a foot or leg site severely limits the child's activity.

Also consider how long the child will be receiving I.V. therapy. If he's scheduled for long-term therapy, plan your venipuncture sites

in advance, and rotate them every 72 hours, or according to hospital policy. Regular rotation reduces the risk of infection, thrombophlebitis, and other complications. *Important:* Avoid a site over a joint, since you'd have to immobilize the joint.

Selecting equipment

Use a small-gauge (21G to 27G) needle or catheter for a child. A small needle's less likely to irritate the vein wall. It'll also look less frightening to the child than a larger needle. For long-term therapy, consider using a catheter instead of a needle, to minimize the risk of vein injury.

You'll administer most pediatric I.V. medications with a volume-control set (although you may use the direct-bolus method under some circumstances). The volume-control set delivers small amounts of medication or fluid over an extended period of time. For greatest accuracy, however, use an infusion pump with the volume-control set. Remember, a child's size and metabolism make him especially susceptible to overdose, fluid overload, or dehydration. Take special care to maintain the correct flow rate, and to accurately record his fluid intake and output. (For information on recognizing and treating I.V. complications, see page 74.)

To learn more about I.V. techniques, consult the NURSING PHOTO-BOOK MANAGING I.V. THERAPY.

Preparing a child for I.V. therapy

You're explaining I.V. therapy to 4-year-old Alan Wolfe, who needs penicillin G potassium (Novopen-G*) I.V. for 2 weeks. He listens attentively and accepts your explanation calmly. You're congratulating yourself for skillful patient teaching, when Alan startles you with an unexpected question: "Will the needle *ever* come out?"

With this simple question, you realize that your patient teaching hasn't been quite complete. Like most nurses, you take some things for granted—the eventual end of therapy, for example. But what's obvious to you may not be so obvious to your patient—especially a young one like Alan. When preparing a child for I.V. therapy, take care to assure the child that the needle will come out as soon as he's well.

Also, keep in mind that a child's likely to have some special fears and concerns. For example, he may believe that the I.V. fluid will poison him. Or, if he doesn't *feel* sick, he may not understand why he needs I.V. therapy, and think that you're punishing him. Encourage him to express his thoughts, and provide appropriate support.

On page 37, we provided

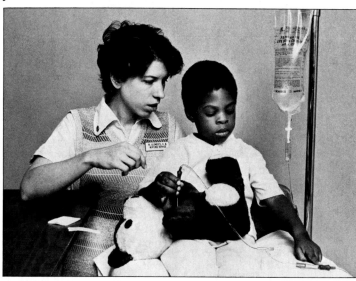

some tips for preparing a child for venipuncture. You'll use most of them when you initiate I.V. therapy, too. But because the child will have a needle or catheter in place for several days or more, he needs additional preparation and continuing support. Make the following guidelines a routine part of patient teaching. *Important:* When preparing the child, don't neglect to include his parents. They can provide additional support and reinforcement.
• Acquaint the child with I.V.

equipment. For example, fill a volume-control set with colored water, and help the child tape the I.V. line to a doll. Playing with the equipment helps the child resolve fears and misconceptions about therapy. (Of course, you won't let him play with real needles.)
• Tell him how his mobility will be affected by I.V. therapy. If he's ambulatory, for example, assure him that he'll still be able to walk and play, using a portable I.V. pole. But, stress the importance of protecting the I.V.

site. Show him an armboard, and explain that you'll apply it to help keep his arm still.

If he's ambulatory, also show him how to push an I.V. pole. Tell him to keep his affected arm below his chest, so the medication flows properly. Urge him to use his other arm for play, eating, and other activities.
• Tell him not to play with his I.V. tubing, flow clamp, or any other part of the equipment.
• Allow him to decorate his I.V. taping with a colorful sticker.
• Encourage him to participate in his own care. This technique helps prevent any regression in his development by giving him a sense of control. Even a young child can hand you tape as you secure the needle or catheter. Point out the drip chamber, and ask him to note how quickly the fluid's dripping. Then, ask him to tell you if he notices any change. (Remember, a child may accidentally jostle open the flow clamp.)

Teach an older child signs of infiltration and phlebitis. Ask him to notify you if such signs occur. With your supervision, he may also learn to pick out venipuncture sites and even to remove a needle or short peripheral catheter from his vein.

*Available in both the United States and in Canada

Protecting an I.V. site

Protecting a child's I.V. site can be a challenge. As you may know from experience, an active child can easily dislodge an I.V. needle, possibly injuring himself. What can you do to minimize this risk?

The first step is securely taping the needle or catheter in place. For details on taping techniques, see the NURSING PHOTOBOOK MANAGING I.V. THERAPY.

The next step is patient teaching. If the child's old enough to follow directions, teach him not to touch the equipment, and ask him to protect the site from jostling. If he's ambulatory, show him how to push his I.V. pole to prevent stress on the line. His cooperation reduces the risk of complications.

If possible, use a catheter instead of a needle. A flexible catheter is less likely to perforate the vein wall.

On this page, you'll see some other protective measures. But no matter which one you choose, remember these points:
• Never tape the protective cover so tightly to the patient's skin that you occlude blood flow.
• Try to use a clear, protective cover so you can frequently examine the I.V. site for complications, such as infection or infiltration. If the cover isn't clear, remove it hourly to inspect the site.

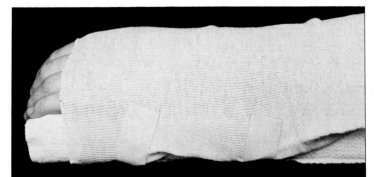

Stockinette and armboard
Obtain some 4″ stockinette and cut a piece that's the same length as your patient's arm. Slip the stockinette over your patient's arm, and place that arm on an armboard. Then, grasp the stockinette at both sides of his arm, and stretch it underneath the armboard. Securely tape the stockinette underneath the armboard, as shown.

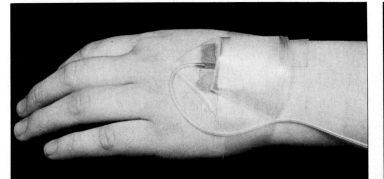

Medicine cup
Take a clean, empty medicine cup made of clear plastic, and cut it in half lengthwise. Using nonallergenic tape, tape the half-cup over the I.V. site. As you can see, the I.V. taping protects his skin from the cup's edges.

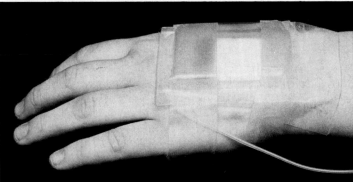

Needle container
If you're using a butterfly needle, make a protective cover out of the needle's plastic container. As you see, this protective device is similar to the medicine cup device.

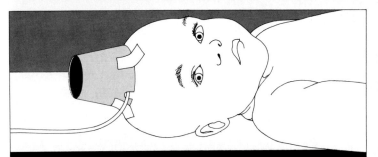

Paper cup
Consider using a small paper cup to protect a scalp site. First, cut off the cup's bottom. Then, cut a small slot through the top rim to accommodate the I.V. tubing. Place the cup upside down over the insertion site, so the I.V. tubing extends through the slot. Then, secure the cup with strips of tape, as shown in this illustration. The opening you cut in the cup allows you to examine the site without disturbing it. *Note:* You may also protect a scalp site by placing a stockinette on the infant's head.

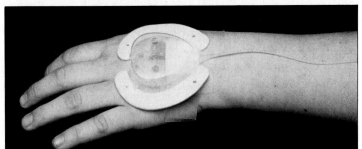

Posey™ I.V. shield
First, peel back the strips covering the adhesive backing on the bottom of the shield. Position the shield over the site, so that the I.V. tubing runs through one of the shield's two slots. Then, firmly press the shield's adhesive backing against the child's skin. You can easily observe the site's condition through the clear plastic shield.

Suppose the shield's too large to fit securely over the site? Cut off the shield's narrow end, just below the two air holes. Now, you can easily shape the shield to your patient's arm.

Parenteral

Nurses' guide to I.V. therapy complications

Caring for a child who's undergoing I.V. therapy? Remain especially alert for possible complications. His size, age, and weight, as well as his higher metabolic rate, make fluid volume calculation more difficult than for an adult. As a result, he's more susceptible to fluid imbalance. In addition, if he's active or uncooperative, he risks injuring himself by dislodging the I.V. needle or catheter.

Read this chart to learn how to recognize and deal with some I.V. therapy complications. (For more information, see the NURSING PHOTOBOOK MANAGING I.V. THERAPY.)

Complication	Possible causes	Signs and symptoms
Dehydration	• Administration of hypertonic solution without adequate hydration • Inaccurate output monitoring, leading to unrecognized fluid loss • Fever • Vomiting • Rapid breathing • Fluid shift into third space	• Low-grade fever • Flushed skin, dry mucous membranes, poor skin turgor • Hypotension • Rapid pulse • Thirst • Weight loss • Alteration in urine output (usually oliguria) • Elevated hematocrit and serum sodium level • Muscle weakness, lethargy
Overhydration	• Congestive heart failure, renal failure, liver failure • Administration of excessive fluids I.V. • Inaccurate intake and output monitoring, leading to unrecognized fluid gain	• Weight gain • Moist rales • Dyspnea • Hypertension • Possible reduced hematocrit • Abdominal cramping • Possible reduced serum sodium level (from dilution) • Muscle weakness • Lethargy
Irritated vein (phlebitis)	• Vein injury, either during venipuncture or from needle movement later • Prolonged use of vein • Use of vein that's too small for the amount or type of solution • Use of a needle or catheter that's too large for the vein • Insufficient dilution of an irritating medication	• Vein is sore, hard, cordlike, and warm to the touch; may look like a red line above the insertion site • Pain along vein • Discoloration at insertion site
Occluded vein	• Scarring of vessel from irritation • Excessive pressure on insertion site, from restraint, protective cover, or taping • Needle or catheter that's too large, occluding the vein • Blood clot, caused by vein irritation or sluggish infusion rate	• Infusion slows or stops • Edema in limb • Possible pain • Discoloration at or distal to the insertion site • Palpable clot in vein. (*Caution:* Don't press on a clot, or you may dislodge it.) • Temperature change distal to insertion site
Perforated vein wall	• Poor insertion technique • Needle movement from child's activity • Inappropriate needle size • Inserting a needle over a joint without proper immobilization	• Possible bleeding • Hematoma formation and warmth at site • Pain

Nursing considerations

- Notify doctor if you suspect dehydration.
- Administer fluids, as ordered. (Make sure the order's appropriate for the patient's weight and condition.)
- Frequently check vital signs and skin turgor to assess the effectiveness of fluid administration.
- Weigh patient at least once daily. If possible, weigh him at the same time, use the same scale, and have him wear the same (or similar) clothing.
- Monitor daily serum electrolyte measurements, as ordered.
- Monitor hematocrit readings, if ordered.
- Closely monitor fluid intake and output for signs of fluid imbalance.

- Notify the doctor if you suspect overhydration.
- Monitor daily serum electrolyte measurements, as ordered.
- Monitor hematocrit readings, if ordered.
- Question any fluid replacement order that appears excessive for your patient's weight and condition.
- Frequently assess vital signs, and intake and output. Remember to include *all* fluid intake; for example, gelatin, ice chips, and formula.
- Weigh your patient daily.
- Check the I.V. infusion rate hourly to make sure it's correct. Minimize the risk of overhydration by using a calibrated volume-control set, and/or an I.V. pump.
- Promptly report temperature and respiratory changes, so the doctor can adjust the infusion rate, if necessary.

- Remove the I.V. needle or catheter, and restart I.V. infusion at another site. Choose a vein that's large enough to accommodate the amount and type of solution.
- Use a needle or catheter that's an appropriate size for your patient, and the amount and type of solution.
- Immobilize the I.V. needle or catheter by securely taping it. Use extension tubing or adapters to reduce stress on the insertion site.
- Use a catheter instead of a needle, especially for long-term I.V. therapy.
- To reduce the need for repeated venipunctures, draw any blood samples the doctor orders immediately after inserting the I.V. needle or catheter. (But never draw blood through an I.V. needle or catheter that's been infusing fluid.)
- Make sure irritating medications are adequately diluted.

- Notify the doctor. *Do not* attempt to irrigate the line.
- Remove I.V. needle or catheter, if ordered, and restart I.V. infusion at another site.
- Be alert for signs of pulmonary embolism, if the occlusion's due to clotting.
- Make sure tape, restraints, and protective covers don't press on insertion site.
- Choose needle or catheter of appropriate size.
- Keep infusion flowing at prescribed rate.

- Remove I.V. needle or catheter.
- Apply pressure for at least 5 minutes, to stop bleeding and prevent hematoma formation.
- Restart I.V. infusion at another site.
- Use a catheter, if possible, or choose a needle that's an appropriate size.
- Avoid sites over joints.
- Restrain the child, if necessary, but only as a last resort.

Learning about subcutaneous injections

As you know, you give subcutaneous injections when the doctor wants the medication to take effect slowly. When injected subcutaneously, medication is absorbed through the patient's adipose and connective tissues. That's why most subcutaneous injection solutions are isotonic, nonirritating, nonviscous, and soluble.

The doctor may order a subcutaneous injection if:
- the prescribed medication is most effective when absorbed through the subcutaneous tissue.
- the patient can't or won't swallow, or is unable to take anything by mouth for any other reason.
- the medication will be destroyed in the gastrointestinal tract.

The doctor probably won't order a subcutaneous injection if your patient's obese, or if his skin tissue is edematous, burned, damaged by previous injections, or diseased. The doctor will also choose another route if your patient's in shock or has occlusive vascular disease with poor perfusion. In either circumstance, circulation is inadequate for proper absorption of medication through the patient's subcutaneous tissue.

Subcutaneous injection tips

When you administer a subcutaneous injection to a child, remember the important points listed below. For a demonstration of proper technique, review the photostory beginning on page 77.
- Choose an injection site on the outside of the upper arm or thigh, the buttocks, or the abdomen's lower quadrants. Test for an adequate fat layer by pinching the skin between your thumb and forefinger. If the fat in the subcutaneous layer seems inadequate, test another site.
- Consider the child's age, weight, and condition when choosing a site. For example, if he has very thin arms, use a site on his buttocks or abdomen instead.
- If your patient receives frequent subcutaneous injections (for example, if he has diabetes and needs daily insulin injections), choose a site according to his rotation schedule. Teach the child and his parents to document each injection site on a calendar.
- If your patient's an infant or a thin child, use a ⅜" or ½" needle. For a larger child, use a ⅝" needle.
- Have another needle available in case your patient moves before you've injected the medication, contaminating the needle. *Note:* If blood backflow contaminates the medication in the syringe, discard it and obtain a new syringe of medication. Blood injected with the medication will irritate your patient's tissue.
- Before giving the injection, introduce a small air bubble into the syringe by pulling back slightly on the plunger. The bubble helps seal the medication in the subcutaneous tissue, and it ensures that the patient gets a complete dose of medication.

Note: Because an insulin syringe is specially designed to deliver a highly accurate dose, this step isn't necessary when you use one.

Parenteral

Learning with Sugar Babe®

Twelve-year-old Roger Simms has recently learned that he has diabetes and needs daily insulin injections. "I hate needles," he tells you resentfully. "Why did this happen to me?"

In addition to fearing daily injections, a diabetic child may feel angry about his condition. How can you help him deal with his feelings, while teaching him how to manage his diabetes? Consider using a teaching aid like the Sugar Babe® doll featured here.

To emphasize the diabetic child's continuing need for exercise, the Sugar Babe doll is dressed in jogging clothes. To help the child learn site rotation, injection sites are clearly marked on her arms, legs, buttocks, and abdomen. Most importantly, her lifelike skin, when punctured by a needle, simulates the feel of needle entry through real skin. (Drainage holes in the doll's feet allow you to drain the doll after water injections.)

The doll comes with a special patient-teaching manual that you or the parents can read with the child. In addition to detailing injection techniques, it provides an easy-to-understand explanation of diabetes. It also contains valuable information on diet, exercise, mixing insulins, rotating injection sites, and testing sugar levels.

Use the doll and manual together to educate the child about his condition. As his skill, knowledge, and confidence grow, he'll gain a sense of control over his condition. And, by learning how to draw water into a syringe and inject it into the doll, he can quickly master injection techniques. Before long, he may be ready to give himself injections. In the following photostory, a young patient demonstrates the correct technique. (For more information about Sugar Babe, write to Sugar Babe, Inc., P.O. Box 3133, Princeton, NJ, 08540.)

Note: Although a child as young as age 5 can learn to give himself injections with the help of you or his parents, most younger children haven't developed the adequate fine-motor coordination necessary for giving an injection.

Evaluating a child's self-injection technique

1 *Gary Devlin, age 11, has just learned how to give himself his daily insulin injection. Now, you're going to watch him perform the procedure, to make sure he does it properly.*

Before he begins, Gary assembles all the equipment he needs and washes his hands. He checks the insulin's expiration date and makes sure the medication's the correct strength and type. Then, he mixes the insulin by slowly rolling—but not shaking— the vial between his palms.

Next, he unwraps an alcohol swab, as shown here, and cleans the vial's rubber stopper.

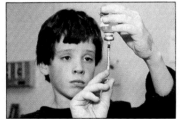

2 Now, Gary removes the needle cap and draws into the syringe an amount of air equal to the insulin dose. Next, with the vial standing upright, he inserts the needle into the vial's rubber stopper and pushes the plunger. By injecting air into the vial, he eliminates its vacuum, making insulin withdrawal easier. He turns the vial and syringe upside down, as shown, and slowly pulls the plunger about 5 units past his dose. Then he lightly taps the syringe so air bubbles rise. Next, he slowly pushes the plunger until the top of its stopper reaches the line marking his exact dose. This action expels the air bubbles.

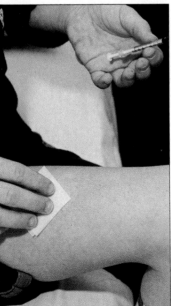

3 After removing the needle from the vial, Gary selects an injection site on his thigh, according to his site rotation schedule. He uses an alcohol swab to cleanse the site, rubbing in a circular motion.

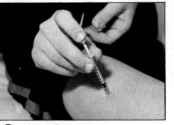

4 Now, Gary pinches the skin at the cleansed site between his thumb and forefinger to isolate the subcutaneous layer. Using a dartlike motion, he quickly inserts the needle into his skin at an angle that's between 45 and 90 degrees, and then releases the pinched skin.

Holding the syringe in one hand, he gently pulls up on the plunger to check for blood backflow. (You may decide against teaching this step if your patient's very young, because he may accidentally pull the needle out of his skin.) Since no blood appears in the barrel, he slowly injects the insulin, as shown.

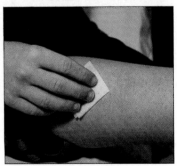

5 Gary places an alcohol swab over the site, and presses lightly as he withdraws the needle. He continues to press on the site for several seconds, as shown. Next, he replaces the needle cap and snaps the needle off the syringe; then he properly disposes of them. He marks the injection site on the calendar you gave him, to help him correctly rotate injection sites.

Finally, he stores the insulin vial in a cool, dark place. You congratulate Gary for his excellent technique. Obviously, you've taught him well.

Parenteral

Learning about I.M. injections

Giving an intramuscular (I.M.) injection to a child? Consider this route's pros and cons. As you probably know, muscles have more blood vessels and fewer sensory nerve endings than other parenteral sites, making I.M. administration relatively safe and effective.

You'll use the I.M. route to:
• achieve a rapid drug effect.
• avoid loss of drug effects from vomiting or gastric activity.
• ensure long-term absorption by forming a medication deposit.
• administer medication to a child who's unconscious, unable to swallow, or uncooperative.
• administer aqueous suspensions, solutions in oil, or medications that don't come in oral form.
• administer medications that are irritating to subcutaneous tissues.

But, when using the I.M. route, also keep these risks in mind:
• You may damage blood vessels, causing bleeding or improper absorption of medication.
• You may damage nerves, causing unnecessary pain or paralysis.
• You may damage bone.

Choosing an intramuscular injection site

Choosing the best intramuscular injection site for your pediatric patient isn't an easy task. You must take a number of factors into consideration; for example, the child's age, weight, and muscle development, the amount of medication you're administering, and the medication's absorption rate.

Now, let's consider the child's age and muscle development. If your patient's under age 3, use the vastus lateralis muscle group for the injection. It's the largest muscle mass in a child of that age and has few major blood vessels and nerves.

For children above age 3, the ventrogluteal and dorsogluteal areas are possible injection sites, because they're also relatively free of major nerves and blood vessels. But before you select either area, make sure the child has been walking for at least 1 year. This ensures that the muscles are sufficiently developed. *Caution:* If the posterior gluteal muscle's poorly developed, you risk injuring the patient's sciatic nerve.

If your patient's older than age 18 months, and you want rapid medication absorption, consider choosing the deltoid muscle. Blood flow is more rapid in the deltoid than in other muscles. But choose this site with caution, because the deltoid isn't fully developed until adolescence. In a younger child, it's small and very close to the radial nerve, which may be injured during needle insertion.

Deltoid: Adolescents (small amounts of medication may be given at this site to a child older than 18 months)

Deep brachial artery
Radial nerve

Ventrogluteal: Over age 3

Iliac crest   Greater trochanter of femur

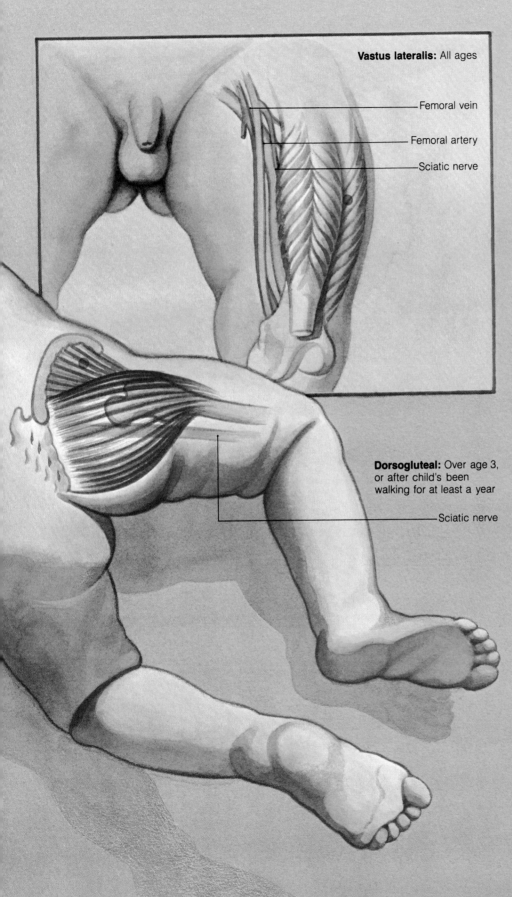

Vastus lateralis: All ages

Femoral vein

Femoral artery

Sciatic nerve

Dorsogluteal: Over age 3, or after child's been walking for at least a year

Sciatic nerve

Giving an I.M. injection

If you have to administer an intramuscular injection to a child, follow these guidelines:
• In determining what size needle to use, consider the child's age, nutritional status, and muscle development; and the drug's viscosity.
• When injecting less than 1 ml of medication, use a tuberculin syringe for accuracy.
• To help the child relax his muscle before the injection, have him concentrate on something else. For example, ask him to pant, count, or wiggle his toes. Encourage him to cooperate by playing Simon Says.
• Tell your patient the injection will hurt, but assure him that the discomfort will last only a short time.
• Ask another nurse to help restrain the child, if necessary. And keep extra medication and equipment available in case the needle or syringe becomes contaminated.
• After you've drawn up the medication, draw up 0.2 cc to 0.3 cc of air into the syringe. Doing so helps clear the needle of medication and prevents medication seepage from the injection site.
• Choose an injection site. (See sites marked in green on illustrations at left. The blue lines on the ventrogluteal illustration show how to place your fingers to locate landmarks.)
• Cleanse the site with an alcohol swab. Use a brisk circular motion that creates friction. For greatest antimicrobial action, allow the alcohol to dry before inserting the needle. This precaution also eliminates the risk that you'll inject alcohol into the child.
• Stretch the skin around the insertion site to make it taut. Doing so displaces subcutaneous tissue, facilitating proper needle insertion.
• Insert the needle at a 90° angle with a quick, dartlike motion to minimize pain. Maintain a firm grip at the lower portion of the syringe.
• Gently pull back on the plunger to confirm correct needle placement. If blood appears in the syringe, withdraw the needle and discard the needle, medication, and syringe. Using uncontaminated medication and equipment, begin the procedure again at another site. If no blood appears, continue the procedure.
• Inject the medication slowly to give the muscle time to accommodate it. Withdraw the needle with one quick motion, at the same angle you inserted it.
• Document the procedure, including the injection site that you used. When administering multiple injections, rotate injection sites. When reusing an injection site, palpate the tissue, and check for edema and erythema. If these conditions exist, try to place additional injections outside the affected area.
• Allow the child to put a brightly colored adhesive bandage strip over the site.

Parenteral

Understanding I.M. injection complications

Improper technique	Possible result	Complications
Using a needle that's too short	Depositing medication into incorrect tissue layer	• Nonspecific injection pain • Sterile abscess • Tissue degeneration • Granuloma • Hypertrophy
Using a needle that's too long	Depositing medication into periosteum; injury to periosteum and/or bone	• Needle tip breaking off in bone • Death of periosteum, resulting in bone growth retardation
Failing to replace needle after drawing up a caustic medication or an iron compound	Medication adhering to outside of needle, causing tissue irritation or discoloration	• Nonspecific injection pain • Local skin and muscle reaction to medication • Infection • Tissue necrosis • Tissue discoloration from iron compounds
Injecting into underdeveloped muscle	Injury to a nerve	• Tingling • Shooting pain down limb • Footdrop (after injection into a dorsogluteal site) • Paralysis
Not locating proper landmarks before injecting	Injury to a nerve, bone, or blood vessel	• Nerve damage (see complications listed immediately above) • Bleeding; hematoma • Needle tip breaking off in bone • Injecting medication into periosteum
Forgetting to check for blood backflow	Injecting medication into a vein or artery	• Speed shock (increased heart rate, shortness of breath, decreased blood pressure, loss of consciousness) • Anaphylactoid reaction to a medication base not intended for venous administration
Neglecting to draw 0.2 to 0.3 cc of air into syringe before injecting	Medication leaking from injection site; incomplete delivery of medication	• Skin irritation • Formation of a hardened area under the skin (sterile abscess) • Tissue necrosis • Decreased effectiveness of medication
Break in aseptic technique	Introduction of microorganisms or other contaminants into muscle layer	• Subcutaneous or muscle abscess • Tissue degeneration • Septicemia
Poor rotation of injection sites	Degeneration of fatty tissue; accumulation of a large medication deposit in muscle	• Malabsorption or no absorption of medication • Tissue degeneration • Nerve damage • Overdose, if increased blood flow to muscle (from exercise or heat application) causes rapid absorption of large medication deposit

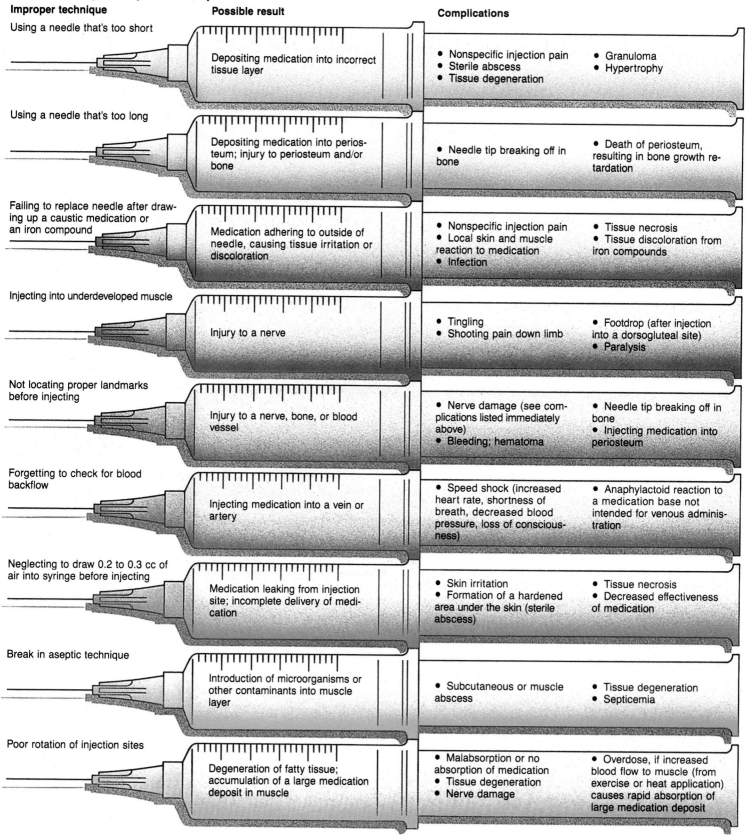

Rectal

You probably know that rectal medications may be ordered for either local or systemic effects. But have you ever considered *why* the doctor may sometimes prefer this route?

Obviously, medications intended for local bowel effects can't be given any other way. And, when used for systemic medications, the rectal route has these advantages:
• It eliminates the risk of aspiration.
• It ensures that the child won't vomit the medication before it's absorbed.
• Digestive enzymes won't destroy the medication, and the medication won't irritate the stomach.
• The liver won't immediately biotransform the medication, since medication absorbed from the lower rectum initially bypasses the portal system.

To learn more, read on.

Learning about suppositories and enemas

Use this chart to learn more about possible uses for suppositories and enemas. Keep these disadvantages in mind: The medication may be completely or irregularly absorbed through the rectum, depending on the child's ability to retain it, and on the presence of feces. And, he'll probably find the procedure uncomfortable and embarrassing.

Description	Uses	Special considerations
Suppository A solid medication in a firm base, such as cocoa butter, that melts at body temperature. May be molded in a variety of cylindrical shapes. Available in small sizes.	Some given for local effect (for example, laxatives, lubricants, and cathartics); others for systemic effect (for example, antipyretics, bronchodilators, and sedatives)	• Don't give a suppository if you suspect damage to the anal sphincters or bowel wall. • To make insertion more comfortable, lubricate the suppository with water-soluble lubricant. • Store suppositories in the refrigerator, to preserve their shape and firmness. • When giving a suppository that's been refrigerated, warn the child that it'll feel cold.
Nonretention enema A medicated or nonmedicated liquid not intended for mucosal absorption	Given for local effect, to cleanse the bowel and eliminate flatus. Rarely, iced solutions are given to reduce high fever.	• Administer with disposable bottle, or through rectal tube. • Unless contraindicated, warm an enema to room temperature before administration. A very warm or cold enema may cause abdominal cramping. • Protect bed linens with a bed-saver pad. • Position a bedpan under the child's buttocks, to collect bowel returns. If your patient's an infant, collect bowel returns on folded diapers or bed-saver pads instead.
Retention enema A nonirritating solution that's usually medicated; intended to be retained for at least 30 minutes, or until absorbed	May be given to soften bowel contents or to provide bulk, or as a general anesthetic. Other types are rarely used for children, although any medicated enema designed for adult use may be given after appropriate dosage adjustment. *Note:* Rarely, a nutrient retention enema may be given.	• Never give a retention enema to a child younger than age 6. He won't be able to retain it. • Give *before* meals, since a full stomach stimulates peristalsis and hastens expulsion. • Don't administer a retention enema if your patient has diarrhea or a fecal impaction (unless the enema was ordered to treat the condition). Either condition interferes with absorption of medication. • Give a small amount of solution through a small rectal tube (see the chart below for guidelines). By doing so, you create less pressure in your patient's rectum, making retention easier.

Nurses' guide to rectal tube administration

Use the chart below as a guide when you give your patient an enema with a rectal tube and bulb syringe. In addition, keep the following points in mind:
• Consider the child's size and age. (As a rule, his size is the more important consideration.) If your patient's small for his age, use the smallest tube suggested below.
• Also consider the properties of the medication you're giving. For example, if you're giving a syrup, choose a tube that's large enough in diameter to easily administer a viscous liquid.
• Check the child's rectum before beginning the procedure. If it's inflamed, notify the doctor before proceeding.

Retention enemas

Age-group	Rectal tube size	Amount of tube to insert	Amount of fluid to introduce
Adolescents	14 to 20 French	3″ to 4″ (7.6 to 10.2 cm)	150 to 200 ml
Children over age 6	12 to 14 French	2″ to 3″ (5.1 to 7.6 cm)	75 to 150 ml

Nonretention enemas

Age-group	Rectal tube size	Amount of tube to insert	Amount of fluid to introduce
Adolescents	22 to 30 French	3″ to 4″ (7.6 to 10.2 cm)	750 to 1,000 ml
Children over age 6	14 to 18 French	2″ to 3″ (5.1 to 7.6 cm)	500 to 1,000 ml
Children over age 2	12 to 14 French	1½″ to 2″ (3.8 to 5.1 cm)	500 ml or less
Infants	12 French	1″ to 1½″ (2.5 to 3.8 cm)	250 ml or less

Rectal

Preparing your patient for a rectal medication

Whenever you administer a rectal medication to a child—particularly an older one who's just becoming aware of his own body—be sensitive to his feelings. He'll probably feel embarrassed at having a stranger insert medication into his rectum. That's why you must remember to always use tact and compassion when performing the procedure.

First, try to maintain as much privacy as possible for your patient. Close all doors and curtains around his bed. Provide a drape, and avoid exposing him unnecessarily.

Then, explain the procedure to him. Speak calmly, and use terms he understands or terms that he uses. Also, explain the procedure to the child's parents. They can help reassure the child and provide support.

Before you begin, allow your patient to become familiar with the equipment and procedure. Tell him what the medication will feel like. For example, if you're administering a suppository, warn the child that he'll feel an urge to defecate. Tell him the procedure may feel uncomfortable, but it won't hurt. Try to relax your patient by giving him a toy to play with. Also, have him take slow, deep breaths to relax his anal sphincter and make insertion easier. Then, continue to reassure your patient after each step of the procedure.

If your patient won't lie still during the procedure, ask a co-worker to help hold him. But restrain the child only as a last resort. Remember, he's already upset, and restraining him may make things worse.

Administering a suppository

1 *The doctor has ordered a 100 mg Tigan (trimethobenzamide hydrochloride) suppository for 7-year-old Linda Bartman to help control her nausea. Make sure you know how to administer it by reading this photostory:*

First, wash your hands and gather the equipment you'll need: the prescribed suppository, a glove or finger cot, water-soluble lubricant, and tissues.

Nursing tip: Suppose the suppository feels too soft to remove easily from the wrapper. Without unwrapping the suppository, hold it under cold running water until it becomes firm.

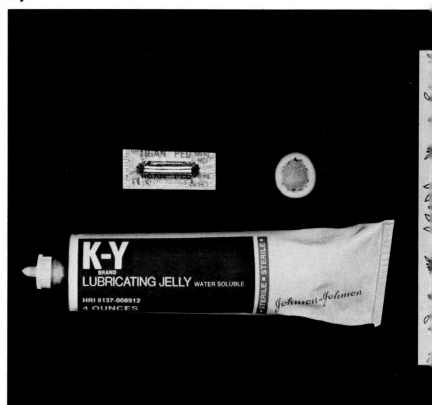

2 Provide as much privacy as possible for your patient. Close her door and draw her bed curtains. Calmly explain the procedure to her, using words she can understand. Also, explain the procedure and the need for the medication to her parents. Check the medication order and your patient's identification band to make sure you're administering the right drug to the right patient. Then, wash your hands.

Now, position Linda on her left side, with her right leg drawn up (Sims' position), so her anal area is exposed. (If your patient's an infant or toddler, place her on her back, with her knees flexed.)

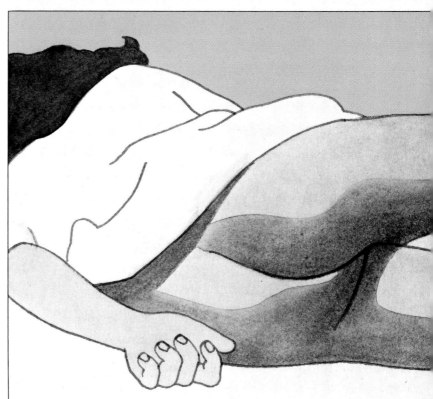

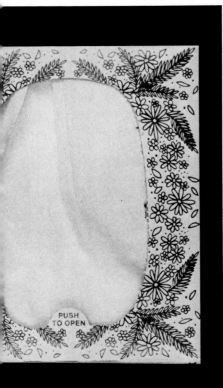

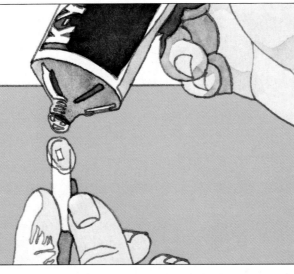

3 Put the finger cot over the index finger on your dominant hand. Or, put a glove on your dominant hand. Then, remove the suppository from its wrapper and lubricate the tapered end.

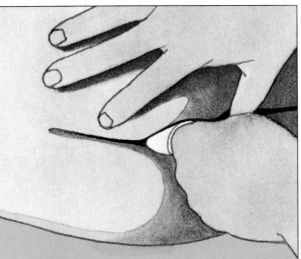

4 Using your ungloved hand, separate Linda's buttocks to expose her anus. Ask her to breathe deeply through her mouth. This helps relax her internal anal sphincter, easing insertion. With your gloved hand, quickly but gently insert the suppository into her rectum, tapered end first. Use your index finger to direct it along the rectal wall until it's past the child's internal anal sphincter. But, make sure you don't push the suppository into a fecal mass; if you do, the medication won't be absorbed properly. Remove the suppository, if possible, and notify the doctor.

Note: If your patient's age 3 or younger, use your little finger to insert the suppository.

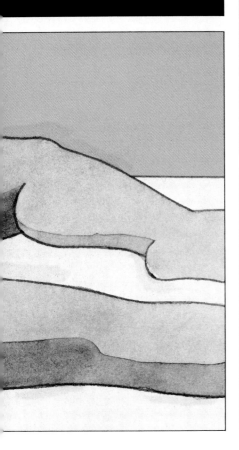

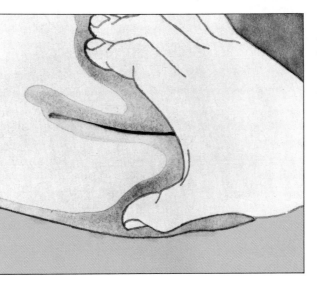

5 Withdraw your finger. Hold your patient's buttocks firmly together for about 10 minutes, until the urge to defecate passes. Wipe excess lubricant from her anus with tissues.

Linda should retain the suppository for at least 20 minutes to allow the medication to be absorbed. If she defecates, check the stool for the suppository. Notify the doctor if all of it was expelled with the stool. *Note:* If you give a suppository to relieve constipation, your patient can defecate as soon as she feels the urge.

Finally, remove and dispose of your glove or finger cot, wash your hands, and document everything, including how long the patient retained the suppository.

Rectal

Using a Fleet* enema for children

1 *Charlie Miles, age 4, is scheduled for bilateral herni-orrhaphy. The doctor's ordered a preoperative sodium biphosphate enema to cleanse his bowel. If you're using the Fleet* ready-to-use enema for children, do you know how to proceed? Read these two pages for guidance.*

First, gather the equipment you'll need: the Fleet enema (contained in a disposable plastic bottle), a bed-saver pad, and a potty-chair or bedpan (not shown). If your patient's not yet toilet trained, obtain a diaper instead of a bedpan.

Warm the enema solution by placing the bottle in a basin of warm tap water for about 20 minutes. Then, remove it from the basin.

2 Next, explain the procedure to Charlie and his parents. Use language they can understand. Use the same term for defecate that the child uses. Tell him why the enema's needed, and what he may feel. If necessary, have a co-worker help restrain the child while you administer the enema.

Note: Don't forget to close the door and the bed curtain to ensure your patient's privacy. The procedure may embarrass him.

Now, wash your hands. Lay down the bed-saver pad to protect the linens. Then, place Charlie in a kneeling position with his head and chest resting comfortably on the bed, as shown here.

Or as an alternative, place him on his left side, with his right leg drawn up (Sims' position), so his anal area is exposed. Have him fold his left arm beneath his head.

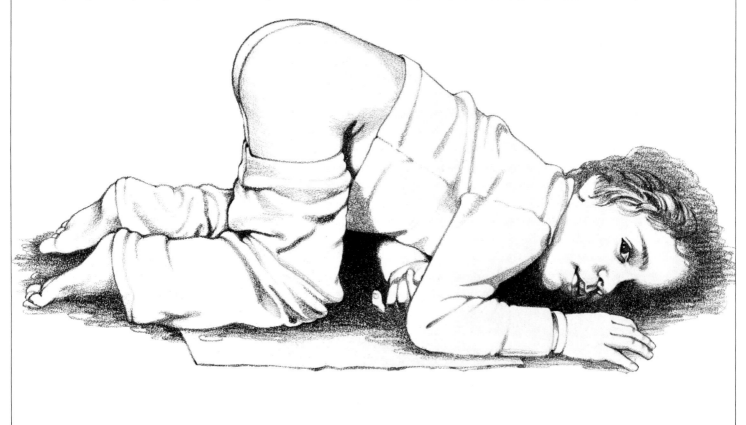

*Available in both the United States and in Canada

3 Take the enema bottle in one hand, and hold it upright. With your other hand, remove the protective shield that's covering the bottle tip. You'll notice that the tip's already lubricated.

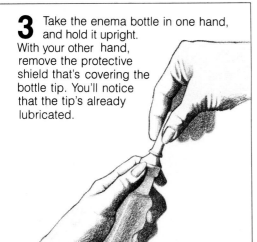

4 Have Charlie take some slow, deep breaths to help him relax. Then, with steady pressure, gently insert the tip of the enema bottle into his rectum. Point the tip of the bottle toward his navel, as shown in this illustration.

Slowly squeeze the bottle to instill the solution into your patient's rectum. Continue squeezing it until nearly all the solution's expelled. Leave a small amount of solution in the bottle so you don't introduce air into the rectum. Don't worry; the bottle contains more than enough solution to be effective.

5 After you've instilled the solution, press Charlie's buttocks together to keep him from expelling the medication. Remove the bottle tip from his rectum. Then, help him into a comfortable position on his side.

Continue pressing Charlie's buttocks together for about 3 minutes until his desire to defecate is strong. Then, place him on the potty-chair, and provide privacy if he desires. Or, if the child's upset, let his parents help him. (If your patient's not toilet trained, diaper him.)

Note: If you're giving an enema to an older child, and you have to examine the bowel returns, allow him to use the bathroom. But, remind him not to flush the toilet.

After you're finished the procedure, dispose of the bed-saver pad and enema bottle, and wash your hands. Document the procedure and the results in your nurses' notes.

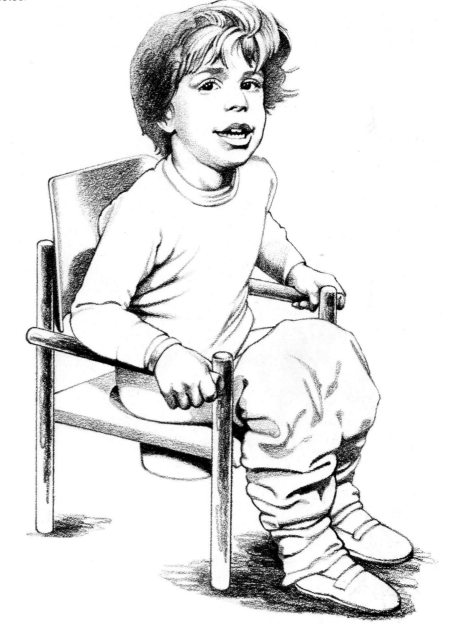

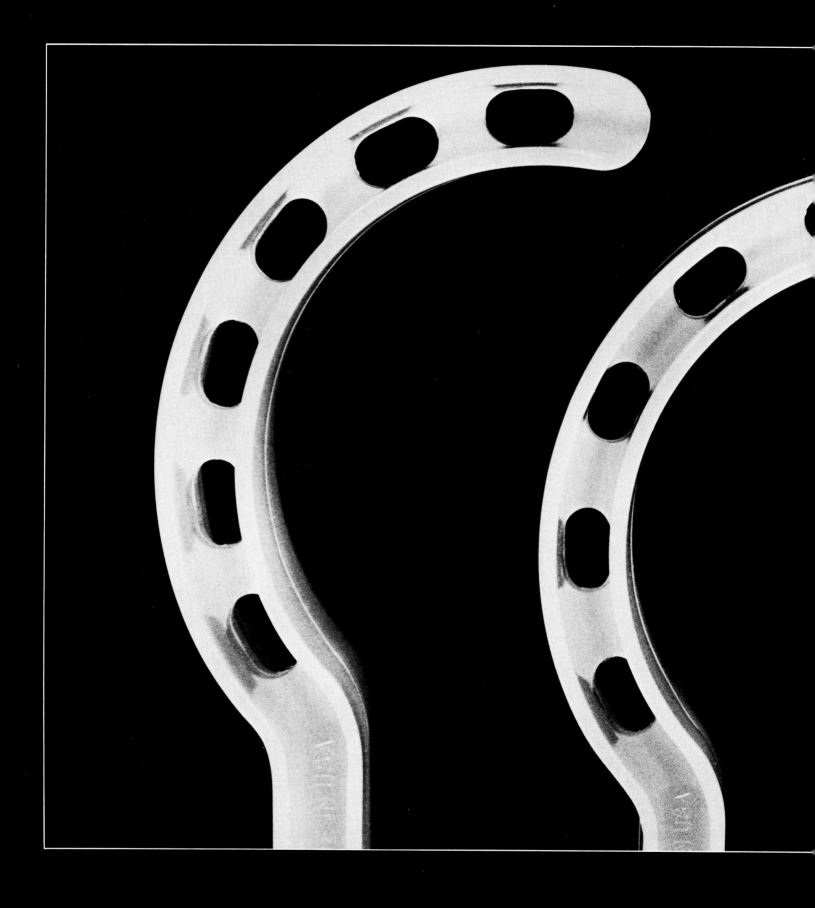

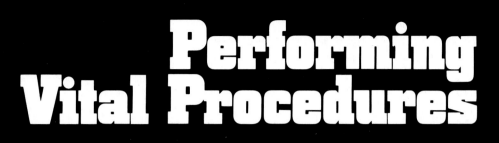

Performing Vital Procedures

Respiratory

Cardiac

Special problems

Respiratory

Do you know that respiratory tract diseases account for about half of the acute illnesses in children under age 17? As a pediatric nurse, you may care for many children with respiratory problems. Are you sure you know all you need to give them top quality nursing care?

On the following pages, we'll provide that information. For instance, we'll show you:
• how a child's respiratory system anatomy differs from an adult's.
• how to combat respiratory arrest.
• how to clear an obstructed airway.
• how to use a hand-held resuscitator.
• how to use a mist tent.

We'll also provide important information on common respiratory disorders, including pneumonia and status asthmaticus. Read this section carefully.

Reviewing pediatric respiratory system anatomy

"My little boy always seems to have a cough or cold. Is this normal?" How many times has a concerned parent asked you a question like this? As a pediatric nurse, you know that upper respiratory system infections and other respiratory problems are common in children, so you can provide some reassurance. But do you know *why* these problems are so common?

Consider a few of the most obvious reasons. A child's relatively short, compact respiratory tract allows bacteria and other microorganisms to travel easily into his lungs. And because a child's immune system isn't well developed, he has fewer defenses against the invaders.

To complicate matters, a child's lungs contain fewer alveoli than an adult's. So, when a child's lungs become congested, he suffers greater loss of gas exchange. Yet, because of his fast metabolism, he needs even *more* oxygen than an adult needs. No wonder a respiratory problem can be so debilitating for a youngster.

Other anatomical differences that distinguish a child's respiratory tract make him especially prone to respiratory problems, such as airway obstruction. Here are a few examples:
• A child's mucous membranes are loosely attached to his airway. As a result, they're easily irritated, which may cause edema and coughing.
• His airway is smaller in diameter than an adult's, and contains a greater proportion of soft tissue, including the soft palate and tongue. All of these factors make airway obstruction more likely if excessive mucus formation or edema occurs for any reason.
• An infant's larynx is located two or three cervical vertebrae higher than an adult's, increasing the risk of obstruction by aspiration.

Keep in mind that even an apparently minor respiratory system problem may become life-threatening. When your pediatric patient has such a problem, treat him with special care.

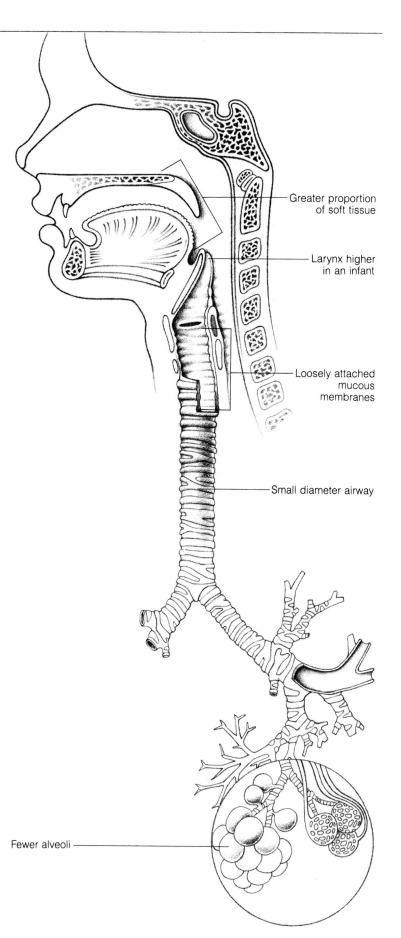

Greater proportion of soft tissue

Larynx higher in an infant

Loosely attached mucous membranes

Small diameter airway

Fewer alveoli

Understanding common respiratory problems

Respiratory problems may affect a child's upper respiratory tract (nose, pharynx, epiglottis, larynx, trachea), or his lower respiratory tract (bronchi, bronchioles, alveoli). Typically, upper respiratory tract problems contribute to airway blockage, resulting in breathing difficulty on *inspiration*. Lower respiratory tract problems, on the other hand, inhibit gas exchange in the lungs. As a result, the patient may have breathing difficulty on *expiration*.

In the following chart, you'll learn more about common pediatric respiratory problems. But some nursing interventions are necessary and appropriate in almost every circumstance. Keep these important general guidelines in mind:
• Always have the necessary equipment for intubation and tracheotomy readily available.
• Keep a hand-held resuscitator nearby.
• If the child can safely swallow, encourage him to drink cool, high-calorie fluids to maintain nutrition and prevent dehydration. But avoid milk and milk products, since they thicken mucus secretions. *Caution:* To reduce the risk of aspiration, *don't* give your patient anything by mouth if he has epiglottitis, or any other condition that's likely to require intubation.
• If ordered, provide fluids I.V., to prevent dehydration and supply nutrients.
• Monitor fluid intake and output, and weigh your patient daily.
• Reduce fever with antipyretics or cool mist delivered by a mist tent, as ordered, or with tepid water sponge baths.
• To relieve breathing difficulties and loosen secretions, provide humidified air with an aerosol mask or mist tent, as ordered.
• Frequently auscultate breath sounds and monitor vital signs, to assess the patient's condition.
• Obtain frequent arterial blood gas (ABG) measurements, as ordered, and stay alert for signs of hypoxia and hypercapnia.

Upper respiratory tract

Problem
Nasopharyngitis (common cold)

Age-group affected
All ages

Description
Infection causing mucosal edema and vasodilation

Cause
Viral (usually rhinovirus)

Signs and symptoms
• Fever possible, especially in infants and young children
• Dry, irritated nose and throat, possibly accompanied by sneezing and coughing
• Irritability and restlessness
• Chills
• Muscle soreness
• Vomiting or diarrhea possible in infants and young children

Nursing interventions
• Promote bed rest while child is feverish. If possible, isolate him from other children.
• Observe your patient for respiratory complications. Watch an infant with special care, because he normally breathes only through his nose.
• If necessary, remove nasal secretions with suction equipment, nasal aspirator, or ear syringe.
• Administer nose drops, as ordered.
• If ordered, obtain a throat culture to test for streptococcal infection.
• Administer antibiotics, if ordered.

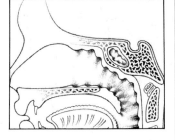

Problem
Acute epiglottitis

Age-group affected
2 to 8 years

Description
Severe infection of the epiglottis and surrounding area; signs and symptoms usually appear suddenly. May follow another upper respiratory tract infection.

Cause
Bacterial (*Hemophilus influenzae*, type B; group A streptococcus; pneumococcus)

Signs and symptoms
• Drooling
• Enlarged, cherry-red, edematous epiglottis
• Dysphagia
• Dyspnea
• Croaking, froglike sound on inspiration; inspiratory stridor
• Retractions
• Fever

Nursing interventions
• Never use a tongue depressor to examine your patient's throat, because you may cause a laryngospasm that will completely obstruct his airway.
• Initially, don't give him anything by mouth, because he may need intubation.
• Administer parenteral fluids, if ordered. If the child can safely swallow, and intubation is unnecessary, enourage him to drink fluids.
• Maintain an open airway. Keep intubation and tracheotomy equipment nearby.
• Reassure your patient, and provide continuing support. Encourage his parents to stay with him, if possible.
• Obtain culture specimens, as ordered.
• Administer antibiotics, as ordered.
• Provide bed rest throughout disease's acute phase.

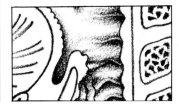

Problem
Acute laryngotracheobronchitis

Age-group affected
Infant to 3 years

Description
Inflamed vocal cords and edema of surrounding tissue, causing laryngeal obstruction. Onset is usually gradual; may initially be mistaken for or may follow other upper respiratory tract infection such as nasopharyngitis.

Cause
Viral (parainfluenza, influenza, measles, respiratory syncytial virus, adenovirus)

Signs and symptoms
• Hoarseness; brassy, barking cough
• Inspiratory stridor
• Increasing inspiratory dyspnea with substernal and suprasternal retractions
• Labored and prolonged expirations
• Diminished breath sounds bilaterally
• Scattered rales and rhonchi
• Soreness in chest
• Pallor or cyanosis
• Irritability, restlessness, exhaustion

Nursing interventions
• Watch your patient for tachycardia, cyanosis, changes in level of consciousness, and diminished breath sounds.
• Obtain nasopharyngeal and blood cultures, as ordered.
• Provide bed rest and continuing emotional support and reassurance.
• Encourage frequent position changes, to promote postural drainage.

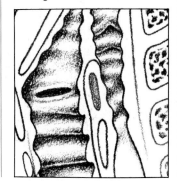

Respiratory

Understanding common respiratory problems continued

Lower respiratory tract

Problem
Status asthmaticus

Age-group affected
Any age

Description
Bronchial asthma attack unrelieved by bronchodilators. Respiratory metabolism is unbalanced; patient shows signs of hypercapnia and respiratory acidosis. May accompany nasopharyngitis or pneumonia. Onset may be rapid or gradual.

Causes
Allergy, infection, metabolic imbalance, emotional stress

Signs and symptoms
• Prolonged expiratory phase with high-pitched wheeze from mucous membrane edema
• Hypoxia and cyanosis
• Tachypnea
• Sternocleidomastoid muscle retraction
• Shallow chest movements from fatigue
• Anxiety and restlessness
• Dyspnea, possibly aggravated by anxiety

Nursing interventions
• Position the patient in high Fowler's position.
• Draw blood specimens for serum electrolyte measurements, as ordered.
• Give sodium bicarbonate I.V., as ordered, to reverse respiratory acidosis.
• Administer bronchodilators I.V., rectally, or with intermittent positive-pressure breathing (IPPB) treatments, as ordered. If the patient can safely swallow, administer oral expectorants, if ordered.
• If ordered, cautiously administer corticosteroids to relieve bronchospasm.
• Be prepared to administer a methylxanthine drug; for example, theophylline (Elixophyllin*), as ordered, to relieve bronchospasm.
• Administer oxygen, if ordered, with caution; high levels may cause respiratory depression.
• Provide extra emotional support.
• Watch for changes in level of consciousness.
• After the crisis, loosen secretions with postural drainage, percussion, and vibration. Teach the child's parents these techniques.

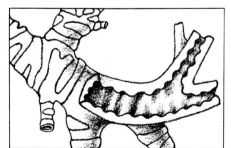

*Available in both the United States and in Canada

Problem
Bronchiolitis

Age-group affected
2 months to 2 years. Most common among infants born prematurely.

Description
Inflammation of bronchioles; obstruction of bronchioles with cellular debris. May begin as a simple upper respiratory tract infection with serous nasal discharge.

Cause
Viral (respiratory syncytial virus, adenovirus, parainfluenza, rhinovirus, *Mycoplasma pneumoniae*)

Signs and symptoms
• Moderate temperature elevation
• Increasing respiratory distress, including paroxysmal hacking cough, dyspnea, and tachypnea
• Irritability
• Nostril flaring
• Intercostal and subcostal retractions
• Palpable liver and spleen from depressed diaphragm
• Shallow respiratory excursion; prolonged expiratory phase
• Fine, moist rales; diminished breath sounds
• Hyperresonance on palpation
• Scattered consolidation on X-ray
• Hypoxia and hypercapnia

Nursing interventions
• Isolate the child, if possible, to avoid spreading infection.
• Promote bed rest, and place patient in high Fowler's position to help him breathe more easily.
• Perform percussion, vibration, and postural drainage to help loosen secretions.
• Be prepared to administer oxygen, if the doctor orders.

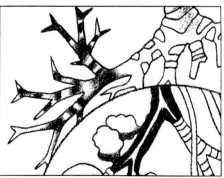

Problem
Pneumonia

Age-group affected
All ages

Description
Lung inflammation. May be preceded by an upper respiratory tract infection.

Causes
Bacterial (pneumococcus, staphylococcus, streptococcus) or viral (mycoplasm, influenza, respiratory syncytial virus, adenovirus, varicella, rubella)

Signs and symptoms
Bacterial
• Rapid onset of fever
• Productive cough
• Dyspnea
• Tachypnea
• Expiratory grunt
• Cyanosis
• Moist rales
• Diminished or absent breath sounds
Viral
• Intermittent fever
• Dyspnea after exertion
• Rubbing pain on inspiration
• Possible abdominal pain, causing confusion with appendicitis
• Dry, hacking cough that may become productive as cellular debris accumulates
• Tachypnea
• Cyanosis
• Diminished or absent breath sounds
Note: Signs and symptoms of bacterial and viral pneumonia are indistinguishable in infants under 4 months.

Nursing interventions
• Obtain sputum culture, as ordered, to identify causative organism.
• Prepare the patient for chest X-rays, as ordered.
• Promote bed rest.
• Perform percussion, vibration, and postural drainage to loosen and remove secretions.
• Administer antibiotics, as ordered, if sputum culture identifies a bacterial cause, or to prevent a secondary infection.

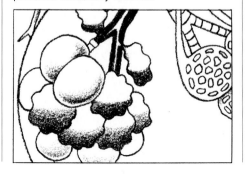

Learning about mist tents

If your pediatric patient's having trouble breathing, the doctor may order him placed in a mist tent (croup tent) like the one featured in the photostory at right.

The mist tent contains a nebulizer that transforms distilled water into mist. The mist is then delivered into a small, plastic tent or canopy that's placed over the child's crib or bed. When inhaled, moist air liquifies and loosens secretions in the child's airway.

You can use a mist tent to administer humidified air or oxygen, as ordered, by connecting the mist tent to either an air compressor or an oxygen source.

What if the doctor orders a *cool* mist for your patient? With some mist tents, you can add ice to a compartment that cools the distilled water. Other types automatically cool or warm the mist. Check to see which type's available at your hospital.

When caring for a child in a mist tent, follow these guidelines:
• Thoroughly explain the procedure to the child and his parents. The enclosed tent may frighten a young child. Try to make therapy a game for him, by encouraging him to pretend he's camping. To allay his anxiety, allow him to keep a special toy next to him. (But, if the child's receiving oxygen, don't let him use any toy that may cause an electrical spark.) Have someone stay with the child as much as possible, to comfort and reassure him.
• Frequently change the child's clothing and bed linen, because they'll quickly become damp inside the mist tent.
• Watch closely for signs of increasing respiratory difficulty, such as a hacking, dry cough; shortness of breath; increasing stridor; more pronounced retractions; or cyanosis.
• Assess the child's vital signs (including his temperature) at least once an hour.
• Thoroughly clean the nebulizer bottle each time you refill it, following the manufacturer's instructions.
• Tuck the tent under the mattress to prevent humidity loss. If the tent doesn't enclose the entire mattress, secure it by folding a bath blanket or sheet across the patient's chest and over the tent's bottom edge. Snugly tuck the blanket or sheet beneath the mattress. (Always place a bath blanket or other cover between the patient's skin and the tent.)
• Document when you placed the child in the mist tent, when you removed him from it, and the oxygen concentration inside the tent (if appropriate). Also, document any changes in his respiratory condition, and note how well he breathes outside the mist tent.

Using a mist tent

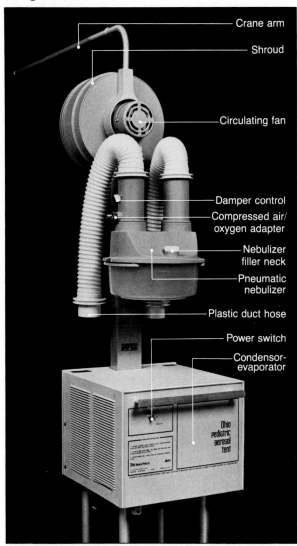

Crane arm
Shroud
Circulating fan
Damper control
Compressed air/oxygen adapter
Nebulizer filler neck
Pneumatic nebulizer
Plastic duct hose
Power switch
Condensor-evaporator

1 *Suppose you're caring for a child with bronchitis. To loosen his secretions and help him breathe easier, the doctor wants him placed in a mist tent with cool, humidified air. To find out how to use one type of mist tent, read the following photostory.*

We're using the Ohio® Pediatric Aerosol Tent shown at left. This device can nebulize up to 5.5 ml of water per minute. Then, it automatically cools and circulates the mist in the disposable plastic canopy (or tent) you'll place around the child's crib or bed.

In addition to the Pediatric Aerosol Tent system, you'll need about 2.5 liters of distilled water, and a source of compressed air. *Note:* If the doctor orders humidified oxygen, you'll need an oxygen source instead.

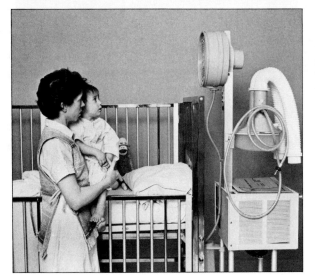

2 Now, explain the procedure to your patient, using words he understands. Position the Pediatric Aerosol Tent system at the head of the patient's crib or bed.

Respiratory

Using a mist tent continued

3 Then, place the crane arm into the opening at the top of the circulating fan. Lock the arm into position so it's level, and position it over the center of the bed.

Slide the three canopy hangers over the crane arm, passing the crane arm through the center loop on each hanger, as shown here. The hangers' loops should point downward.

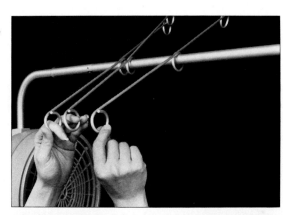

4 Next, unpack the canopy from its wrapper. Unfold it, smoothing out as many wrinkles as possible. Then, hang the canopy by attaching the rubber bands that come with it to the loops on the hangers. Make sure the side of the canopy with three openings is facing the circulating fan. Zippered pockets on each side allow easy access to the child.

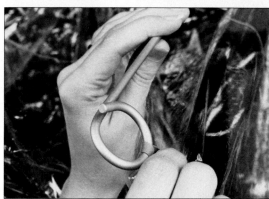

5 Stretch the large center opening in the canopy over the shroud (the plastic cover around the circulating fan), as the nurse is doing here. Make sure the edges of the opening fit snugly into the groove around the shroud.

Now, stretch the canopy's two smaller openings over the two plastic duct hoses. Make sure the canopy's openings fit snugly over each hose.

6 Now you're ready to fill the nebulizer. Remove the cap from the nebulizer's filler neck, and pour the water into the nebulizer reservoir, as the nurse is doing here. Take care not to pour more than 2.5 liters of water into the reservoir. (The proper level is marked on the reservoir.) Replace the cap on the filler neck.

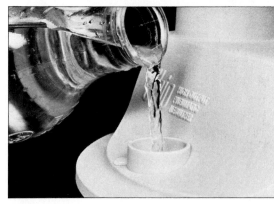

7 Place the canopy over the child's bed. Leave one side open until after you've turned the machine on and checked the mist flow. Plug the machine's power cord into a nearby electrical outlet.

Using an air hose, connect the adapter on the nebulizer to the flowmeter that regulates the amount of compressed air. Make sure all connections are tight.

Important: Set the flowmeter to deliver air at the rate of 10 liters per minute. Doing so prevents carbon dioxide from building up inside the canopy.

Now, you're ready to turn on the machine. Since the doctor ordered cool mist, push the power button up to the COOL position, as shown.

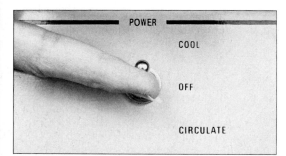

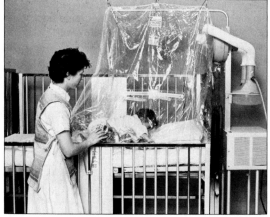

8 After the mist begins filling the canopy, pull down the open flap. Stay with the child for about 10 minutes to check the mist's density. (He should be barely visible inside the tent.) If the density's okay, tuck the canopy beneath the bed mattress. Prevent leaks by covering the canopy sections that don't fit beneath the mattress with a folded sheet or bath blanket.

Suppose the mist isn't dense enough? To change the density, adjust the nebulizer's damper control, or adjust the airflow knob.

Check the water level in the nebulizer reservoir at least once every 4 hours, or check it when you're changing the child's clothing or assessing his vital signs.

Finally, document the procedure in your nurses' notes. Include any problems you encountered.

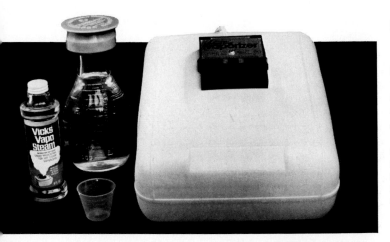

Using a vaporizer

1 *If your patient suffers from nasal or bronchial congestion, the doctor may order a vaporizer containing a medication like camphor or eucalyptus oil to make her more comfortable. Here's how to assemble it:*

After confirming the doctor's order, assemble this equipment: a vaporizer, the prescribed medication, and 1,000 ml distilled water. Explain the treatment to the child.

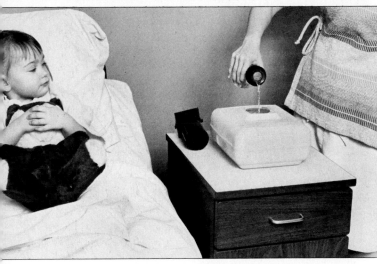

2 Pour in the distilled water until it reaches the level marked on the unit. Then, plug in the unit.

Now, measure the correct medication dose (check the medication label for instructions). Add the medication to the cup at the top of the vaporizer. When the water vaporizes, the steam will diffuse the medication into the air.

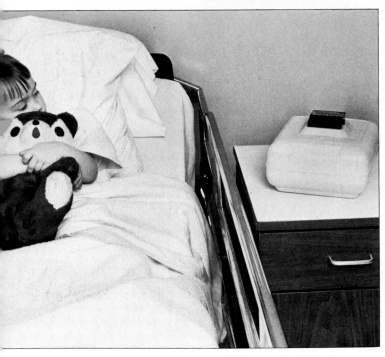

3 Position the patient so she's comfortable, and caution her against playing with the vaporizer. Put the vaporizer within several feet of her. Be sure the stream's directed toward your patient so she can inhale the medicated steam easily. But don't put it so close that the steam burns her. For safety, place it on a table. Position the table so no one trips over the vaporizer's cord.

Make sure the unit's working properly. Then document the procedure in your nurses' notes.

Periodically check your patient and the vaporizer. Also, check your patient's bed linen. If it's damp, you've probably placed the vaporizer too close. Reposition it, and replace the bed linen. Continue to use the vaporizer, as indicated or prescribed. Replace the vaporizer's water, as needed.

Using a nasal inhalation device

If your patient suffers from an allergy like hay fever, the doctor may prescribe flunisolide (Nasalide) to relieve persistant rhinitis. The self-care aid on the next page will help your patient learn to correctly administer the drug. But remember, no aid is a substitute for personal patient teaching. Explain the procedure to your patient and his parents, and answer their questions. Make sure they know:
• the name of the drug, its intended effects, and its possible side effects.
• the prescribed dose and frequency.
• the procedure for assembling and cleaning the device. (Stress the importance of keeping the device clean, to prevent it from becoming a source of infection.)

Take care to warn the patient against overusing the drug. If it proves ineffective, tell him to notify his doctor. Also, caution him against using any other drugs (including over-the-counter drugs) without the doctor's permission. *Note:* Flunisolide is not recommended for children under age 6.

For more information on inhalation drugs and devices, see the NURSING PHOTOBOOK GIVING MEDICATIONS.

Respiratory

Self-care

How to use a nasal inhalation device

1 **Dear Patient:**
The doctor wants you to use a nonaerosol medicated spray, called _____ to relieve your runny nose. Carefully read the directions on the bottle's label, and use the spray exactly as the doctor or nurse explained. The pictures on this page will remind you exactly what to do.

First, take these pieces of equipment out of their box. As you see, the pump is in a plastic bag, to keep it clean.

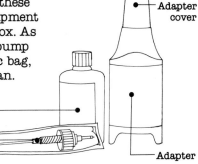

Adapter cover

Solution bottle

Pump

Adapter

2 Next, take off the solution bottle's cap, and remove the pump from its bag. Tightly screw the pump into the bottle. Now, take the adapter, and remove its cover. Pointing the adapter *away* from you, slide the solution bottle into the bottom of the adapter. Make sure the solution bottle fits snugly.

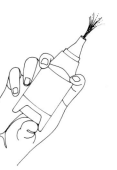

Hold the adapter in your hand, as shown above, and continue to point it away from you. Using a pumping motion, repeatedly push the bottle into the adapter with your thumb, until a fine spray mist appears. (You may have to pump five or six times.) This motion primes the pump. (You *don't* have to prime the pump each time you use the medication. But do prime the pump again after taking the equipment apart for cleaning. Also, you may need to prime the pump if you haven't used this medication for 5 days or more.)

3 Gently blow your nose to clear your nostrils. (Or, clear your nostrils with medication the doctor's given you.) Then, bend your head slightly forward, and put the tip of the adapter into one nostril. Press your other nostril closed with a finger, as shown here.

With one quick, firm motion, pump the solution bottle; sniff gently at the same time. Do this one more time, if the doctor directs.

Then, repeat this step for the other nostril.

4 Now, remove the adapter tip from your nose, and tip your head slightly back for a moment. This allows the medication to spread across the back of your nose. Put the adapter cover back on the adapter tip.

Keep the adapter cover on the adapter tip when you're not using it. If the adapter tip becomes clogged, take the bottle out of the adapter, unscrew the pump from the bottle, and soak *only the pump* in warm water. Then, dry the pump, and put everything back together, as already shown on this page. Prime the pump again.

Important: Don't use this equipment set for more than 5 months. Also, tell the doctor if the medication doesn't help.

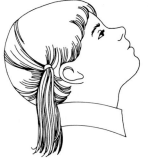

Learning about respiratory insufficiency

When a patient's lungs are unable to meet his body's metabolic needs, respiratory insufficiency results. The insufficiency may be caused by central nervous system (CNS) depression, neuromuscular paralysis, or an airway obstruction. In infants and children, respiratory insufficiency precedes respiratory arrest—which, in turn, precedes cardiac arrest.

As you probably know, two types of respiratory insufficiency exist: *sudden onset* and *slow onset*. Sudden onset respiratory insufficiency is usually associated with an airway obstruction caused, for example, by a foreign body or anaphylaxis. In such a case, the signs and symptoms are obvious: gasping, choking, coughing—from partial obstruction—and stridor, cyanosis, and apnea, if the obstruction's complete.

Slow onset respiratory insufficiency, on the other hand, is usually caused by:
- CNS depression from injury
- gradual respiratory deterioration caused by neuromuscular paralysis
- a chronic respiratory disease.

As a result of injury, or any of these diseases, the patient becomes poorly ventilated. If untreated, poor ventilation leads to acidosis, periods of apnea, and respiratory arrest (cessation of breathing).

Recognizing danger signs

Because the signs and symptoms of slow onset respiratory insufficiency are subtle and gradual, you'll need to count on your assessment skills to recognize them. First, familiarize yourself with your patient's baseline vital signs, paying particular attention to respiratory depth, regularity, and character. Then, be alert for these signs and symptoms of respiratory insufficiency:
- nasal flaring (in infants up to age 3)
- chest retraction (substernal, suprasternal, or intercostal)
- expiratory grunting (heard with or without a stethoscope), wheezing, or prolonged expirations
- increasing respiratory rate (but not depth)
- dyspnea on exertion
- cyanosis of lips and nailbeds.

In addition, watch for nonspecific signs of respiratory insufficiency, such as fatigue, poor muscle tone, loss of appetite, mood changes (including euphoria or depression), pallor, slow blanching, high blood pressure, tachycardia, cool extremities, and gray-blue skin mottling (if your patient's Caucasian or Oriental).

Of course, the signs and symptoms of respiratory insufficiency are also signs and symptoms for many other disorders. If you suspect respiratory insufficiency in your patient, request an order for arterial blood gas (ABG) measurements. If ABG measurements indicate hypoxia and hypercapnia, your patient has respiratory insufficiency. Act quickly to prevent respiratory arrest.

First, check your patient's airway for obstruction. If he has an airway obstruction, you may be able to restore normal breathing by simply clearing his airway. (For details on clearing an obstructed airway, see the following photostory.)

But, if your patient's respiratory insufficiency isn't caused by an airway obstruction, you may need to immediately begin artificial respiration, either by mouth or with a hand-held resuscitator. Beginning on page 97, we'll show you how to use one.

As you work, do your best to keep your patient and his family as calm as possible. Explain what you're doing, and provide emotional support. Remember, anxiety increases the child's oxygen needs.

Keep in mind that cardiac arrest may follow respiratory insufficiency. If your patient suffers cardiac arrest, begin cardiopulmonary resuscitation (CPR) at once. To review pediatric CPR technique, carefully study the information and photos beginning on page 105.

Clearing a child's airway

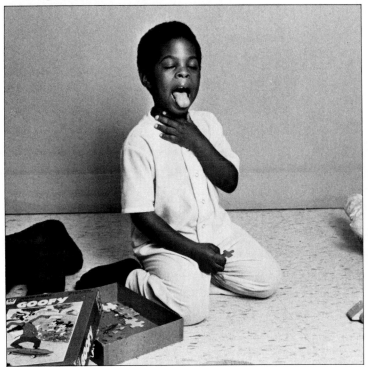

1 Picture this situation. You're on your way to the hospital cafeteria after a busy morning. As you walk through the children's playroom, you see 4-year-old Alan Wolfe with a small toy in his mouth. Before you can warn him to remove it, he clutches his throat and begins coughing. Do you know what to do? If you're unsure, follow these steps:

First, determine if Alan's airway is obstructed by asking, "Can you speak?" If he verbally responds, even with a "no," let him continue to cough.

If he doesn't respond, or can't relieve the obstruction with forceful coughing, suspect airway obstruction and call for an anesthesiologist or nurse anesthetist. Then, act quickly to implement the following steps. Remember, if Alan's airway remains obstructed for 3 to 5 minutes, he may suffer irreversible brain damage.

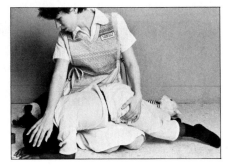

2 Now, kneel on the floor and place Alan over your thighs, as shown here. Make sure his head is down, and he's bent at the waist. Support him with one hand. *Caution:* Never bend the child's head over the edge of a table or bed. You may seriously injure him.

Respiratory

Clearing a child's airway continued

3 Using the heel of your hand, deliver four sharp back blows over Alan's spine, between the scapulae, as the nurse is doing here.

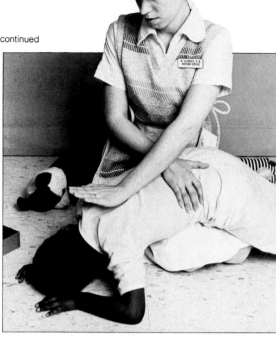

4 If the toy's still lodged in Alan's airway, get ready to deliver chest thrusts. Supporting Alan's head and back, roll him onto the floor in a supine position. Straddle him, and open his shirt.

To position your hands for chest thrusts, run your middle finger from Alan's umbilicus toward his head, and feel for the bony xiphoid notch. Estimate 1½″ to 2″ (3.8 to 5.1 cm), or approximately two finger-widths above this point. You'll deliver chest thrusts here.

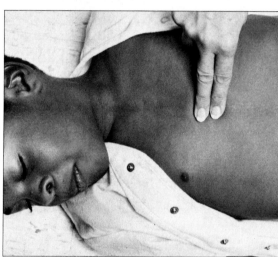

5 With the heel of your hand, exert pressure downward, depressing Alan's chest 1″ to 1½″ (2.5 to 3.8 cm) four times in rapid succession.

If the toy's not dislodged, roll the child back onto your thighs, as shown in step 2, and deliver four more back blows. If this doesn't work, roll the child onto his back again, and deliver four chest thrusts. Continue this sequence until the toy's expelled.

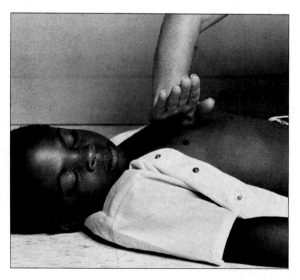

6 Now the child's unconscious. You've given him repeated back blows and chest thrusts and attempted ventilation, but the airway's still blocked. What's next?

With your patient supine, open his mouth by lifting his tongue and lower jaw forward. Support his lower jaw with your fingers, and place your thumb over his tongue, as shown here.

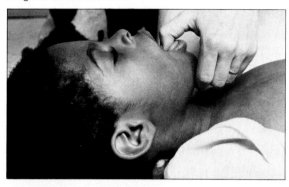

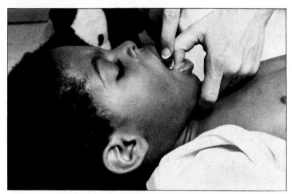

7 Can you see the foreign body? If so, insert the index finger of your other hand along the inside of his cheek. With a hooking motion, try to dislodge the foreign body and lift it out. Take care not to force the object deeper into his airway.

Important: Never attempt to remove a foreign body you can't see. You may push it deeper into the airway and cause further damage. Instead, prepare to assist with an emergency tracheotomy, if the toy's located at carina trachea level or above. If the toy's descended to a mainstem bronchus, prepare for bronchoscopy or emergency surgery.

If you're able to remove the foreign body, use a two-finger sweeping motion to clear Alan's airway of any remaining vomitus, mucus, or blood. Once you've cleared the airway, check for breathing. If he still isn't breathing, tilt his head back slightly and begin artificial respiration. (For details on cardiopulmonary resuscitation, see the information beginning on page 105.)

When breathing's restored, have the doctor check Alan, even if he appears normal. The foreign body may cause airway edema and lead to further obstruction.

Document the incident in your nurses' notes.

Clearing an infant's airway

1 *In the preceding photostory, you learned how to clear a child's airway. But suppose you encounter an infant with an airway obstruction. Do you know how to act? Read this photostory carefully.*

Note: In an infant, consider cyanosis an indication of complete airway obstruction.

To position an infant for back blows, lay him prone on your forearm, as shown, with one of his legs on each side of your arm. Make sure his head is lower than his chest and abdomen. To support his head, cradle his jaw in your cupped hand, as the nurse is doing here. (Take care not to obstruct his nose with your hand.) Support your forearm by slightly elevating your thigh.

[Inset] Now, using the heel of your hand, deliver four rapid blows over his spine, between his scapulae.

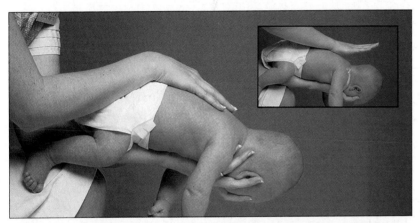

2 If his airway remains blocked, turn him to a supine position on your forearm. Remember to support his head and neck as you turn him, and to position his head lower than his chest and abdomen. Now, while continuing to support him on your forearm and elevated thigh, find the correct hand position for delivering chest thrusts.

To do so, draw one imaginary line between his nipples, and another up from his umbilicus. You'll give chest thrusts at the point where the lines intersect.

Using your fingertips, deliver four

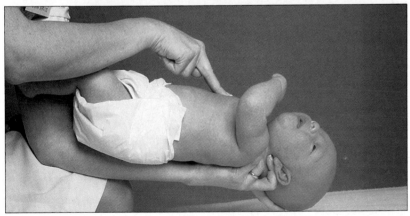

chest thrusts ½" to 1" (1.3 cm to 2.5 cm) deep, as the nurse is doing here. (More forceful thrusts may injure the infant.)

If this action fails to dislodge the object, continue to alternate back blows and chest thrusts until the object's dislodged. If the infant loses consciousness, try to ventilate him. Then attempt to remove the object with your fingers, but only if you can *see* it. If you're unsuccessful, prepare the infant for an emergency tracheotomy, bronchoscopy, or surgery.

Document the entire episode.

Learning about hand-held resuscitators

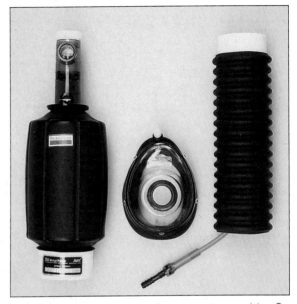

Caring for a child with a respiratory system problem? Be prepared to use a hand-held resuscitator if his condition worsens.

Why? Because a pediatric resuscitator, when used correctly, ventilates the patient more effectively than mouth-to-mouth respirations. The resuscitator also gives you the option of administering oxygen (when needed), and may eliminate the need for intubation. In infants and children, intubation can easily damage the airway or stimulate reflex bradycardia.

As you know, hand-held resuscitators come in three sizes: infant (250 cc air capacity), pediatric (500 cc air capacity), and adult (1,000 cc air capacity). Infant resuscitators have round masks; pediatric and adult resuscitators have oblong ones. Each type of mask is designed to cover the patient's nose and mouth. It should fit snugly, so no air escapes when you squeeze the bag.

You may be familiar with several different types of hand-held resuscitators. In the following photostory, we'll feature a Hope® II self-inflating resuscitator bag, shown above.

Because of this bag's elasticity, the system refills independently of the gas flow. Whether or not the bag's connected to oxygen, the intake valves at the bag's ends allow rapid reinflation following compression. When the bag's attached to oxygen, these valves mix the oxygen with air, allowing the system to deliver an oxygen concentration of up to 55%. Except in an emergency, this bag's not recommended for severely hypoxic patients.

However, when you surround the intake valves with the gas reservoir accessory, you can deliver between 70% and 90% oxygen. *Note:* Some self-inflating bags have built-in reservoirs.

And finally, when you use a self-inflating bag, make sure it has a pop-off safety valve that'll release air when the pressure's too great.

Respiratory

How to use a hand-held resuscitator

1 *Nine-year-old Amy Freeman was admitted to your unit for neurologic observation after an automobile accident. When you enter her room to administer evening medication, you find her gasping for air. Although her heart rate's slow, you suspect respiratory, not cardiac, distress. She'll need artificial ventilation immediately. Since you knew respiratory distress might occur, you have a hand-held resuscitator (such as the Hope® II pediatric resuscitator) accessible in the patient's room. Here's what to do.*

Open Amy's airway immediately. To do this, place her flat on her back. Then, lift her neck slightly so her head tilts back, and her chin points upward.

Note: Avoid hyperextending a child's neck. Doing so may cause her pliable trachea to collapse, obstructing her airway.

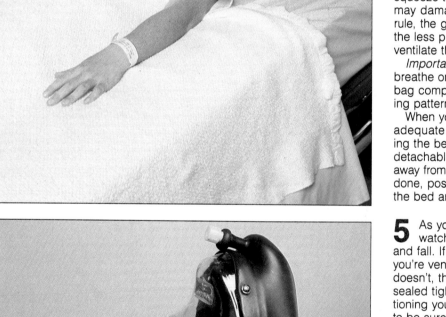

2 If Amy still isn't breathing after you position her head, quickly call for help. (But don't leave her to do so.) Then, prepare to use the hand-held resuscitator. If necessary, assemble it by attaching the mask to the bag, as the nurse is doing here.

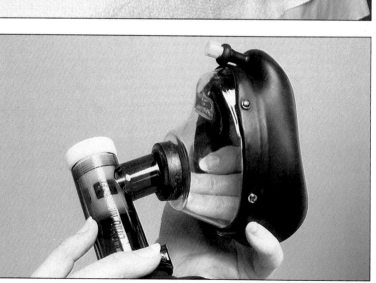

3 Now, place the mask over Amy's mouth and nose. Make sure the nose portion covers the bridge of her nose, and the base is between her lower lip and chin. To ensure a tight seal, place your thumb and several fingers over the mask, as the nurse is doing in this photo. Use the rest of your hand to maintain her head in the correct position by lifting Amy's chin upward.

Nursing tip: If the seal isn't tight, try turning the mask around. Place the nose portion over the chin and the base at the nose.

4 With your other hand, gently squeeze the bag approximately once every 5 seconds. (Squeeze the bag every 3 seconds if your patient's an infant.) Don't squeeze the bag forcefully, or you may damage her lungs. As a rule, the greater the bag's capacity, the less pressure you need to ventilate the patient's lungs.

Important: If your patient tries to breathe on her own, coordinate bag compressions with her breathing pattern.

When you have time, ensure an adequate working area by removing the bed's headboard (if it's detachable) and pulling the bed away from the wall. When that's done, position yourself between the bed and the wall.

5 As you compress the bag, watch for Amy's chest to rise and fall. If it does, you'll know you're ventilating her lungs. If it doesn't, the mask may not be sealed tightly enough. Try repositioning your hands and check to be sure your patient's still in the correct position.

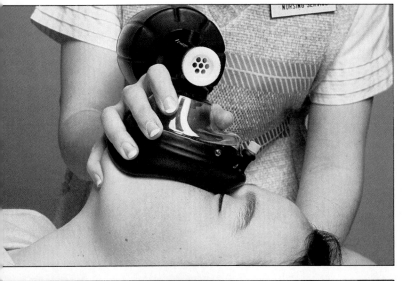

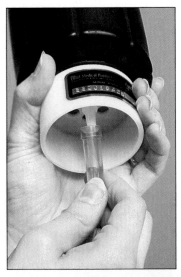

6 If your patient appears cyanotic, connect the resuscitator to the oxygen wall unit. Attach one end of the oxygen tubing to the bottom of the bag, as shown, and the other end to the nipple adapter on the flowmeter. You may want to add an oxygen reservoir to the resuscitator, if one's available. Of course, some bags have the reservoir built in.

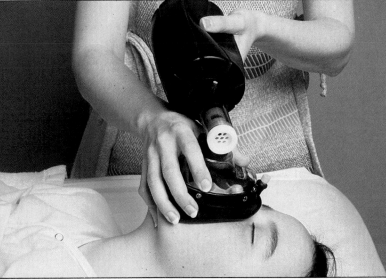

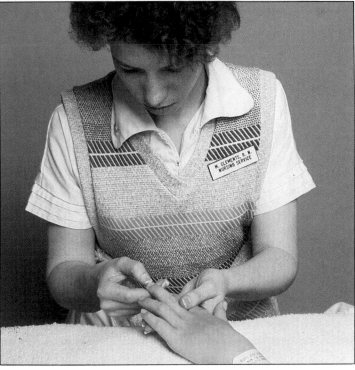

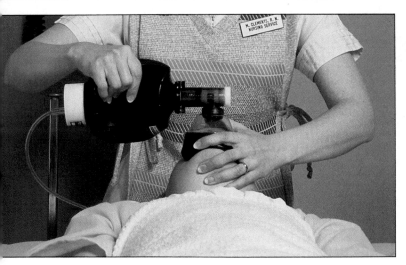

7 Continue to manually ventilate Amy's lungs until she's breathing spontaneously, or the doctor or nurse anesthetist evaluates her need for intubation and continued mechanical ventilation. Remember, when bag breathing is prolonged, your patient may suffer gastric distention. (As you continue ventilating her lungs, watch her abdomen for signs of distention.) Be ready to help insert a nasogastric (NG) tube, if necessary, to remove gas from her stomach.

When help arrives, check Amy's lips and fingernails to see if the color has improved. If her blood oxygen level is inadequate, her skin color will be bluish. (If your patient's black, the inside of her lips and eyelids will be bluish.)

Finally, document everything in your nurses' notes.

Cardiac

Reviewing prenatal cardiac anatomy

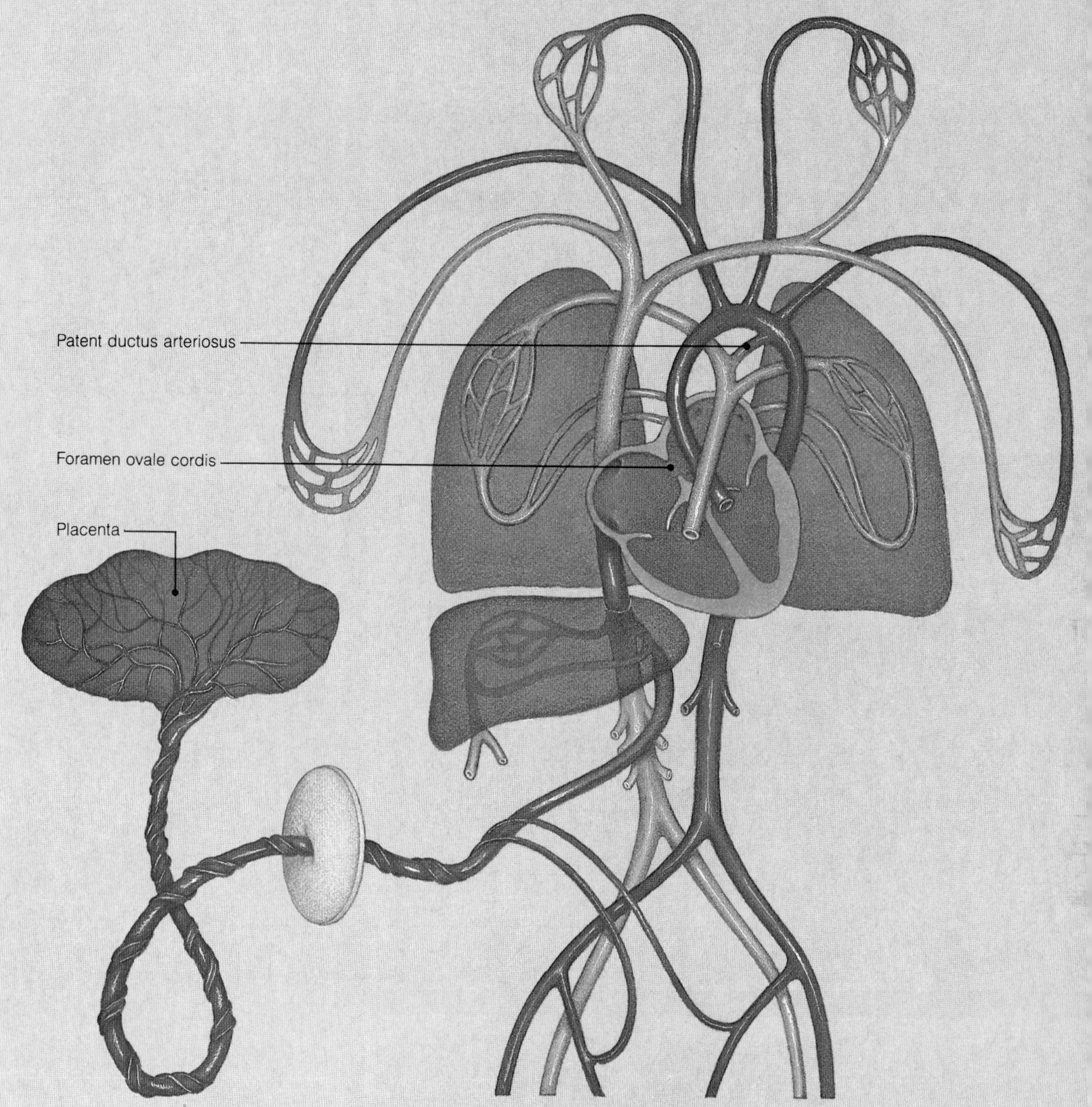

How skilled are you at assessing abnormal heart sounds? Do you know how to differentiate an innocent from an organic murmur? When to listen for clicks and snaps? How a murmur's pitch, sound, and location may relate to a congenital heart defect?

And what about heart disease and defects? Do you know what signs and symptoms may indicate aortic stenosis, tetralogy of Fallot, or rheumatic heart disease? Are you prepared to piece together nonspecific signs and symptoms from your observations and the child's history?

Study the following pages carefully. You'll find them helpful and informative. In addition, review the photo sequence on giving cardiopulmonary resuscitation (CPR) to a child or infant. And remember, pediatric CPR is more specialized than adult CPR. To avoid performing the procedure improperly and possibly injuring the child, obtain CPR training from a certified instructor.

Patent ductus arteriosus

Foramen ovale cordis

Placenta

As you know, the heart is a hollow, muscular double-pressured pump that circulates blood through the body with strong rhythmic contractions. The heart's low-pressure right side receives unoxygenated blood from the body and delivers it to the lungs for reoxygenation. In turn, the heart's high-pressure left side receives oxygenated blood from the lungs and delivers it to all body parts. Keep in mind that pressure differences in the upper and lower chambers cause the heart's valves to open, allowing blood passage. Heart-muscle contraction, with subsequent valve closure, spurs the passage.

But, when a deformity within the heart—caused by improper development or disease—obstructs or alters the normal blood-flow pattern, a serious and possibly life-threatening condition results.

To understand how these deformities occur in infants and children, let's briefly review cardiac development. Use the illustration above to identify major prenatal structures.

The heart is the first functional organ in the embryo. In a matter of weeks, the heart progresses from a simple tube that supplies blood to the embryo, to a complex four-chambered organ that pumps blood through the fetus. Simply speaking, the heart undergoes more changes in less time than any other organ in the body.

Of course, the fetus uses the placenta instead of its lungs as its oxygen source. For this reason, fetal blood circulation, unlike adult blood circulation, depends on three major structures:
• the placenta, which exchanges gases and metabolic wastes
• a patent foramen ovale cordis, which allows passage of maternally oxygenated blood from the right to the left atrium
• a patent ductus arteriosus, which allows blood passage between the pulmonary artery and aorta.

These structures reduce blood flow into the unexpanded lungs and shunt oxygenated blood into the systemic circulation.

In addition, equality between pulmonary and systemic vascular resistance influences blood flow. This means that the *systemic* vasculature carries a *large* volume of fetal blood from the heart to the placenta and systemic circulation, and back again. The *pulmonary* vasculature carries a *small* volume of blood from the heart to the unexpanded lungs, and back again.

Remember that at birth, the infant's lungs expand. This leads to a rapid decrease in pulmonary vascular resistance, and an increase in oxygen tension. As a result, shunting through the ductus arteriosus stops and the structure gradually closes. And, as pulmonary blood flow increases, the foramen ovale cordis also closes. When these changes are complete, normal postnatal circulation begins.

Is all this important to understanding cardiac disorders? Yes. Because sometimes the heart doesn't complete all the changes necessary to accommodate circulation.

When congenital deformities or acquired disease prevents normal cardiopulmonary function in an infant or child, a careful history and thorough assessment are the best ways to identify the disorder. Always be alert for signs of improper oxygenation, such as cyanosis, fingertip clubbing, and labored breathing. Also, watch for signs of inadequate cardiac output, such as an infant pulse rate faster than 160 beats per minute, murmurs, easy fatigability, and arrhythmias.

Keep in mind that a patient with a heart defect may be asymptomatic for one of these reasons:
• The defect isn't severe enough to cause symptoms.
• The defect hasn't yet created significant hemodynamic changes.
• The heart has compensated for the deformity with only slight hemodynamic changes.

Identifying abnormal heart sounds

Assessing your patient's heart sounds? If so, you may hear more than sounds identifiable as S_1 through S_4. When the heart sounds you hear are abnormal or unusual, or vary in rate, rhythm, or intensity, you may be listening to a benign alteration in normal heart sound (innocent murmur), or a rheumatic or congenital murmur (organic murmur).

Turbulent blood flow through the normal heart and great vessels may cause *innocent* murmurs, which are loudest in anxious, febrile, or thin-chested children. These murmurs usually disappear when the child reaches adulthood and are not clinically significant.

Organic heart murmurs, on the other hand, indicate heart or great vessel abnormalities, such as dilation, constriction, partial obstruction, and increased blood flow.

Whenever you hear a heart murmur, regardless of type, be sure to document it according to these guidelines:
• *Timing:* Identify the murmur by its occurrence in the systolic or diastolic phase. Keep in mind that an early systolic murmur is also called an ejection murmur, and a murmur heard throughout systole is called a pan- or holosystolic murmur.
• *Sound:* Describe the quality of the murmur as blowing, harsh, musical, or rumbling.
• *Pitch:* Identify the frequency of the murmur as high or low.
• *Location:* Name the auscultation location where you hear the murmur best: aortic, pulmonic, tricuspid, or mitral. (For a review of cardiac auscultation areas, turn to page 25.)
• *Radiation:* List the bordering structures in which the murmur is also heard.
• *Loudness:* Employ this rating system to describe the volume of the murmur: 1—barely heard; 2—faint but distinct, heard when the patient's in any position and after exercise; 3—moderately detectable; 4—loud; 5—very loud; 6—heard before stethoscope comes in contact with chest. *Note:* Murmurs given a 4, 5, or 6 rating are accompanied by a thrill (palpable vibration).
• *Intensity:* Identify the part of the respiratory cycle during which the murmur is most distinct. If more distinct on inspiration, describe it as crescendo. If more distinct on expiration, call it decrescendo. If equally distinct throughout the cycle, describe it as crescendo-decrescendo.

As you probably know, intensity and loudness vary between periods of activity and periods of rest, as well as from patient to patient. For this reason, they've been excluded from the descriptions at right. However, be sure to include the information in your nurses' notes. That way, you'll have a more accurate record of your patient's condition.

A murmur heard during **systolic ejection** is harsh, rough, and high pitched. It may be heard over the pulmonic or aortic area, and indicates pulmonary or aortic stenosis, respectively.

A **midsystolic** murmur is harsh, rough, and high pitched. If heard over the aortic and suprasternal notch areas, it may indicate aortic valve disease; if heard over the pulmonic area, it may indicate pulmonary stenosis.

A **late systolic** murmur has a high-pitched blowing sound. It's best heard over the apex, and indicates mitral valve insufficiency.

A **holosystolic** murmur heard over the *mitral* area indicates mitral insufficiency. It has a high-pitched, blowing sound.

A **holosystolic** murmur heard over the *tricuspid* area indicates tricuspid insufficiency. It has a high-pitched, blowing sound.

An **early diastolic** murmur heard over the *left sternal border* (not the aortic area) indicates aortic insufficiency. It has a high-pitched, blowing sound.

An **early diastolic** murmur heard over the *pulmonic* area indicates pulmonary insufficiency. It has a high-pitched, blowing sound.

A **mid-to-late diastolic** murmur heard over the *mitral* area indicates mitral stenosis. It has a low-pitched, rumbling sound.

A **mid-to-late diastolic** murmur heard over the *lower left sternal border* indicates tricuspid stenosis. It has a low-pitched, rumbling sound.

Cardiac

Recognizing clicks and snaps

When you listen to your patient's heart, you may hear a systolic click or opening snap. These heart sounds are considered abnormal and may indicate a heart defect.

A click may occur at any time during the systolic phase of the cardiac cycle. Exactly when you hear it determines what the click is called. However, an opening snap occurs only when the heart is in the diastolic phase. To learn more about clicks and snaps, study this chart carefully.

Type of sound	Timing	Location	Possible indications
Ejection click	Onset of systolic ejection	Aortic area, with patient in left lateral position	Aortic stenosis, aortic insufficiency, coarctation of the aorta, aneurysms of the ascending aorta, hypertension with aortic dilation
		Pulmonic area, with patient in left lateral position	Pulmonic stenosis, pulmonary hypertension
Non-ejection click	Mid- to late systole	Mitral area, with patient in left lateral position	Prolapsed mitral valve syndrome
Opening snap	Early diastole	Fourth intercostal space, at left sternal border	Mitral stenosis
		Second intercostal space, at right sternal border	Tricuspid stenosis

Nurses' guide to congenital heart defects

Are you aware that about 8 out of every 1,000 children are born with heart defects? And, among premature infants, the incidence increases two to three times or more, depending on birth weight. So, as a pediatric nurse, you need to know the basics about these serious disorders.

Generally, heart defects are classified into two groups: cyanotic and acyanotic. Here's how they differ.

As you know, the heart's powerful left side normally produces significantly higher pressure than its right side. A cyanotic defect alters this situation, causing abnormally high pressure in the heart's *right* side. This condition, combined with other abnormalities associated with some defects, may permit shunting of unoxygenated blood from the heart's right side to its left side. The subsequent flow of unoxygenated blood from the left ventricle to the body causes cyanosis.

Acyanotic defects, on the other hand, don't produce these abnormal pressure changes. So, a septal defect, for example, permits shunting of oxygenated blood from the heart's high-pressure *left* side to its low-pressure *right* side. Because the left ventricle still ejects oxygenated blood to the body, no cyanosis results. But keep in mind that an acyanotic defect may *become* cyanotic if its effects worsen.

Clearly, either type of defect may threaten your patient's health—and even his life. Your skill at recognizing early signs and symptoms is crucial. Read the following chart to learn more about common congenital heart defects.

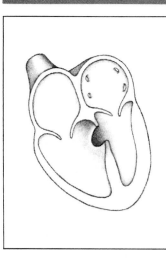

Ventricular septal defect (VSD)
Abnormal opening in the ventricular septum, allowing blood to shunt between the left and right ventricles. Most common congenital heart disorder; occurs more often in premature than in full-term infants.

Characteristics
• Causes oxygenated blood from left ventricle to mix with unoxygenated blood in right ventricle (left-to-right shunt)
• Acyanotic, unless very large, or coupled with other disorder causing right-to-left shunt
• Usually asymptomatic at birth; becomes evident after 2 weeks of age
• May improve, or close spontaneously approximately 6 months after birth
• If opening fails to close 1 to 2 years after birth, may cause pulmonary valve obstruction
• May act as life-saving safety valve when coupled with other severe heart defects, such as transposition of the great vessels
• If opening's large, may result in cardiac complications, such as congestive heart failure and bacterial endocarditis
• Large VSD may eventually cause pulmonary vascular disease and pulmonary artery hypertension

Signs and symptoms
• Overactive precordium, especially after feeding
• Within 6 weeks after birth, harsh systolic murmur heard best in third and fourth left intercostal spaces; associated with palpable thrill. Murmur may be only sign of disorder.
• Increased right ventricular and pulmonary artery pressure
• If condition's severe: poor growth development; labored breathing; and frequent feeding pattern (hungry infant wakes, feeds vigorously, becomes dyspneic, slows and stops feeding, sleeps a short time, wakes and repeats cycle)

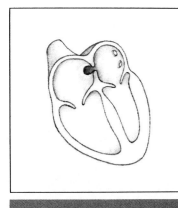

Atrial septal defect (ASD)

Opening or gap between the left and right atria, allowing left-to-right shunting of blood between chambers. Condition caused by delayed or improper closure of foramen ovale cordis or atrial septal wall. More common in females. Classified into three types: ostium secundum, located in the fossa ovalis cordis (most common); sinus venosus, located in upper atrial septum; and ostium primum, located in lower atrial septum.

Characteristics

• May go unrecognized because of sign and symptom subtlety
• May cause atrial arrhythmias, secondary to right atrial overload
• May interfere with conduction system
• May cause pulmonary hypertension, if defect is severe
• May act as a life-saving safety valve if associated with a severe heart defect, such as transposition of the great vessels
• May result in complications, such as pulmonary thrombosis or embolism; bronchopulmonary infections; and pulmonary artery rupture
• May close spontaneously within 1 year after birth

Signs and symptoms

• Soft, pulmonic midsystolic murmur heard at second or third left intercostal space
• In infants, dyspnea on exertion, fatigue, orthopnea
• In older children with a large defect, frail, delicate appearance; left precordial bulge

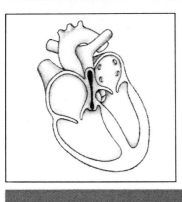

Pulmonary stenosis

Narrowing of pulmonic valve usually resulting from altered or distorted pulmonary valve cusps or right ventricular outflow obstruction. Classified into three types: valvular, subvalvular, and supravalvular.

Characteristics

• Usually acyanotic and asymptomatic, unless defect's severe
• Associated with a history of maternal rubella
• Causes increased right ventricular pressure, to overcome obstruction.

This, in turn, elevates right atrial pressure, leading to increased systemic venous blood pressure.
• May result in right ventricular failure
• Low or normal pulmonary artery pressure

Signs and symptoms

• Dyspnea
• Fatigue
• Extremity coldness, peripheral cyanosis
• Subjective complaints (such as tiring easily) that increase with age

• Precordial pain possible
• In valvular pulmonary stenosis, systolic ejection murmur associated with a thrill (best heard at upper left sternal border). If defect's severe, murmur may radiate over precordium and back.
• If right ventricular end diastolic pressure increases, right ventricle hypertrophy occurs
• To relieve respiratory distress, child may assume squatting position

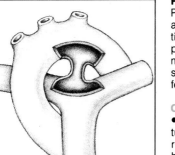

Aortic valvular stenosis

Narrowing of aortic valve or left ventricular outflow obstruction. More common in males.

Characteristics

• Acyanotic, unless defect's severe
• Usually asymptomatic in infants and children
• Severe obstruction causes increased left ventricle pressure to maintain aortic pressure. This condition may lead to left ventricle hypertrophy.

Signs and symptoms

• In infants, atypical systolic murmur and possible intractable congestive heart failure
• Systolic ejection click followed by systolic ejection murmur and a thrill felt at the second right intercostal space or suprasternal notch
• Irritability
• Tachycardia
• Dyspnea and fatigue on exertion
• Angina pectoris
• Syncope
• Pale skin
• Narrow pulse pressure

• Weak peripheral pulses
• Possible abdominal pain
• Diaphoresis
• Epistaxis

Patent ductus arteriosus (PDA)

Patent duct between the descending aorta and pulmonary artery bifurcation, allowing shunting from the pulmonary artery to the aorta. Normally, ductus arteriosus closes shortly after birth. More common in females.

Characteristics

• Associated with history of prematurity, first trimester maternal rubella, coxsackievirus infection, or birth at high altitude
• Acyanotic; usually asymptomatic

• May be accompanied by coarctation of aorta
• May cause pulmonary congestion, especially in premature infants
• May lead to complications, such as congestive heart failure, ductus arteriosus aneurysm (causing blood to dissect between duct walls), spontaneous aneurysm rupture, and recurrent respiratory infections

Signs and symptoms

• Continuous murmur with characteristic machine-like quality, loudest at second and third left intercostal spaces. Murmur may obscure S_2 heart sound and be only sign of disorder.
• Dyspnea on exertion
• Precordial asymmetry; in infants, overactive precordium
• Widened pulse pressure
• Full or bounding pulses
• Pulmonary artery hypertension with right-to-left shunt, and right atrial and ventricular hypertrophy

Cardiac

Nurses' guide to congenital heart defects continued

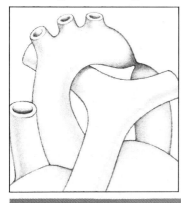

Coarctation of the aorta

Constriction of the aorta. More common in males. Classified into two types; preductal and postductal. Defect may occur anywhere on aortic arch.

Characteristics
- Acyanotic
- Symptoms usually occur in either early infancy or adulthood (20 to 30 years of age)
- Collateral circulation may develop around defect, minimizing pressure changes
- If condition's severe, may lead to complications, such as congestive heart failure, endocarditis, cerebral hemorrhage, aneuryms, and premature arteriosclerosis secondary to hypertension
- Frequently associated with bicuspid aortic valve

Signs and symptoms
- Elevated blood pressure and bounding pulses proximal to defect, hypotension, and weak or absent pulses distal to defect
- Dizziness
- Fainting
- Headache
- Epistaxis
- Cold feet
- Systolic ejection click heard at base and apex of heart. Associated with systolic or continuous murmur between scapulae.
- Pulmonary hypertension
- Aneurysm proximal to defect

Tetralogy of Fallot

Combination of four defects: ventricular septal defect (VSD), overriding aorta, pulmonary stenosis, and right ventricular hypertrophy

Characteristics
- Unoxygenated blood is shunted through VSD
- Oxygenated and unoxygenated blood is mixed in left ventricle and pumped out aorta, causing cyanosis
- Pulmonary stenosis restricts blood flow to lungs and increases right ventricular pressure
- Defects may cause complications such as iron deficiency anemia, polycythemia, coagulation disorders, paradoxical embolism, cerebral infarction, and abscesses

Signs and symptoms
- Cyanosis
- Loud systolic ejection murmur heard along left sternal border. May diminish or obscure pulmonic S_2 component.
- Finger and toe clubbing
- Dyspnea
- On palpation, possible cardiac thrill at left sternal border
- In newborn: intense cyanosis after patent ductus arteriosus closes; severe dyspnea on exertion; syncope; limpness; and occasional convulsions. If defect is untreated, it may be fatal.
- To compensate for respiratory distress, child may assume characteristic squatting position
- Respiratory distress and fatigue during feeding
- Growth retardation

Truncus arteriosus

Failure of embryonic arterial trunk to separate into aorta and pulmonary artery. Resulting single vessel overrides ventricles and carries blood for both pulmonary and systemic circulation.

Characteristics
- Ventricular septal defect (VSD) always present
- Common trunk may have 2 to 6 valve cusps
- Usually fatal within 6 months if untreated

Signs and symptoms
- Cyanosis
- Systolic murmur about 1 month after birth
- Fatigue
- Dyspnea
- Failure to thrive
- Parasternal lift
- Loud decrescendo diastolic murmur possible
- Ejection click
- S_2 has only one component, because of single valve in common trunk
- Tachypnea
- Rales
- Recurrent respiratory infections
- Wide pulse pressure possible
- Congestive heart failure, usually indicating rapid physical decline
- Hepatomegaly possible

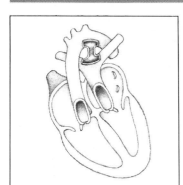

Transposition of great vessels

Aorta leaves right ventricle; pulmonary artery leaves left ventricle. Usually associated with ventricular septal defect (VSD), atrial septal defect (ASD), and/or patent ductus arteriosus (PDA). More common in males.

Characteristics
- Associated with history of maternal diabetes
- Causes unoxygenated blood to flow through right atrium and ventricle and out aorta to systemic circulation. Oxygenated blood flows from lungs to left atrium and ventricle and out pulmonary artery to lungs.
- May cause premature contractions and escape beats
- May be fatal unless VSD, ASD, or PDA develops as safety valve for two independent circulations

Signs and symptoms
- Cyanosis. (In infants with large PDA or VSD, cyanosis is minimal.)
- High birth weight possible
- Signs of congestive heart failure, such as severe dyspnea, within 12 to 24 hours after birth
- Poor sucking reflex
- Systolic murmur, if VSD is present
- Hepatomegaly
- Metabolic acidosis from hypoxia. (Hypothermia intensifies signs of acidosis.)

Learning about rheumatic heart disease

When we talk about rheumatic heart disease, we're referring to permanent cardiac damage caused by rheumatic fever. Specific cardiac damage may include pancarditis (myocarditis, pericarditis, and endocarditis) and valvular disease. In some cases, cardiac damage caused by severe pancarditis may result in congestive heart failure and death.

What causes rheumatic fever? Authorities suspect a Group A beta-hemolytic streptococcal infection. The disease is most common in children between ages 5 and 15, and seems to have a familial tendency. It occurs most frequently in lower socioeconomic groups, possibly because of contributing environmental conditions.

As you know, diagnosing rheumatic fever in its early stages isn't easy. Why? Because many of the early signs and symptoms are vague and nonspecific. Consider these examples: fever between 100.4° F. to 102.2° F. (38° C. to 39° C.); mild or occasionally severe anemia; lassitude; irritability; nausea; weight loss; and pallor. Other nonspecific signs and symptoms of rheumatic fever may include abdominal pain, spontaneous nosebleeds, and dyspnea on exertion.

On the other hand, specific signs and symptoms of the disease may include one or all of the following:

• *History of streptococcal infection* (cold, sore throat, or impetigo) a few days or up to 6 weeks earlier
• *Sydenham's (or rheumatic) chorea* that develops up to 6 months after a streptococcal infection. Chorea is characterized by mild to severe involuntary muscle contractions. This type of chorea usually resolves without causing residual neurologic damage.
• *Polyarthritis* causing swelling, redness, and pain in patient's large joints, such as knees, ankles, elbows, hips, and wrists
• *Skin lesions,* such as erythema marginatum (nonpruritic, macular, transient rash producing red lesions with blanched centers), and subcutaneous nodules 3 mm to 2 cm in diameter. (Usually found near tendons or bony prominences; or joints, especially the elbows, knees, wrists, and knuckles.) These lesions may indicate carditis.

Understanding carditis

Carditis is the most destructive sign of rheumatic fever and may affect the pericardium, myocardium, endocardium, or heart valves, particularly the mitral valve. Pericarditis, for example, causes a friction rub, as well as pain and effusion.

Myocarditis produces characteristic lesions called Aschoff's bodies, as well as cellular swelling and interstitial collagen fragmentation. These changes cause formation of progressively fibrotic nodules—and interstitial scars.

Endocarditis, by far the most serious form of carditis, causes valve leaflet swelling, erosion along leaflet lines, and valvular blood, platelet and fibrin deposits which form beadlike vegetation on heart valves (see the illustration).

Because of damage caused by carditis, your patient may experience signs of congestive heart failure, such as upper

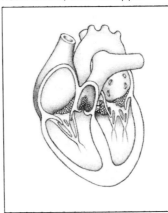

right quadrant pain, tachycardia, a hacking nonproductive cough, edema of the extremities, and significant mitral and aortic murmurs. The most common of these murmurs include:

• systolic murmurs from mitral regurgitation.
• midsystolic murmurs due to stiffening and swelling of mitral leaflet.
• occasional diastolic murmurs from aortic regurgitation.

How can rheumatic fever be managed *before* it causes permanent damage? The goal is threefold: *eliminate the streptococcal infection* by administering penicillin or erythromycin (if the patient has a penicillin hypersensitivity); *relieve signs and symptoms* of joint pain, inflammation, and fever, by giving salicylates such as aspirin; and *prevent recurrence* by continuing prophylactic antibiotic therapy for at least 5 years, or until patient reaches age 25. (Since the chance of recurrence decreases with age, antibiotic therapy beyond age 25 usually isn't necessary.)

In addition, be sure to provide complete bed rest for your patient, as ordered. When the doctor says it's okay (usually after 5 weeks), your patient can progressively increase his physical activity.

Cardiopulmonary resuscitation: Know the basics

As a nurse, you know that your ability to perform cardiopulmonary resuscitation (CPR) can mean the difference between life and death for your patient. You also know that recommended standards for performing CPR change frequently, as more effective techniques are developed. Your responsibility is to get up-to-date CPR instruction from a qualified instructor— and then to *keep* up-to-date by reviewing your skills with an instructor at least once a year. Also, stay informed of your hospital's current CPR policy.

But for a procedure as vital as CPR, yearly reviews aren't enough. Don't wait until a cardiac emergency occurs to try out your skills. Instead, test yourself with mock cardiac arrest drills. By practicing beforehand, you increase your ability to respond calmly and effectively when a real crisis occurs. In addition, these drills may help you identify some of your own limitations, so you can deal with them before someone's life is at stake.

Suppose, for example, your jaw joints tend to lock when you open your mouth wide. You'll

want to know about this limitation—and learn how to cope with it—before an emergency arises.

You can also explore the easiest way to maintain an airtight seal around a child's nose and mouth. (You may need to devise several different techniques, depending on the child's size.)

And, when providing chest compressions, you can determine what position's most comfortable for you. Depending on your own size, you may work most effectively kneeling on the bed, standing by the

side of the bed, or standing on a small stool.

Reviewing CPR technique

Use the following three pages to review currently accepted pediatric CPR technique. (Again, don't use these photostories as a substitute for hands-on training.)

The technique shown beginning on page 106 applies to children weighing more than 50 kg (about 110 pounds). As you'll see, it's basically the same as adult CPR. But if your patient weighs less than 50 kg, use the photostory on page 108 as a guide.

Cardiac

Reviewing cardiopulmonary resuscitation

1 *Let's say your patient, 11-year-old Al Barnes, has congestive heart failure. As you're caring for him, he suddenly stops breathing. When you can't feel a carotid pulse, you know he needs immediate cardiopulmonary resuscitation (CPR). Do you know what to do? Study this photostory to review basic technique.*

Begin by calling for help. (But never *leave* your patient to seek help.) Then, make sure Al's lying on a firm surface. Because of Al's history, you have a CPR board handy. Quickly put it under him, as shown.

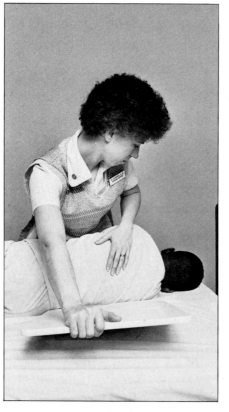

2 When you're administering unassisted CPR, you must provide both respirations and chest compressions. Here's how to proceed:

Open Al's airway by lifting and tilting his neck slightly upward, and his head back. To help maintain this position, keep one of your hands under Al's neck, as the nurse is doing here.

Important: Never hyperextend a child's neck. Doing so may collapse his airway.

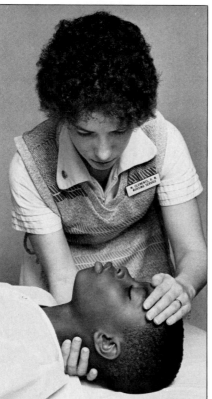

3 To provide artificial respirations, place your mouth over Al's mouth. Get a tight seal. Then, with your free hand, pinch his nose shut. Deliver four small breaths. Never breathe forcefully into a child's lungs. Doing so may overinflate them.

Watch Al's chest as you provide artificial respirations. If it doesn't rise and fall as you breathe into his airway, you're not inflating his lungs. To correct the problem, try repositioning his head and neck, as described in step 2. If you still can't inflate his lungs, suspect an airway obstruction. Take immediate steps to clear his airway; then try again. (For details on managing an airway obstruction, see pages 95 through 97.)

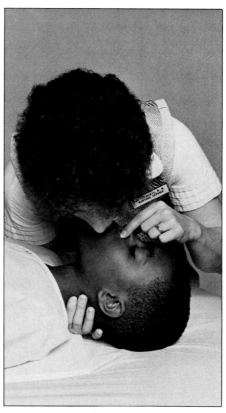

4 Before proceeding, quickly check for breathing and a carotid pulse. If you feel no pulse and your patient's still not breathing, position yourself for chest compressions by kneeling or standing beside him.

To determine where to place your hand, first locate midsternum. To do this, open his shirt and position one finger on the suprasternal notch (top of the sternum) and another finger on the xiphoid process, as shown. Midsternum lies halfway between your two fingers. Because your patient's a child, you'll give chest compressions halfway between midsternum and the xiphoid process.

Important: Never give chest compressions directly over his xiphoid process, or you could lacerate his liver or heart.

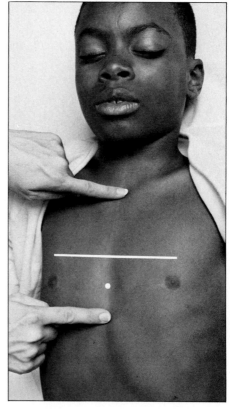

5 Interlock your fingers and place the heel of one hand at the proper spot on your patient's sternum. Cock your wrists, so your fingers don't touch the chest wall.

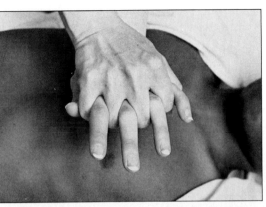

6 Then, lean forward so your shoulders are directly over his sternum and your arms are at a 90° angle to his chest, as shown. Maintain the 90° angle for proper pressure placement. But take care not to deliver *forceful* chest compressions—too much pressure may cause myocardial injury or sternal fracture.

Compress his sternum 1" (2.5 cm); then, briefly release all pressure. When the sternum returns to its normal position, the heart's chambers refill. Repeat this procedure until you've compressed his chest 15 times. Work smoothly, quickly, and rhythmically, making sure compression and relaxation times are equal. To maintain proper rhythm, count aloud—"one, two, three, four, five"—up to 15. Perform this compression/relaxation sequence at a rate of 80 per minute. *Important:* Don't remove your hands from his chest when you release pressure, or you may lose correct hand placement.

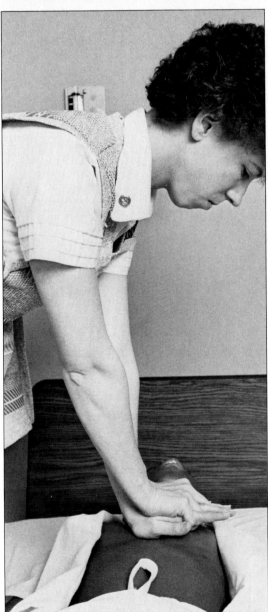

7 For CPR to be effective, Al *must* continue receiving artifical respirations, too. After giving 15 chest compressions, reposition his head as shown in step 2, and give him *two* small breaths in rapid succession. Don't give his lungs time to empty completely between breaths. Remember to watch his chest to see if it rises and falls.

Because you're giving CPR unassisted, you'll continue steps 6 and 7 at a rate of two breaths per every 15 chest compressions (2:15). Try to make the transitions between compressions and respirations as quick and smooth as possible. *Important:* Before beginning each new series of chest compressions, take care to relocate proper hand position.

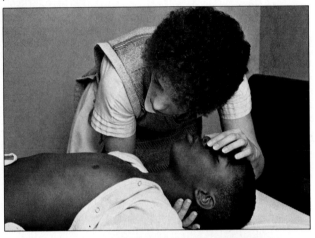

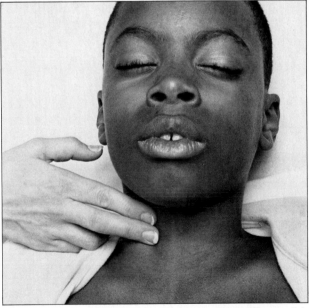

8 After performing CPR for 1 minute, check Al's carotid pulse. If it's still absent, continue CPR until advanced life support equipment and drugs arrive, or until someone relieves you. After the crisis is over, thoroughly document the event.

For details on giving two-person CPR, see the NURSING PHOTOBOOK GIVING CARDIAC CARE.

Cardiac

Providing CPR for a small child

1 *Suppose an infant or small child needs cardiopulmonary resuscitation (CPR)? For any child who weighs less than 50 kg (110 pounds), follow these steps:*

If your patient appears to be unconscious, quickly check for breathing and brachial pulse. If you can't detect breathing or a pulse, position him supine on a firm surface. Or, if he's a small infant, you can support him on one arm, as shown here. Notice how the nurse is able to tilt his head backward, at the correct angle. Remember not to hyperextend his neck.

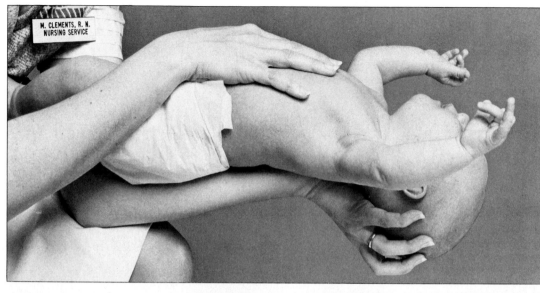

2 For a larger infant or a child, position his head and neck by placing one hand under his shoulder blades and lifting slightly as you gently push back on his forehead.

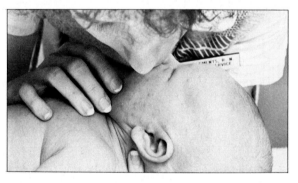

3 No matter which way you've positioned your patient, next cover his nose and mouth with your mouth, and give four small puffs of air. Take care to deliver only air from your mouth; air delivered from your lungs will exert too much force on his lungs.

Next, check for a pulse. If none is present, prepare to give chest compressions.

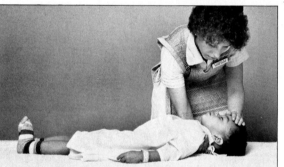

4 Place just the tips of your index and middle fingers at midsternum, as shown, and compress your patient's chest ½" to 1" (1.3 to 2.5 cm). More forceful compression may damage his lungs and heart. *Caution:* Take care to place your fingertips precisely; improper fingertip placement may result in liver, lung, or heart damage.

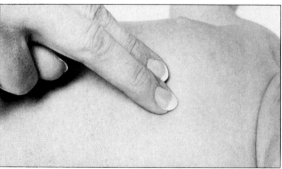

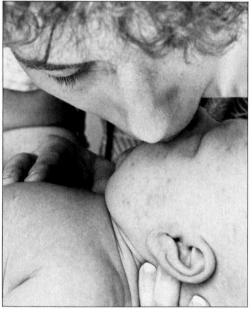

5 Because an infant's smaller than a child, you can easily perform artificial ventilation and chest compression without changing your position. This permits you to provide CPR at the ideal ratio: one breath per five chest compressions (1:5). To do so, quickly perform five chest compressions, while counting aloud to five. Deliver a breath on the upstroke of the fifth compression. You should be giving the infant a breath every 3 seconds, while maintaining a compression rate of at least 100 per minute. You'll continue to provide CPR until help arrives with emergency drugs and equipment.

After the crisis is over, remember to thoroughly document everything.

Nurses' guide to pediatric emergency cardiac drugs

Does your pediatric patient need emergency cardiac drug therapy? If so, the doctor will choose the drug, dose, and route best suited to your patient's needs. For your easy reference, here's a list of cardiac drugs commonly administered to children. For more information on these and other drugs, refer to the NURSING DRUG HANDBOOK™ or the NURSE'S GUIDE TO DRUGS™

ATROPINE SULFATE

Indications
- Sinus bradycardia
- Heart block

Pediatric dosage
I.V. bolus: 0.01 to 0.03 mg/kg

Contraindications
- Tachycardia
- Glaucoma
- Bladder disorders

Side effects
Tachycardia; flushing; dry, warm skin; increased respirations; restlessness; irritability; disorientation; depression; urinary retention; thirst; headache; constipation

Special considerations
- Watch heart rate and rhythm to determine drug effects. Doctor may order an additional dose or switch to another drug.
- Watch for side effects and report signs of drug toxicosis.
- Store drug in a light-protected container.

CALCIUM GLUCONATE
(10% solution)

Indication
- Cardiac arrest

Pediatric dosage
I.V. bolus: 20 to 30 mg/kg
I.V. drip: 200 to 700 mg/kg/24 hours

Contraindications
- Ventricular fibrillation
- Hypercalcemia
- Renal calculi

Side effects
Tingling sensations; sense of oppression or heat waves; syncope; slight blood pressure drop; vasodilation; bradycardia; cardiac arrhythmias; cardiac arrest; chalky taste; hypercalcemia; polyuria; renal calculi; venous irritation

Special considerations
- Monitor electrocardiogram (EKG) readings.
- Make sure I.V. bolus rate does not exceed 1 ml/min. Stop infusion if patient complains of discomfort.
- Frequently monitor blood calcium levels. Report abnormalities.
- Watch for signs of hypercalcemia (especially after giving large doses to a patient with renal failure).
- Do not administer by scalp vein, because severe tissue necrosis and sloughing may result if extravasation occurs.
- Do not infuse through an I.V. line containing sodium bicarbonate, or the drug will precipitate.

DIGOXIN SK-Digoxin, Lanoxin*

Indications
- Congestive heart failure
- Atrial fibrillation or flutter
- Paroxysmal atrial tachycardia
- Supraventricular tachyarrhythmias

Pediatric dosage
Premature/newborn
Loading dose
I.V. bolus: 25 to 40 mcg/kg/day in 3 divided doses
Maintenance dose
I.V. bolus: 20% to 30% of total loading dose divided into two equal doses and given 12 hours apart
Less than 2 years
Loading dose
P.O.: 60 to 80 mcg/kg/day in 3 equal doses
Maintenance dose
P.O.: 20 to 25 mcg/kg/day in two equal doses given 12 hours apart
Over 2 years
Loading dose
P.O.: 40 to 60 mcg/kg/day
I.V.: 20 to 40 mcg/kg/day
For either route, give ½ dose immediately, then ¼ dose every 8 hours for two doses.
Maintenance dose
P.O.: 10 to 15 mcg/kg/day divided into two equal doses and given every 12 hours
I.V.: 8 to 12 mcg/kg/day divided into two equal doses and given every 12 hours

Contraindications
- Coronary occlusion or angina in the absence of congestive heart failure
- Hypersensitivity to cardiotonic glycosides, or signs of toxicity
- With caution, if the patient has ischemic heart disease; acute myocarditis; ventricular tachycardia; hypoxia or myxedematous states; Stokes-Adams syndrome; carotid sinus syndrome; emphysema; heart blocks; impaired renal or hepatic function

Side effects
Changes in heart rate and rhythm; irritability of heart muscle and conduction system; anorexia, nausea, and vomiting; excessive salivation; abdominal pain and diarrhea; headache; fatigue; general malaise; disorientation; visual disturbances; skin reactions such as pruritis, urticaria, and facial edema

Special considerations
- Take apical pulses for 1 minute. Withhold drug and notify doctor if apical pulse rate is less than 90 to 100 beats per minute, or according to specific order.
- Monitor the digitalis-toxic patient for arrhythmias.
- Monitor fluid intake and output.
- Watch for signs of hypokalemia. Monitor serum potassium levels.
- Observe for these positive responses to drug: improved heart rate and rhythm, improved respirations, weight reduction, and diuresis.

DOBUTAMINE HYDROCHLORIDE
Dobutrex

Indications
- Short-term parenteral therapy to strengthen heart muscle contractions (inotrophic effect)
- Heart failure, caused by organic heart disease or heart surgery

Pediatric dosage
I.V. infusion: 2.5 to 15 mcg/kg/min. Dilute reconstituted vial in at least 250 ml 5% dextrose and water or normal saline solution. Adjust rate according to response.

Contraindications
- Idiopathic hypertrophic subaortic stenosis
- With caution if patient has uncontrolled atrial fibrillation. Administer a digitalis preparation before giving dobutamine hydrochloride to control ventricular response.

Side effects
Increased heart rate; elevated blood pressure; increase in ectopic ventricular beats. Rarely, nausea, headache, chest pain, or shortness of breath.

Special considerations
- Correct hypovolemia, if applicable, before giving drug.
- Continuously monitor blood pressure and heart rate.
- Do not give with alkaline solutions.
- Do not administer sodium bicarbonate through an I.V. line containing dobutamine hydrochloride.
- Use solutions containing dobutamine hydrochloride within 24 hours.
Note: Solutions containing dobutamine hydrochloride may be discolored, but this doesn't affect potency.

DOPAMINE HYDROCHLORIDE
Intropin*

Indications
- Cardiogenic shock
- Hypovolemic shock associated with trauma, septicemia, open heart surgery, renal failure, congestive heart failure

Pediatric dosage
I.V. infusion: 2 to 10 mcg/kg/min. May be increased to no more than 20 mcg/kg/min.

Contraindications
- Uncorrected tachyarrhythmias
- Pheochromocytoma
- Ventricular fibrillation
- With caution if patient has occlusive vascular disease, cold injuries, diabetic endarteritis, arterial embolism
- With caution for pregnant adolescent
- With caution if patient is receiving MAO inhibitors

Side effects
Cardiac arrhythmias; palpitations; widening of QRS intervals; headache; dizziness; pallor; sweating; nausea; vomiting; restlessness; tremors, weakness; respiratory difficulty; anginal-type pain; hypotension

Special considerations
- Closely observe patient, monitoring his cardiac conduction continuously, his blood pressure every 5 minutes, and his urine output hourly. Notify doctor if you observe any changes.
- Check infusion site frequently for extravasation. If extravasation occurs, doctor may infiltrate site, using 5 to 10 mg of phentolamine hydrochloride (Regitine) with 10 to 15 ml normal saline solution.
- Use infusion pump.
- Mix dopamine hydrochloride with I.V. solution just before administration.
- Don't mix dopamine hydrochloride with other drugs.

EPINEPHRINE HYDROCHLORIDE
Adrenalin Chloride

Indications
- Cardiac and circulatory failure
- Hypotensive states
- Allergic reactions including anaphylactic shock
- Angioneurotic edema
- Status asthmaticus

Pediatric dosage
I.V.: 0.1 to 1.0 mcg/kg/min as 1:50,000 solution. Regulate rate by response.

Nurses' guide to pediatric emergency cardiac drugs continued

EPINEPHRINE HYDROCHLORIDE
Adrenalin Chloride
(continued)

Contraindications
• Shock other than anaphylactic, ventricular fibrillation, and narrow angle glaucoma
• With extreme caution if patient has degenerative heart disease

Side effects
Cerebral hemorrhage; cardiac arrhythmias; palpitations; widened pulse pressure; precordial pain; headache; nervousness, vertigo, tremor; sweating, nausea; weakness; dizziness; tachycardia

Special considerations
• Don't expose to light, heat, or air.
• When preparing to give drug intravenously, first take baseline blood pressure and pulse. Then, after initiating therapy, closely monitor the patient every minute until desired effect is reached; then, every 2 minutes until he stabilizes. After he stabilizes, monitor blood pressure every 15 minutes.
• If patient has a sharp increase in blood pressure, give rapid-acting vasodilators, as ordered.

ISOPROTERENOL HYDROCHLORIDE Isuprel*

Indications
• Cardiac standstill
• Stokes-Adams and carotid sinus syndromes
• Bradycardia
• Atrioventricular (AV) heart block

Pediatric dosage
I.V. infusion: 1 mg in 100 ml of 5% dextrose in water. Give at 0.1 to 0.5 mcg/kg/min. Adjust rate to patient's response.

Contraindications
• Tachycardia caused by digitalis intoxication
• Preexisting arrhythmias
• With caution if patient has coronary insufficiency, diabetes, hyperthyroidism, congestive heart failure, or ventricular irritability

Side effects
Tachycardia; palpitations; bronchial edema; flushing; headache; arrhythmias; chest pain; tremors; anxiety; fatigue; nausea and vomiting

Special considerations
• Closely monitor patient's heart rate and rhythm, central venous and arterial blood pressures, arterial blood gases, and urinary output. If heart rate exceeds 130 beats per minute, slow down or discontinue infusion.

• Administer with an infusion pump.

LIDOCAINE HYDROCHLORIDE
Xylocaine*

Indications
• Ventricular tachycardia
• Acute ventricular arrhythmias

Pediatric dosage
I.V. bolus: 1 mg/kg. May be repeated, but not to exceed 3 mg/kg/day.
I.V. infusion: 1 gm in 250 ml 5% dextrose in water, at 20 to 40 mcg/kg/min.

Contraindications
• Hypersensitivity to amide-type local anesthetics
• Adams-Stokes syndrome
• Complete or second-degree heart block
• With caution if patient has liver or severe kidney disease or damage; congestive heart failure; marked hypoxia; severe respiratory depression; shock

Side effects
Dizziness, restlessness, apprehension, tinnitus, visual disturbances, hearing loss; vomiting; difficulty breathing or swallowing; twitching, tremors, convulsions; hypotension; cardiovascular collapse; cardiac conduction disorders; bradycardia; cardiac and respiratory arrest; numbness in extremities, lips, or tongue

Special considerations
• Monitor patient's heart rate, rhythm, and blood pressure during administration.
• Watch for side effects and notify the doctor if any occur.
• If toxic signs, such as dizziness, appear, stop infusion at once. Continued infusion could lead to convulsions and coma.
• When administering by I.V. infusion, use an infusion pump.
• For antiarrhythmic therapy, never use lidocaine hydrochloride with epinephrine hydrochloride (Adrenalin Chloride) added.

PROPRANOLOL HYDROCHLORIDE Inderal*

Indications
• Supraventricular, atrial, and ventricular arrhythmias
• Hypertension
• Angina

Pediatric dosage
I.V. bolus: 0.01 to 0.15 mg/kg/dose. Give bolus dose slowly. Dose may be repeated every 6 to 8 hours.

Contraindications
• Sinus bradycardia
• Heart block other than first degree
• Cardiogenic shock
• Right ventricular failure
• Bronchial asthma
• With caution if patient has renal or hepatic dysfunction; left ventricular heart failure; acute myocardial infarction; arrhythmias induced by digitalis toxicosis; respiratory disease
• With caution after cardioversion
• With caution if patient's diabetic

Side effects
CHF or circulatory collapse; hypotension; cardiac disturbances, including bradycardia, angina, asystole, AV heart block; GI disturbances; CNS disturbances, including hallucinations, uncoordinated movements, syncope, dizziness, insomnia, confusion, and depression; rashes; peripheral vascular insufficiency; bronchospasms, wheezing; blood sugar abnormalities

Special considerations
• Take apical pulse rate before administration. If pulse is below 50 beats per minute, withhold drug and notify doctor.
• Auscultate patient's lungs for rales and his heart for gallop rhythm during administration. If found, notify doctor.
• Have atropine sulfate on hand to counteract possible bradycardia.
• Observe diabetic patient for insulin shock. (Propranolol hydrochloride masks characteristic signs of hypoglycemia, including tachycardia and sweating.)
• When stopping therapy, gradually slow infusion rate.

SODIUM BICARBONATE

Indications
• Cardiac arrest
• Metabolic acidosis

Pediatric dosage
Cardiac arrest
I.V. bolus: 2 to 4 mEq/kg. Subsequent doses based on arterial blood gas (ABG) measurements. Not to exceed 8 mEq/kg/day.

Contraindications
• No contraindications for life-threatening emergencies

Side effects
GI disturbances, such as abdominal cramps, anorexia, nausea, and vomiting; dizziness, convulsions; thirst; diminished respirations; with overdose, alkalosis, hypernatremia, hyperosmolarity

Special considerations
• May be added to I.V. solution, unless solution contains epineprine hydrochloride or norepinephrine.
• Do not infuse through I.V. line containing lactated Ringer's solution (or any other solution containing calcium), or the drug will precipitate.
• Obtain ABG and serum electrolyte measurements during administration, and report changes.
Note: Sodium bicarbonate may cause tissue sloughing if extravasation occurs.

VERAPAMIL HYDROCHLORIDE
Calan, Isoptin

Indications
• Treatment of supraventricular tachyarrhythmias including paroxysmal supraventricular tachycardia
• Temporary control of rapid ventricular rate, accompanying atrial flutter, or atrial fibrillation

Pediatric dose
Newborn to 1 year
Initial dose
I.V. bolus: 0.1 to 0.2 mg/kg
Repeat dose
I.V. bolus: 0.1 to 0.2 mg/kg 30 minutes after first dose
1 year to 15 years:
Initial dose
I.V. bolus: 0.1 to 0.3 mg/kg
Repeat dose
I.V. bolus: 0.1 to 0.3 mg/kg 30 minutes after first dose. Not to exceed 10 mg per single dose.
Note: Administer all I.V. bolus doses over at least 2 minutes.

Contraindications
• Congestive heart failure (CHF). Drug greatly exacerbates condition.
• Severe hypotension or cardiogenic shock
• Second or third degree heart block
• Sick sinus syndrome
• Patient receiving beta-adrenergic blocking drugs *I.V.*

Side effects
Brief hypotension, usually transient and asymptomatic; bradycardia including AV blocks; paradoxical increase in ventricular rate in atrial fibrillation or atrial flutter

Special considerations
• Monitor blood pressure for signs of hypotension. Patient may complain of dizziness or headache.
• Frequently monitor heart rate.
• Do not administer beta-adrenergic drugs I.V. within 4 hours after giving verapamil hydrochloride. These drugs depress myocardial activity and slow AV conduction.

*Available in both the United States and in Canada

Special problems

What is a special pediatric problem? It may be a seizure disorder, burn, multiple trauma, or a complication resulting from poison ingestion. To deal with these problems, you'll need to know what to look for, what to expect, and what immediate action to take. In addition, you'll need to know how to help the patient and his family cope.

On the next few pages, we'll explain the procedures and equipment, as well as the skills you'll need to meet these special challenges. We've also included home care aids with tips on poison-proofing the home and preventing accidental burns.

Understanding seizures

When we talk about a seizure, we're referring to abnormal electrical discharges from the brain's neurons. And, depending on the location and number of these discharges, a seizure may cause unconsciousness, convulsive movements, or motor, sensory, or behavioral abnormalities.

In children, the risk of seizure is greatest between birth and age 2; between ages 5 and 7; and at the onset of puberty, when girls are at greater risk than boys.

As you probably know, recurring seizures, called epilepsy, are divided into two groups: partial (electrical discharges occur in a localized area of the brain) and generalized (discharges occur simultaneously in both brain hemispheres). In some patients, partial seizure activity may develop into a generalized seizure.

Within these groups, several specific seizure types exist. The following information will familiarize you with these types. But remember, your patient may exhibit a seizure that deviates from the standard descriptions, or he may experience several seizure types simultaneously.

Partial seizures

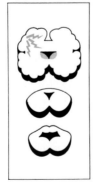

● **Elementary (focal) seizures** may have motor or sensory components, depending on discharge location. *Partial motor seizures* produce tonic (muscle stiffening) and clonic (rapid alternate muscle contraction and relaxation) movements of a body part, such as the face, arm, leg, or thumb. In some cases, partial motor seizures spread, and may include one entire side of the body. (These are sometimes called jacksonian seizures.) They may also immediately precede a major motor tonic-clonic seizure (grand mal seizure).
● **Partial sensory seizures** produce tingling, numbness, or warmth in a body part; or visual, auditory, olfactory or taste disturbances.
● **Complex partial seizures,** sometimes called temporal lobe or psychomotor seizures, are characterized by 1 to 2 minute periods when the patient appears to be staring or daydreaming with rapidly fluttering eyelids. He may fall to the ground. In addition, the seizures may produce automatism (repetition of inappropriate acts) such as lip smacking, chewing, and running in circles. Postictal (postseizure) confusion may accompany the staring episodes.

Generalized seizures

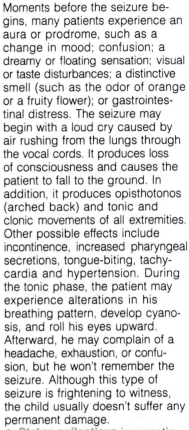

● **Absence seizures** (petit mal or lapse seizures) produce brief (10 to 30 second) lapses of awareness. Like complex partial seizures, they make the patient appear to be staring or daydreaming. Although the patient's eyelids flutter rapidly, he doesn't fall, or experience automatisms or postictal confusion. He'll resume normal activity without being aware of the attack. Some patients experience 10 or more seizures a day.
● **Myoclonic seizures** are characterized by brief involuntary muscular jerks of the body or extremities, which may occur rhythmically.
● **Infantile spasms** develop before the child reaches age 1. The seizures produce sudden brief muscle spasms which may affect one part of the body, such as an arm or leg, or affect the body symmetrically. All but 10% of affected infants suffer mental retardation.
● **Akinetic (atonic) seizures,** or drop attacks, result from a sudden loss of muscle tone. The patient loses consciousness and may fall to the ground. But some patients exhibit only head-nodding that lasts just a few seconds.
● **Major motor tonic-clonic (grand mal) seizures** begin abruptly and last several minutes.

Moments before the seizure begins, many patients experience an aura or prodrome, such as a change in mood; confusion; a dreamy or floating sensation; visual or taste disturbances; a distinctive smell (such as the odor of orange or a fruity flower); or gastrointestinal distress. The seizure may begin with a loud cry caused by air rushing from the lungs through the vocal cords. It produces loss of consciousness and causes the patient to fall to the ground. In addition, it produces opisthotonos (arched back) and tonic and clonic movements of all extremities. Other possible effects include incontinence, increased pharyngeal secretions, tongue-biting, tachycardia and hypertension. During the tonic phase, the patient may experience alterations in his breathing pattern, develop cyanosis, and roll his eyes upward. Afterward, he may complain of a headache, exhaustion, or confusion, but he won't remember the seizure. Although this type of seizure is frightening to witness, the child usually doesn't suffer any permanent damage.
● **Status epilepticus** is a continuous seizure state in which seizures occur in rapid succession, without the patient regaining consciousness between them. While this condition may be seen with any seizure type, it's usually associated with major motor tonic-clonic seizures. A continuous tonic-clonic seizure is an acute medical emergency and must be stopped immediately before cerebral hypoxia causes irreversible brain damage.
● **Febrile convulsions** aren't usually associated with epilepsy. They may be inherited and usually occur between age 6 months and 3 years. They rarely occur after age 7. The convulsions usually occur in a previously well patient whose temperature suddenly rises to at least 102° F. (38.9° C.). They may produce seizurelike tonic-clonic movements that last less than 10 minutes. Most febrile convulsions are generalized, although some have only partial effects.

Special problems

Taking seizure precautions

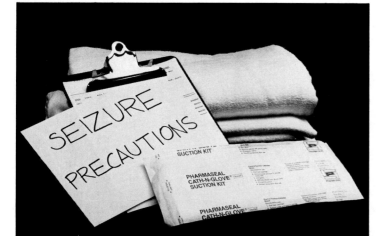

1 *Your patient, 11-year-old Al Barnes, has a history of seizures. Because you know that he may have a seizure at any time, you'll want to take seizure precautions. Here's what to do:*

First, gather the equipment you'll need: suction kit containing a catheter large enough to provide emergency oral and/or nasal suctioning; blankets or bumper pads for the bed rails; a seizure documentation sheet including space for the information detailed on page 114; a sign stating SEIZURE PRECAUTIONS; and tape (not shown).

Also, place a prefilled syringe containing an anticonvulsant medication ordered for emergency use in your patient's medication drawer. Or, tape an ampule of anticonvulsant medication to a syringe and place them in the medication tray.

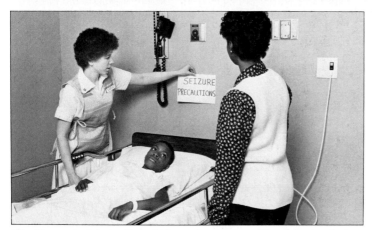

2 Then, explain to Al and his mother what you're doing and why. Stress that these precautions will help ensure Al's safety. Also be sure to ask if he's wearing an orthodontic appliance. If it's removable, tell him and his mother that, as a seizure precaution, he may have to remove it. Suggest that she alert the dentist or orthodontist of the situation.

Tape the seizure precaution sign directly above the head of the bed. This alerts everyone who comes into Al's room to watch for any signs of seizure activity.

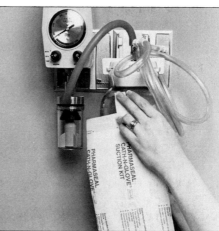

3 Next, tape the suction kit to the suction bottle or the wall above the bed. Remember, if your hospital doesn't have a central suctioning system, you'll also need a portable suction machine. Position the machine close to your patient's bed.

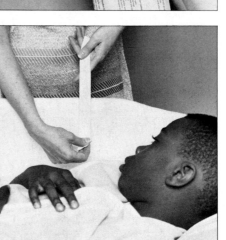

4 Wrap bath blankets around the bed's side rails. Secure the blankets with tape, as the nurse is doing here.

If you're using commercially-made bumper pads, tie them securely to the side rails.

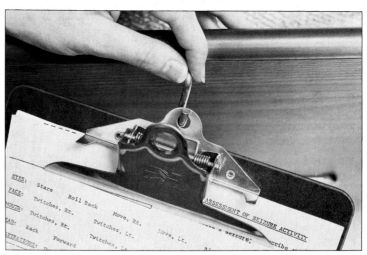

5 Fasten the seizure documentation slip on a clipboard and hang it on your patient's bed. Or, tape the seizure documentation slip above his bed.

Document the seizure precautions taken, including any patient teaching, in your nurses' notes.

Finally, before Al leaves the hospital, familiarize him and his family with the seizure precautions on page 117.

Coping with a seizure

1 *Because Al Barnes is seizure-prone, you've taken all the necessary seizure precautions as shown in the preceding photostory. Now, suppose he has a seizure. Do you know what to do? Read what follows for guidelines:*

As you're performing Al's morning care, he suddenly rolls his eyes upward and arches his back. You realize he's having a seizure. Doing your best to stay calm, you prepare to take the following steps.

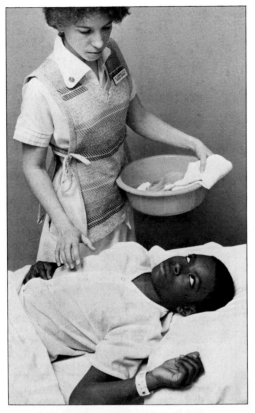

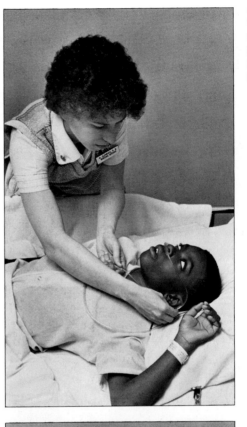

3 If your patient's cyanotic, administer oxygen with a nasal cannula (as shown) or a nasal catheter.

2 First, place Al on his back, if he's not already in this position. Then, raise the bed's padded side rails, as the nurse is doing here. Work quickly. Call or signal for help, but *don't leave your patient.*

Note: If your patient's not in bed, gently place him in a supine position on the floor. If possible, place a blanket under his head.

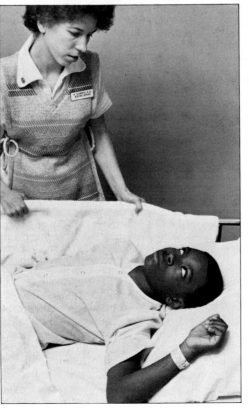

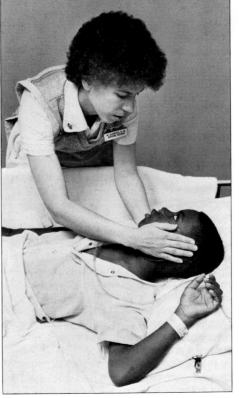

4 Now, loosen Al's pajama top. To maintain a patent airway and reduce the risk of aspiration, try to turn his head to one side, as shown. But never *force* his head in any direction.

Wipe any saliva or vomitus from his mouth. If necessary, use the suction catheter to suction between his lips and between his cheeks and teeth. *Important:* Never attempt to force *anything* (including a tongue depressor) between your patient's teeth, if they're already clenched. Doing so may cause injury.

Special problems

Giving a tepid water bath continued

6 Wrap a washcloth around your hand, tucking in all loose ends. Moisten the washcloth and squeeze out the excess water so the cloth's still wet, but not dripping.
Nursing tip: To keep your patient from becoming chilled, place a warm water bottle against her feet.

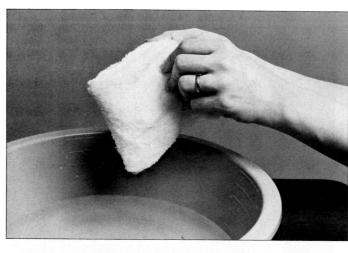

7 Ask Mrs. Morgan to fold back the bath blanket so you can sponge Joanie's chest, abdomen, and legs. As you work, follow the path of her large blood vessels. Use long, soothing strokes, applying gentle friction to the skin.

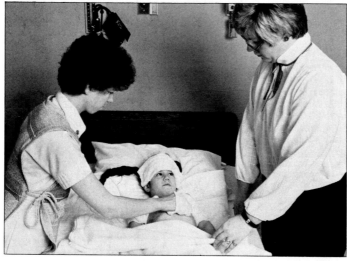

8 Another way to give a tepid-water bed bath is to wrap the patient's arms and legs with towels or washcloths moistened in tepid water. Place moistened towels across the patient's chest and abdomen, as well as under her back. Be sure to cover skin areas that come in contact with each other, such as the axilla, with moistened washcloths. Also, cover her groin and forehead. As the towels and washcloths become warm, replace them with newly moistened ones.

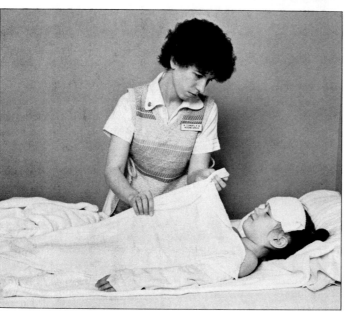

9 When 30 minutes have elapsed, remove the washcloths and towels. Dry her thoroughly with a clean towel. Then, help her into a clean, light gown, as shown here. Replace the bed linens, if necessary, and properly dispose of the equipment.

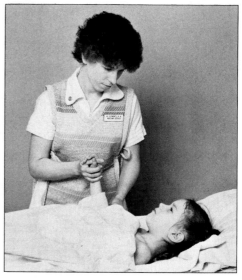

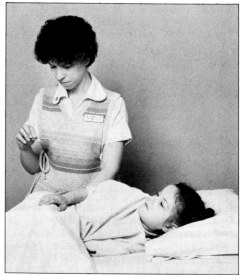

10 In 30 minutes, take Joanie's temperature. If she still has a fever and doesn't appear chilled, wait for her skin to warm up. Then, repeat the procedure.

Suppose the tepid water bath doesn't lower her temperature. Consider using a temperature control system, such as a hyper-hypothermia blanket. (For details on using this system, see the NURSING PHOTO-BOOK COPING WITH NEUROLOGIC DISORDERS.)

Document the procedure and your patient's reaction to it, including her temperature readings, in your nurses' notes.

Teaching the patient and family about seizure precautions

How do you care for a child with a seizure disorder? That depends on the type of seizure disorder, its severity, the patient's age, and his physical and mental condition. As you know, you'll be responsible for observing, assessing, and documenting his condition as well as taking precautions to ensure his safety.

One of these precautions is helping your patient and his family understand and cope with his disorder. Find out what they know about his seizure disorder. Then, clear up any misconceptions they may have. *Note:* Always include the child in your discussions about his condition, unless he's too young to comprehend what you're saying.

During your talks with the child and his family, be sure to emphasize that the child will be able to attend school and participate in most sports and other activities appropriate for his age, including swimming and riding a bicycle (under supervision), playing baseball, tennis, and bowling. But, for safety, advise him to avoid contact sports; for example, football and wrestling, until all seizure activity is well controlled.

Keep in mind that the parents may feel responsible for their child's condition. Encourage them to openly discuss their feelings and assure them that they are not the cause of their child's seizure disorder. Don't hesitate to share your thoughts and feelings with them. Remember, this will help build rapport with them.

Explain to the child and his family that you'll need their assistance in helping the child stay seizure-free. For starters, stress the importance of maintaining the prescribed medication schedule. (For details on anticonvulsant medications, see the following information and chart.)

Then, teach parents about specific precautions they should take, using the following

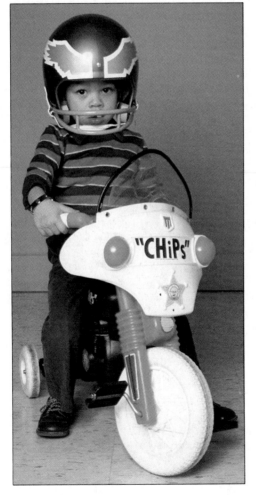

points as a guide. Emphasize that these precautions must be ongoing.
• Remove sharp objects, such as pencils and sharp toys, from your child's room.
• Familiarize yourself with the child's seizure history. If he falls or jerks forward when he has a seizure, make sure he wears a protective helmet as shown below, until his seizures are controlled by medication.
• Work out a medication schedule that's convenient for you. For example, you may find it easier to administer medication at mealtimes and bedtime. And remember, your child must continue taking the medication even after the disorder's controlled. If he stops taking his medication, the seizures may recur.
• Make sure the child always wears a Medic Alert™ bracelet or necklace, as shown in the photo. Or, be sure the child carries a card with him detailing the important information about his condition.
• If your child's small, stay with him when he's on the toilet or in the bathtub.
• Treat the child as normally as possible. For example, don't be afraid to punish him when his behavior merits it.
• If the child's in school, inform the school nurse and the child's teacher of his condition. Include important details, such as the type of seizure, medication and dosage, and what to do when the child has a seizure. Suggest that the teacher or school nurse educate the child's classmates about seizures. That way, if the child has a seizure at school, his classmates may be less frightened and more understanding.
• Keep a record of the child's seizure activity and medication schedule, and notify the doctor of any changes in his condition.
• Contact the Epilepsy Foundation of America, 1818 L Street NW, Washington, DC 20036, for additional information.

Nurses' guide to anticonvulsant drugs

Has the doctor ordered an anticonvulsant drug for your patient with a seizure disorder? If he has, one of your responsibilities is to teach your patient—and his family—about the drug.

First, familiarize yourself with the drugs detailed in the following chart. Then, using easy-to-understand terms, explain these important points to the child and his parents:
• what the prescribed drug is called and what it's used for.
• what specific side effects it may cause.
• what special precautions the child must observe while taking the drug. For example, tell him to avoid activities requiring alertness and good psychomotor coordination (such as riding a bike) until the doctor assesses his response to the drug.
• why initial doses may vary from the maintenance dose. Explain that finding the appropriate dose and dosage for the child may take time. Encourage the child and parents not to become discouraged if the drug doesn't immediately control the child's seizures. The doctor will periodically check the child's blood to determine the therapeutic serum drug level.
• why taking the drug on schedule is so important. Remember, noncompliance with the medication schedule is one of the most common reasons for seizure recurrence.

In addition, warn them to tell the doctor about any other drugs—including over-the-counter products—the child may use. They may interact adversely with the anticonvulsant drug. Also, advise them to inform any other doctor or dentist about anticonvulsant therapy.

If the child develops any side effects (for example, a sore throat, unexplained bruising, or fluid retention), tell his parents to notify the doctor at once. But warn them *never* to stop the drug abruptly, unless the doctor directs them to do so.

For more information on anticonvulsant drugs, see the NURSING DRUG HANDBOOK™ or the NURSE'S GUIDE TO DRUGS™

Special problems

Nurses' guide to anticonvulsant drugs continued

Phenytoin sodium
Dilantin*

Indications
Grand mal, psychomotor seizures, or febrile seizures; status epilepticus of the grand mal type; and nonepileptic seizures following head trauma or Reye's syndrome

Pediatric dosage
Loading dose
I.V. bolus: 15 mg/kg/dose (not to exceed 50 mg/min.)
Maintenance dose
P.O. or I.V.: 4 to 8 mg/kg/24 hours in one or two daily doses

Side effects
Ataxia; slurred speech; confusion; dizziness; insomnia; nervousness; twitching; headache; gingival hyperplasia; blood dyscrasias; hypotension; ventricular fibrillation; nystagmus; diplopia; blurred vision; vomiting; toxic hepatitis; scarlet fever or measles-like rash; bullous, exfoliative or purpuric dermatitis; lupus erythematosus; hirsutism; toxic epidermal necrolysis; periarteritis nodosa; lymphadenopathy; hyperglycemia; osteomalacia; hypertrichosis

Interactions
• These drugs cause *decreased* phenytoin sodium (Dilantin*) activity: alcohol; folic acid (Folvite*); loxapine succinate (Loxitane).
• These drugs cause *increased* phenytoin sodium (Dilantin*) activity and toxicity: oral anticoagulants; antihistamines; chloramphenicol; diazepam (Valium*); diazoxide (Hyperstat*); disulfiram (Antabuse*); isoniazid (Hyzyd); phenylbutazone (Butazolidin*); phenyramidol hydrochloride; salicylates; sulfamethizole (Sulfasol); valproate sodium (Depakene Syrup).
• Tricyclic antidepressants in high doses may precipitate seizures, necessitating dosage adjustment.

Precautions
• Contraindicated in phenacemide (Phenurone) or hydantoin hypersensitivity; bradycardia; sinoatrial (SA) and atrioventricular (AV) node block; Stokes-Adams syndrome.
• Use cautiously in hepatic or renal dysfunction; hypotension; myocardial insufficiency; respiratory depression; and in debilitated patients or patients receiving other hydantoin derivatives.

Nursing considerations
• If administering phenytoin sodium parenterally, never use a cloudy solution.
• If giving direct I.V. push, flush tube with 5 ml normal saline solution before and after drug administration. If unable to give direct I.V. push, mix with normal saline solution at a concentration of 100 mg/20 ml and administer over 10 minute period using a separate I.V. administration set. Don't mix with 5% dextrose in water, as precipitation occurs. *Caution:* Rapid I.V. push may cause cardiac arrhythmias and cardiac arrest.
• Avoid I.M. administration route, as drug may precipitate at injection site, causing tissue necrosis and pain. I.M. route will also cause erratic blood levels.
• Warn child that drug may discolor his urine pink, red, or reddish-brown.
• Tell parents to help the child maintain good oral hygiene and to schedule regular dental exams for him, to minimize effects of gingival hyperplasia.
• Shake liquid suspension well before giving.
• Encourage parents to schedule follow-up evaluations every 4 to 6 weeks, to check for blood dyscrasias.

Primidone
Mysoline*

Indications
Grand mal, psychomotor, and focal seizures

Pediatric dosage
Children up to 8 years
P.O.: 125 mg daily. Increase by 125 mg weekly, up to maximum of 1 g daily, divided q.i.d.
Children over 8 years
P.O.: 250 mg daily. Increase by 250 mg weekly up to maximum of 2 g daily, divided q.i.d.

Side effects
Blood dyscrasias; drowsiness; ataxia; emotional disturbances; vertigo; hyperirritability; fatigue; diplopia; nystagmus; eyelid edema; anorexia; nausea; vomiting; polyuria; morbilliform rash; alopecia; edema; thirst

Interactions
• Phenytoin sodium (Dilantin*) causes increased phenobarbital effect resulting from stimulated conversion of primidone to phenobarbital.

Precautions
• Contraindicated in phenobarbital hypersensitivity.
• Contraindicated in porphyria.
• Use primidone cautiously with phenobarbital (Luminal*).

Nursing considerations
• Tell patient and family to schedule a complete blood cell count (CBC) and routine blood chemistry tests every 6 months, to check for blood dyscrasias.
• Shake liquid suspension well.

Carbamazepine
Tegretol*

Indications
Psychomotor, temporal lobe, grand mal, and mixed seizure patterns

Pediatric dosage
Children under 12 years
P.O.: 10 to 20 mg/kg daily in 2 to 4 equal doses
Children over 12 years
P.O.: 200 mg b.i.d. on first day. May increase by 200 mg per day, in equal doses at 6 to 8 hour intervals. Adjust to minimum effective level when control achieved. Usual maintenance dose is 800 mg to 1,200 mg daily. Don't exceed 1 g total daily dose in patients between 12 and 15 years old and 1,200 mg P.O. daily in patients over 15 years.

Side effects
Dizziness; vertigo; drowsiness; fatigue; ataxia; congestive heart failure; hypertension; hypotension; conjunctivitis; dry mouth and pharynx; blurred vision; diplopia; nystagmus; vomiting; abdominal pain; diarrhea; anorexia; stomatitis; glossitis; urinary frequency or retention; albuminuria; glycosuria; elevated blood urea nitrogen (BUN) level; abnormal liver function test; water intoxication; rash; urticaria; diaphoresis; fever; chills; blood dyscrasias

Interactions
• Troleandomycin phosphate (Tao) and erythromycin (E-Mycin*) may increase carbamazepine blood levels.
• Propoxyphene hydrochloride (Darvon) may increase carbamazepine levels. Use another analgesic.

Precautions
• Contraindicated in patients with bone-marrow depression, or hypersensitivity to carbamazepine or tricyclic antidepressants.
• Use cautiously if patient has cardiac, renal, or hepatic damage or increased intraocular pressure.

Nursing considerations
• Tell parents to schedule complete blood cell count, platelet and reticulocyte counts and serum iron levels weekly for first 3 months, then monthly. If bone marrow depression develops, stop drug, as ordered. Also, have them schedule urinalysis, BUN, and liver function tests every 3 months.
• Recommend periodic eye examinations for the child.

*Available in both the United States and in Canada

Phenobarbital
Luminal*

Indications
All forms of epilepsy, febrile convulsions

Pediatric dosage
Loading dose
I.V.: 3 to 5 mg/kg/dose. May repeat every 10 to 15 minutes up to total of 20 mg/kg. I.V. injection rate should not exceed 60 mg/min.
Maintenance dose
P.O.: 4 to 6 mg/kg daily, divided into two doses

Side effects
Lethargy; headache; dizziness; nausea; vomiting; rash; urticaria; angioedema; paradoxical excitability

Interactions
• Alcohol and other central nervous system depressants, including narcotic analgesics cause excessive central nervous system depression.
• MAO inhibitors potentiate barbiturate effect.
• Rifampin (Rifadin*) causes decreased barbiturate level.
• Primidone (Mysoline*) causes excessive phenobarbital blood levels.
• Valproic acid (Depakene) may cause increased phenobarbital levels.

Precautions
• Contraindicated in patients with barbiturate hypersensitivity, porphyria, hepatic dysfunction, respiratory disease with dyspnea or obstruction, or nephritis.
• Use cautiously in chronically ill patients or in patients with hyperthyroidism, diabetes mellitus, or anemia.

Nursing considerations
• Use I.V. injection for emergency treatment and administer slowly under close supervision. Monitor respirations and blood pressure.
• Monitor for signs of barbiturate toxicosis, such as coma, asthmatic breathing, cyanosis, clammy skin, and hypotension. *Important:* Overdose can be fatal.

Clonazepam
Clonopin

Indications
Petit mal seizures and petit mal variants; akinetic and myoclonic seizures

Pediatric dosage
Children up to 10 years or 30 kg
P.O.: 0.01 to 0.03 mg/kg daily (not to exceed 0.05 mg/kg daily), divided into 2 or 3 equal doses, and given every 8 hours. Increase dosage by 0.25 to 0.5 mg every third day to a maximum maintenance dosage of 0.1 mg to 0.2 mg/kg P.O. daily.
Children over 10 years
P.O.: 1.5 mg daily, divided into 3 doses. Dosage may be increased by 0.5 mg to 1 mg every 3 days, as needed. Maximum recommended daily dose is 20 mg.

Side effects
Blood dyscrasias; drowsiness; ataxia; behavioral disturbances; increased salivation; diplopia; nystagmus; constipation; gastritis; appetite changes; abnormal thirst; sore gums; dysuria; enuresis; nocturia; urinary retention; rash; respiratory depression

Interactions
• None significant

Precautions
• Contraindicated in hepatic disease; sensitivity to chlordiazepoxide hydrochloride (Librium*), diazepam (Valium*), or any other benzodiazepine drugs; acute narrow-angle glaucoma.
• Use with caution if patient has chronic respiratory disease, impaired renal function, or open-angle glaucoma.

Nursing considerations
• Monitor patient for oversedation.
• Tell patient and family to schedule complete blood cell count (CBC) and liver function tests, as ordered.

Ethosuximide
Zarontin*

Indications
Petit mal seizures

Pediatric dosage
Children 3 to 6 years
P.O.: 250 mg daily or 125 mg b.i.d. May increase by 250 mg every 4 to 7 days, up to 1.5 g daily.
Children over 6 years
P.O.: Initially, 250 mg b.i.d. May increase by 250 mg every 4 to 7 days, up to 1.5 g daily.

Side effects
Blood dyscrasias; drowsiness; fatigue; dizziness; ataxia; irritability; hiccups; euphoria; lethargy; myopia; nausea; vomiting; diarrhea; gingival hypertrophy; weight loss; cramps; tongue swelling; anorexia; epigastric and abdominal pain; vaginal bleeding; urticaria; pruritic and erythematous rashes; lupus erythematosus; hirsutism

Interactions
• None significant

Precautions
• Contraindicated in hypersensitivity to succinimide derivatives.
• Use cautiously if patient has hepatic or renal disease.

Nursing considerations
• Instruct parents to schedule complete blood cell count (CBC) every 3 months.
• When used alone in patient with mixed types of seizures, drug may increase frequency of grand mal seizures.
• May cause positive direct Coombs' test.

Valproic acid
Depakene

Indications
Simple and complex absence seizures (including petit mal), mixed seizures (including absence seizures), and sometimes in major motor (grand mal, tonic-clonic) seizures

Pediatric dosage
P.O.: Initially, 15 mg/kg daily divided b.i.d. or t.i.d.; then may increase by 5 to 10 mg/kg daily at weekly intervals up to maximum of 30 mg/kg daily, divided b.i.d. or t.i.d.

Side effects
Inhibited platelet aggregation; thrombocytopenia; increased bleeding time; sedation; emotional upset; depression; psychosis; aggression; hyperactivity; behavioral deterioration; muscle weakness; tremors; nausea; vomiting; indigestion; diarrhea; abdominal cramps; constipation; increased appetite and weight gain; anorexia; pancreatitis; enzyme elevations; toxic hepatitis; alopecia.
Caution: Because drug is usually used in combination with other anticonvulsants, side effects may not be caused by valproic acid alone.

Interactions
• Valproic acid may cause increased phenobarbital levels.

Precautions
• Use cautiously if patient has hepatic dysfunction.

Nursing considerations
• Tell parents to schedule liver function studies, platelet count and prothrombin time before starting drug therapy, and every 2 months afterward.
• If patient develops tremors, reduce dosage as ordered.
• To reduce GI side effects and produce uniform blood drug levels, advise patient to take drug with food or milk.
• May produce false positive test for ketones in urine.
• Available as palatable red syrup. Keep out of reach of children. *Note:* Because syrup is more rapidly absorbed, its peak effect occurs within 15 minutes.
• To avoid mouth and throat irritation, don't allow child to chew capsules. Also, don't mix syrup with carbonated beverages.

*Available in both the United States and in Canada

Special problems

When a child ingests poison: What to do

You're covering for a co-worker in the emergency deparment, when 10-year-old Kathy Hudson is wheeled in, accompanied by her mother. Obviously distraught, Mrs. Hudson tells you that Kathy may have swallowed a bottleful of Valium* (diazepam), which was prescribed for Mrs. Hudson to help relieve anxiety.

In order to properly manage Kathy's condition, you and your co-workers will be working as a team to stabilize her vital signs, assess her level of consciousness, and begin any emergency therapy needed. Do you know how to proceed?

Begin by making sure her airway's patent. Then, take her vital signs, and continue to monitor them throughout treatment. (Watch closely for any signs of shock, such as cold, clammy skin, decreased urinary output, increased respiratory rate, restlessness, change in level of consciousness, and diaphoresis. If you see any of these signs, or your patient complains of nausea or dizziness, notify the doctor.)

As you work, remember to reassure your patient as much as possible. Explain each procedure to her as it's performed, even if she doesn't seem to comprehend what you're saying. If she has questions, answer them.

In addition, reassure your patient's mother (and any other family members present). Provide frequent reports about the child's condition.

To combat the poison's effects, you'll need to take steps to:
• identify the type and amount of poison
• decrease absorption
• increase elimination.

To learn how to proceed, study the information that follows.

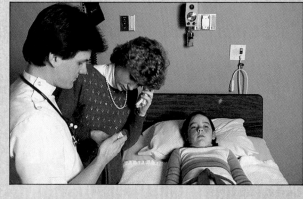

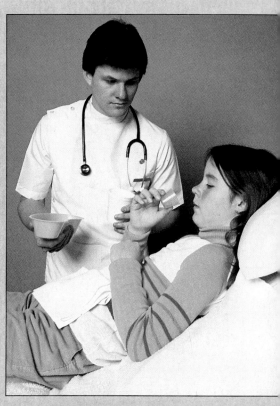

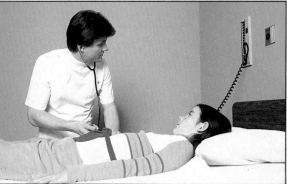

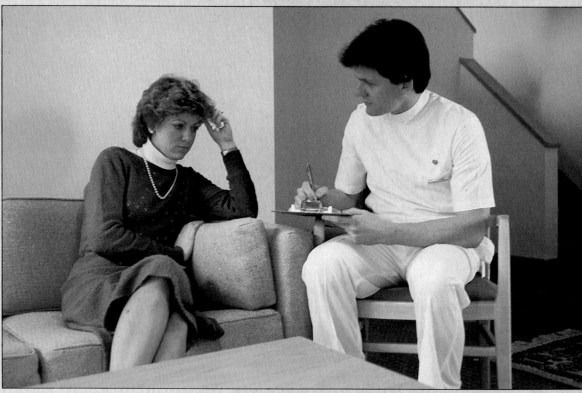

*Available in both the United States and in Canada

Identifying the poison

Gather as much information about the poison as possible. Ask the patient's family members, friends—or the patient herself—what she swallowed or inhaled, where, when, and how much. If the poison came in a bottle or can, ask what was on the label and have the container brought to the hospital. If the poison was a plant or seed, ask to see a sample.

Nursing tip: If you don't know what the patient swallowed, observe for burns in and around her mouth; smell her breath for unusual odors; and examine her hands and clothing for stains and residue.

Also find out what first aid—if any—was administered before the patient arrived at the hospital. And remember, all the facts you accumulate will help you and the doctor determine the best method for decreasing absorption.

Note: Some drugs, such as acetaminophen (Tylenol*) can be removed from the patient's blood only by dialysis. That's one reason why finding out which drug she ingested is vital.

Decreasing absorption

You may decrease poison absorption by inducing vomiting or by performing gastric lavage, depending on the poison ingested. But these methods are contraindicated for some poisons. For example, never induce vomiting if your patient's swallowed a corrosive substance, such as alkali, mineral acid, or lye. Such a substance will sear her mucous membranes as it's vomited. Also, if she aspirates the vomited substance, it will burn her respiratory tract. If less than 1 hour's elapsed since ingestion, prepare to perform gastric

lavage, as ordered. (See the NURSING PHOTOBOOK PERFORMING GI PROCEDURES.) After an hour or more, gastric lavage probably won't be helpful. Concentrate on supporting vital functions.

Important: Don't induce vomiting or perform gastric lavage if your patient's ingested strychnine or a petroleum distillate such as kerosene or mineral oil (unless advised to do so by your poison control center).

If the poison ingested isn't one of those mentioned above, and if your patient's alert and has an intact gag reflex, empty her stomach by inducing vomiting. To do so, you may administer ipecac syrup or apomorphine hydrochloride, as ordered, or stimulate the gag reflex. Note: Do not induce vomiting with salt water, because too much salt may cause hypernatremia.

If you're administering ipecac syrup, be sure to follow 15 ml of syrup (5 ml if patient is under 1 year) with about 200 ml of water. Expect vomiting to occur within 20 minutes. If it doesn't, repeat the dose and wait 30 minutes. If vomiting still doesn't occur, perform gastric lavage, if ordered. Important: If absorbed, ipecac syrup may cause cardiac arrhythmias.

To stimulate the gag reflex, have your patient drink about 100 ml water or milk. Then, touch her posterior pharynx with a blunt object, such as a tongue depressor. Expect vomiting to occur almost immediately.

In some cases, the doctor may order apomorphine hydrochloride (0.1 mg/kg subcutaneously) to empty your patient's stomach and promote upper intestine reflux. Before you administer this drug, be sure to have

her drink about 200 ml water. After administering apomorphine hydrochloride, expect vomiting to occur in approximately 5 minutes.

Note: Apomorphine hydrochloride is rarely used because it depresses the central nervous system (CNS). After the patient vomits, you'll give a narcotic antagonist such as naloxone (Narcan*) as ordered, to combat CNS depression.

When the child's stomach is empty, administer activated charcoal (such as Charcocaps), as ordered. Keep in mind that activated charcoal given after induced vomiting decreases poison absorption from the gastrointestinal tract more effectively than either activated charcoal or vomiting alone. Important: Activated charcoal inactivates ipecac syrup. Don't give activated charcoal before the patient's vomited the ipecac syrup.

Do not use the universal poison antidote (burned toast, tea, Milk of Magnesia®) to decrease poison absorption. Recent studies indicate that it may be harmful.

Increasing elimination

After you've decreased absorption, you'll want to hasten elimination. In most cases, you'll administer a saline cathartic, as ordered. However, if renal excretion is the predominant route of elimination for the ingested poison, and if renal function is intact, the doctor may order forced diuresis.

After the crisis, ask Mrs. Hudson to supply you with any other information she has about the incident. Document everything, including the poison ingested and the treatment given. If you suspect drug abuse or attempted suicide, refer the child and her parents to an appropriate social agency.

*Available in both the United States and in Canada

Special problems

Home care

How to protect your child from poisoning

Dear Parent:
If your child eats or drinks anything that may be poisonous, immediately call your local poison control center for help. Write the phone number here _____ and on a label stuck to the phone. Keep ipecac syrup handy, in case the poison control center instructs you to induce vomiting. To reduce the risk of accidental poisoning, follow these guidelines:

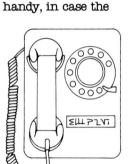

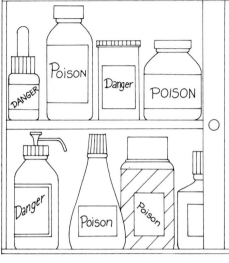

Place poison identification stickers on all household poisons, such as cleaning solutions, polishes, weed spray, and bug killers. Lock them up, or store them on the top shelf of a closet or cabinet—out of reach. (Take care to store them away from food or eating utensils.) After using any of these poisonous products, *immediately* return them to the safe storage place.

Keep cosmetics, such as nail polish, perfume, and hand cream, as well as all aerosol containers, out of your child's reach.

Teach your child that everything within reach isn't good to eat. To prove the point, give him a taste of something unpleasant-tasting (such as vinegar) on the tip of your finger—but be sure to warn him that it *doesn't* taste good.

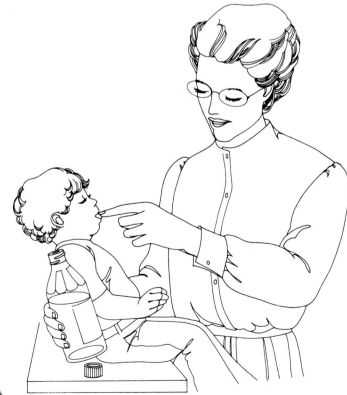

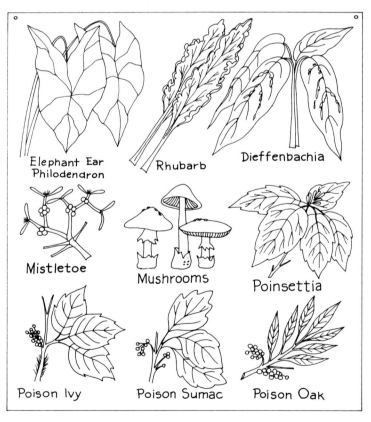

Elephant Ear Philodendron   Rhubarb   Dieffenbachia

Mistletoe   Mushrooms   Poinsettia

Poison Ivy   Poison Sumac   Poison Oak

Learn how to identify poisonous plants, and remove any you may find in your home or yard. Remember, many common houseplants, including poinsettias, are poisonous when eaten.

Keep your purse out of your child's reach. And be sure to tell guests about this precaution. Keep in mind that your child may associate a purse with gum and candy. But remember, many people also keep medicine, perfume, and chemical sprays in their purses.

Always keep products in original containers. For example, never store paint, gasoline, or kerosene in a glass, or in a milk or soda bottle. In addition, never allow your child to play with containers that contained household cleaners, polishes, or pesticides. Discard the empty containers in a location where your child or pet can't find them.

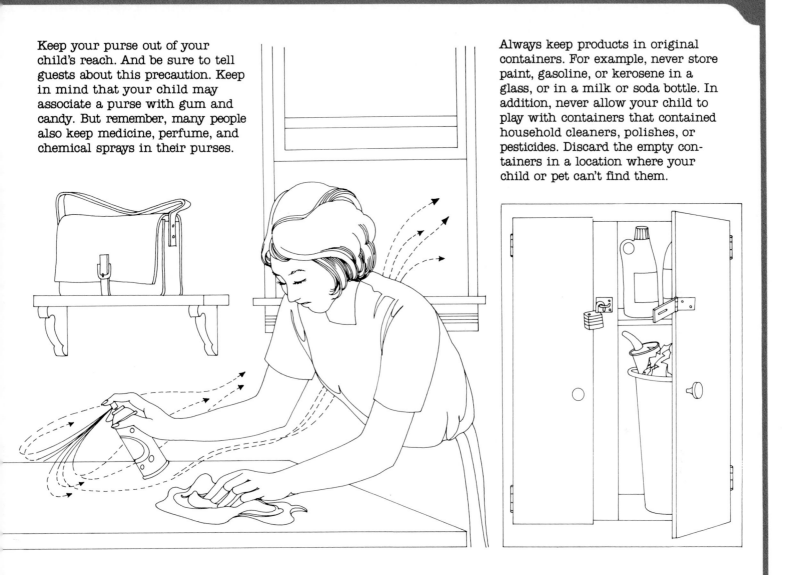

Use cleaning fluid, spray paint, or other poisons only in rooms with adequate ventilation, and avoid breathing vapors. Always follow label directions for protecting eyes and skin. And never mix household poisons together. Doing so may produce toxic or lethal gas.

When dealing with medicine, including vitamins and other over-the-counter drugs, follow these special precautions:
- Lock up all medicines.
- Keep all medicine in child-resistant safety containers. Also, look for safety closures on over-the-counter medicines.
- Never use medicine from an unlabeled bottle. Secure loose labels with transparent adhesive tape, and replace torn ones.

- Give medicine *only* to the person designated on the prescription label.
- If your child takes a specific medicine, check with the doctor before giving him another medicine, even an over-the-counter product like aspirin.
- Never give medicine to your child—or take it yourself—in a dark room. And, when measuring medicine, always pay particular attention to what you're doing.
- Call all medicines by their proper names, and never refer to them as candy.
- Do not take medicine in front of your child. He may try to imitate you and take some himself.
- Flush unused and outdated medicine down the toilet. Then, rinse and discard the container in a location where it's out of reach of your child or pet.

Special problems

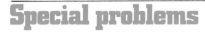

Learning about poison treatment

Do you know what emergency treatment procedures to take when you're caring for a patient who's ingested or inhaled poison? You and your co-workers will work as a team to perform these steps as quickly as possible:
• Make sure his airway's open.
• Closely monitor him for signs and symptoms of respiratory or cardiac depression or arrest. Begin I.V. therapy or other emergency procedures, as needed.
• Identify the poison, and gather as much information about the poisoning as possible.
• Refer to your hospital's updated copy of the National Poison Center Network® Poison Treatment Chart for information on counteracting the poison. Or, contact your local poison treatment center.
• Assist the doctor in poison treatment procedures.
• Obtain specimens of blood, urine, and gastric contents for analysis. Properly label the specimens, and immediately send them to lab.
• Get a complete medical history from the patient (if possible) or his family.

The following chart will give you specific instructions for treating some of the more common types of pediatric poisoning. Study it carefully.

Poison type	Signs and symptoms		Diagnostic indicators
SALICYLATES • Aspirin • Methyl salicylate (Wintergreen Oil)	• Changes in level of consciousness; for example, lethargy, restlessness, disorientation, and coma • If less than 150 mg/kg of aspirin was ingested: deep, rapid respirations; thirst; nausea; tinnitus; hyperventilation; vomiting; and profuse sweating • If more than 150 mg/kg of aspirin was ingested: convulsions, dehydration, decreased sensorium, respiratory failure,	cardiovascular collapse • If methyl salicylate was ingested: wintergreen odor evident around mouth, metabolic acidosis, respiratory alkalosis • Increased body metabolism, prolonged prothrombin time, platelet dysfunction • Hyperglycemia or hypoglycemia possible.	• Blood tests to determine serum salicylate level, body metabolism, prothrombin time, and platelet dysfunction (if present) • Urinalysis to determine acetone and salicylate levels, and pH value
CAUSTICS *Acids* • Metal-cleaning fluid • Some bleaches *Alkalies* • Highly concentrated detergent • Toilet-bowl cleaner • Oven cleaner • Insecticide	• Burning pain in mouth, throat, and stomach experienced immediately after ingestion • Burns around mouth, lips, and tongue possible • Lip edema, drooling • Vomiting • Cramps • Vascular collapse • Possible pulmonary necrosis or glottic edema, caused by aspiration	• Changes in levels of consciousness; for example, lethargy, restlessness, disorientation, and coma • Bloody diarrhea • Several days to a few months after ingestion, esophageal perforation (possibly with mediastinitis or pneumomediastinum) and gastric perforation (possibly with peritonitis)	• Esophagoscopy to determine extent of internal damage
HYDROCARBONS • Kerosene • Lighter fluid • Paint thinner • Gasoline • Furniture polish • Floor wax	• Mucous membrane irritation • Vomiting • Bloody diarrhea • Perianal excoriation • Coughing, gagging, dyspnea, cyanosis, and rales	• Changes in level of consciousness; for example, lethargy, restlessness, disorientation, and coma • Fever possible	• Within 24 hours of ingestion, chest X-rays to identify signs of pneumonia
IRON • Iron tablets • Vitamins with iron	• Orange-brown or burgundy-colored urine on challenge with 50 mg/kg deferoxamine mesylate (Desferal*) • Thirty minutes to 2 hours following ingestion: bloody diarrhea, drowsiness, and fever • Four to 6 hours following ingestion: shock and metabolic acidosis	• Six to 24 hours following ingestion: temporary improvement in signs and symptoms followed by recurrence of symptoms. Signs of liver impairment may also appear. • Twenty-four to 48 hours following ingestion: progressive vascular collapse, convulsions, and coma	• Blood tests to determine elevated serum iron and iron-binding capacity
ACETAMINOPHEN • Tylenol* • Anacin-3	• Between 12 to 24 hours following ingestion: nausea; vomiting; and diaphoresis • Between 24 to 36 hours following ingestion: hepatotoxicity (liver enlargement, tenderness, and jaundice), hyperbilirubinemia, hyperammonemia, and prolonged prothrombin time	• As late as 5 days following ingestion: signs of hepatotoxicity, including upper right quadrant tenderness, and elevated serum glutamic-oxaloacetic transaminase (SGOT), serum glutamic-pyruvic transaminase (SGPT), and serum bilirubin levels.	• Blood tests about 4 hours following ingestion to determine acetaminophen blood level. Concentration in blood plasma greater than 200 mg/ml 4 hours after ingestion, or greater than 50 mg/ml 12 hours after ingestion, may indicate liver damage. • Liver biopsy to determine liver cell necrosis
ORGANOPHOSPHATES • Insecticides, especially those containing parathion or malathion	• Increased salivation • Increased bronchial secretions • Miosis • Blurred vision • Abdominal cramping • Slurred speech	• Muscle fasciculation • Flaccid paralysis • Headache • Rhinorrhea • Respiratory distress • Coma, convulsions	• Serum cholinesterase to determine elevated cholinesterase and white blood cell count • Fasting blood sugar to determine presence of hyperglycemia • Urinalysis to determine presence of albuminuria

*Available in both the United States and in Canada

Nursing interventions

• When a toxic dose greater than 150 mg/kg of a salicylate has been ingested, remove drug from stomach by inducing vomiting or by performing gastric lavage. Administer activated charcoal (Charcocaps) after poison removal.
• If child's dehydrated and has a temperature higher than 101° F. (38.3° C.), use a hyper-hypothermia blanket or tepid water bath to lower temperature.
• Be prepared to administer vitamin K (Aqua-Mephyton*), as ordered, to help relieve bleeding caused by hypoprothrombinemia.

• Administer oxygen, as needed.
• Monitor urinary pH. If patient's acidotic, give 2 to 4 mEq/kg of sodium bicarbonate, to increase urinary pH.
• Administer potassium, as ordered, to replace potassium loss and allow urine alkalinization.
• If patient has a serum salicylate level of 100 to 150 mg/100 ml, or has oliguria, anuria, or heart disease, prepare him for dialysis, as ordered. If he responds poorly to sodium bicarbonate or experiences seizures or coma, dialysis may also be indicated.

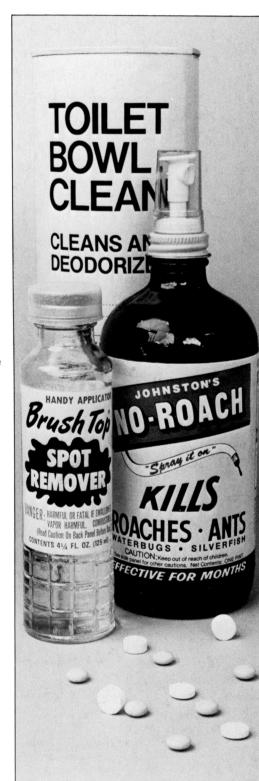

• Do not perform gastric lavage or induce vomiting.
• Prepare the patient for hospital admission.
• If caustic burns are present, don't give the patient anything by mouth.
• If caustic burns aren't evident, and the child can safely swallow, give him one to two glasses of milk to neutralize the poison. If you don't

have milk, give one or two glasses of water instead. *Caution:* Don't neutralize the poison with acid or alkaline products, because an adverse chemical reaction may cause thermal burns.
• Closely evaluate and assess the patient, and prepare him for esophagoscopy, if ordered.
• Administer analgesics, as ordered.

• Do not induce vomiting or perform gastric lavage unless child ingested a potentially lethal dose. Don't give the child anything that may cause spontaneous vomiting.
• Administer humidified oxygen, bronchodilators, and antibiotics, as ordered.

• If the child ingested a potentially lethal dose, and he's alert, administer ipecac syrup to induce vomiting. If he's not alert, assist doctor with cuffed endotracheal tube insertion and gastric lavage.
• If patient has central nervous system, liver, or renal involvement, support vital functions.

• If the child ingested 1 g or more of ferrous sulfate, induce vomiting with ipecac syrup.
• Administer sodium bicarbonate orally to help relieve abdominal discomfort, prevent intestinal erosion, and decrease iron absorption.
• Administer deferoxamine mesylate (Desferal*), as ordered, if patient has any of the following signs and symptoms of severe poisoning: coma, shock, or serum iron level exceeding the iron-binding capacity. But don't give deferoxamine mesylate if signs and symptoms indicate only mild

poisoning. Such signs and symptoms include: vomiting and diarrhea, and burgundy-colored urine after challenging with 50 mg/kg of deferoxamine mesylate.
• If patient develops oliguria or anuria and is receiving deferoxamine mesylate, dialysis may be indicated. Be prepared to assist, as needed. *Important:* Ferrous sulfate must be bound to deferoxamine mesylate for dialysis to be successful.

• Be sure to differentiate acetaminophen overdose from Reye's syndrome and alpha-antitrypsin deficiency in children, and drug abuse and Wilson's disease in adolescents.
• Within 4 hours after ingestion, induce vomiting with ipecac syrup or perform gastric lavage, as ordered.
• Don't force fluids or give drugs to cause diuresis. The kidneys can't eliminate acetaminophen from the blood.

• If patient's acetaminophen level is likely to cause liver damage, contact the Rocky Mountain Poison Center (1-800-525-6115) for details on administering acetylcysteine (Mucomyst*) as an antidote.
• Do not administer activated charcoal (Charcocaps) because it binds with acetylcysteine and reduces the antidote's effectiveness.
• Do not administer enzyme reducers, such as phenobarbital (Luminal*) or alcohol.

• Induce vomiting with ipecac syrup or perform gastric lavage, as ordered.
• To remove poison from skin, wash area thoroughly with copious amounts of running water.
• Administer atropine sulfate, according to doctor's orders.

• Give 20 to 50 mg/kg pralidoxime chloride (Protopam*) I.M. or I.V., as ordered, over 1 hour, to reactivate the blood's cholinesterase.
• Administer oxygen and provide respiratory support, as needed.

Special problems

Understanding lead poisoning

Although lead is contained in a variety of products, this heavy metal is most commonly associated with paint—both interior and exterior. And, of course, paint covers everything from buildings to furniture.

Potential lead poisoning sources are everywhere. For example, water coming through lead pipes, juice kept in an improperly fired ceramic pitcher coated with lead-based glaze, and lead-based paint chips sometimes found in older buildings—all these sources may cause lead poisoning.

What happens when a child ingests lead? For starters, his body absorbs about 10% to 15% of the metal and slowly excretes the rest. Most of the absorbed lead is retained in the child's bones; smaller quantities are stored in bone marrow, soft tissues, and red blood cells.

Suppose the child ingests a lead-based paint chip that's one-fifteenth the size of a dime—and does so daily for several months. In this situation, his body will begin to absorb the lead faster than it's excreted. When this occurs, large amounts of lead accumulate and eventually reach a toxic level. However, the child may ingest lead for 3 to 6 months *before* any signs and symptoms of lead poisoning appear.

Unless lead poisoning is identified and treated, and the source eliminated, toxic lead levels in the body may cause serious complications such as mental retardation and seizures.

Taking action
What can you do? Learn to identify these subtle and nonspecific signs and symptoms of lead poisoning:
- lethargy
- irritability
- clumsiness
- ataxia
- anorexia
- vomiting
- intermittent abdominal pain
- constipation

If your patient has a severe case of lead poisoning, he may also have cortical atrophy, increased intracranial pressure, refractory convulsions, and anemia.

In addition, be alert for any factors that may predispose the child to the risk of lead poisoning; for example, low socioeconomic status or inadequate adult supervision. A child who habitually ingests non-food items is also at risk.

Be sure to gather as much information as possible about the family's socioeconomic, cultural, and environmental background. Find out where the child plays, how water is supplied to the family's home, and how the family stores food and beverages. Also, obtain a careful medical history. Be sure to screen all family members for lead toxicosis. If environmental factors seem to be involved, recommend that the family encourage neighbors to be checked too. Keep in mind that identifying and eliminating the lead source is essential to the child's recovery. You may also prevent others from accidentally ingesting the lead.

If you suspect a child has lead poisoning, check him for an elevated lead level in the blood. As you may know, an elevated blood lead level indicates that lead's been ingested recently. Your next step is to determine the extent of metabolic injury sustained from the lead. To do this, you'll check for elevated free erythrocyte protoporphyrin (FEP) level.

Suppose your patient has lead poisoning. Then, depending on the patient's condition, the doctor will order a chelating agent, such as edetate calcium disodium (Calcium Disodium Versenate*) or dimercaprol (BAL in Oil*) administered parenterally for several days. Both agents bind the lead, producing a stable, soluble complex that's easily excreted by the patient's kidneys. But remember, when administered improperly, these agents can also be toxic.

Helping your patient and his family understand burns

Three-year-old Gaston Dunn is transferred to your unit from the emergency department. Several hours earlier, he accidentally pulled a pot of hot soup onto his chest. From his admission assessment sheet, you learn that he has first- and second-degree burns over 10% of his body. Although the doctor's explained Gaston's condition to the patient and his parents, they seem anxious and confused.

You can help ease their anxiety by doing your best to reassure them about the child's condition. Remember, the patient and his parents may not have understood what the doctor discussed with them. In fact, they may ask *you* about Gaston's burns.

Begin your explanation by telling the Dunns that the terms *first, second,* and *third degree* refer to the burn's severity. Stress that a first-degree burn is the least severe. Tell them the doctor determines the burn's severity by assessing:
- the burn's size and depth
- the child's age
- the type or cause of the burn; for example, a chemical, electrical current, or hot liquid
- the amount of respiratory involvement. (The doctor assumes respiratory involvement if the child has chest, head, or neck burns, or has inhaled hot gases.)
- the child's past and present medical history.

In addition, tell the Dunns about any special equipment Gaston may have in place, such as an indwelling (Foley) catheter, I.V. line, or nasogastric (NG) tube. Also, describe any medication he's receiving, and dressings (if any) that have been applied. So that you're prepared to explain the specifics about Gaston's condition, refresh your own knowledge of burn injuries by reviewing the information and illustration on these pages.

Determining a burn's severity
A first-degree burn is also called a superficial partial-thickness burn because it involves only one or two skin layers. Some possible causes of this type of burn include overexposure to the sun and brief contact with a hot liquid (scald). Usually, the burned area will appear pink or red, with a slightly swollen, dry surface, and without blisters. The area will be painful to the touch and sensitive to temperature changes.

A second-degree burn may also be called a deep partial-thickness burn. A second-degree burn always involves at least two skin layers. Possible causes of this type of burn include:

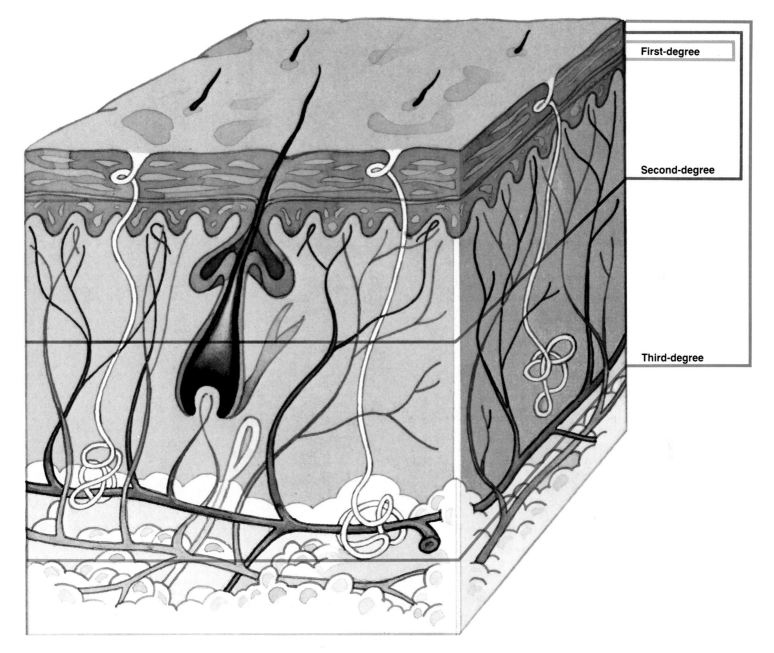

First-degree

Second-degree

Third-degree

- immersion in hot liquid, such as hot bath water
- brief contact with intense heat; for example, by touching a stove's burner
- contact with a hot object, such as a hot coffee pot.

The affected skin will appear pink or red and considerably swollen, and will develop large thick-walled blisters. In addition, it's extremely painful when touched.

A third-degree burn is also called a full-thickness burn because it involves all skin layers. In addition, it extends to underlying tissue, blood vessels, and nerves. Possible

causes of a third-degree burn include the following:
- direct contact with flame
- prolonged contact with a hot surface, such as a stove burner
- chemicals
- electrical current.

Expect the burned skin to be extremely swollen, and white, red, brown, or black in color. It'll also have a waxy texture. You'll find the wound insensitive and leathery to the touch. In some cases, the skin may also be blackened, indicating tissue necrosis or charred tissue.

Providing support
No one needs to tell you that a burned child needs extra support and comfort. But don't forget his parents—they need support, too. Remember, they probably feel guilty about the accident. Do your best to reassure them, and let them express any guilt they feel. If appropriate, suggest ways they can prevent such accidents in the future, and give them a copy of the home care aid on page 129. Document your patient teaching, as well as the details of Gaston's injury and treatment, in your nurses' notes.

Special problems

Burn care: Some reminders

Whether you work in a doctor's office, clinic, or hospital, you'll have to care for a burned child sooner or later. Chances are, you'll see the child even before the doctor does. Will you know what to do?

First, you must assess the child's injuries and determine whether he has first-, second-, or third-degree burns. Then, depending on your assessment, provide the following emergency treatment.

First-degree burn. Moisten sterile 4″x4″ gauze pads in cool sterile water, and place them over the burn. Leave them in place for about 20 minutes (replacing them as necessary, to cool the skin). If necessary, secure the pads with roller gauze, as shown in the first photo. Then, remove the pads and pat dry the burned skin—taking care not to create friction. If necessary to protect the burn, cover it with dry sterile gauze pads and secure them with tape or roller gauze (see second photo). Don't apply tape directly to the burned skin. By covering the burn, you help prevent wound contamination and reduce pain.

Second-degree burn. Follow the same procedure as for a first-degree burn. In addition, observe these precautions:
• Don't pack the area in ice.
• Don't apply any lotions or ointments, unless ordered.
• Don't break blisters or remove dead tissue. Protect blisters with a dressing.
• Elevate a burned extremity above heart level.

Third-degree burn. Consider this an emergency. If you're not already in a hospital, arrange to have the child taken to one immediately. Then, follow these guidelines:
• Don't remove charred clothing.
• Keep the patient as quiet as possible. Because third-degree burns may lead to shock, don't even let him walk.
• Elevate affected extremities above the patient's heart level.

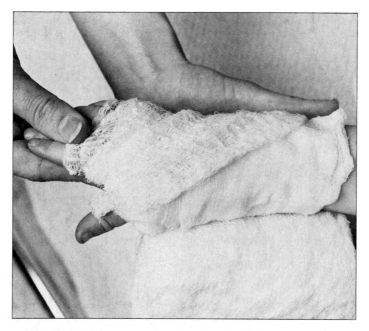

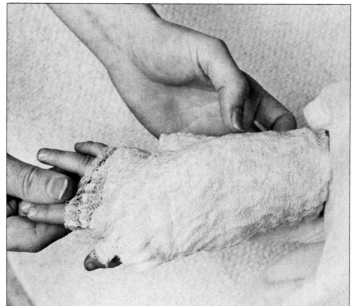

• If his head, throat, or chest is burned, sit or prop him up. Closely monitor his respirations, and continually assess airway patency. Remember, swelling and edema may close his airway, so keep emergency equipment nearby.
• Relieve pain by applying sterile gauze pads moistened in cool sterile water to the burn. But never apply ice or ice water to the burn—you may cause or intensify shock.
• Don't apply any lotions or ointments to the burn, unless ordered.

Document all care given, along with any information you gathered about the accident. If your patient's going to the hospital, send a copy of your notes with him. (For more information on burn care, see the NURSING PHOTOBOOK DEALING WITH EMERGENCIES.)

Preventing burn injuries

Last Wednesday afternoon, 20-month-old Jamie Downing was playing in the kitchen while her mother made lunch. Reaching to open the refrigerator door, Mrs. Downing turned her back for only an instant—but an instant was too long. While her mother wasn't looking, Jamie grabbed a cord dangling from the counter, and pulled a crock of steaming soup down on herself. Parts of her face, shoulders, and chest were severely scalded.

Scald burns can cause severe scarring, especially of the face. Although the injury may heal quickly, disfiguring scar tissue develops within several months. Even expert plastic surgery may not completely repair the damage.

Consider it your job to educate parents about a few common-sense precautions they can take to protect their children from accidental burns. The following home care aid offers suggestions. See that your patient's parents get copies—before it's too late.

Save $1.00 off each NURSING PHOTOBOOK™

Choose your first book. Examine it for 10 days FREE!

Subscribe to the NURSING PHOTOBOOK series and save $1.00 on every volume. That's a significant savings on the entire series. And now you can select your own introductory volume from the books shown or listed.

The NURSING PHOTOBOOK series

Aiding Ambulatory Patients • Assessing Your Patients • Attending Ob/Gyn Patients • Caring for Surgical Patients • Carrying Out Special Procedures • Controlling Infection • Coping with Neurologic Disorders • Dealing with Emergencies • Ensuring Intensive Care • Giving Cardiac Care • Giving Medications • Helping Geriatric Patients • Implementing Urologic Procedures • Managing I.V. Therapy • Nursing Pediatric Patients • Performing GI Procedures • Providing Early Mobility • Providing Respiratory Care • Using Monitors • Working with Orthopedic Patients

This is your order card. Send no money.

Please send me _____
for a 10-day, free examination. If I decide to keep this introductory volume, I agree to pay $14.95, plus shipping and handling. I understand that I will receive another PHOTOBOOK approximately every other month, each on the same 10-day, free-examination basis. There is no minimum number of books I must buy, and I may cancel my subscription at any time simply by notifying you.

G3-PB

I don't want the series. Just send me _____
I will pay $15.95 for each copy, plus shipping and handling. Please send me _____
copies and bill me.

G3-SP

Name _____

Address _____

City _____ State _____ Zip _____

Price subject to change. Offer valid in U.S. only. Pa. residents please add 6% sales tax.

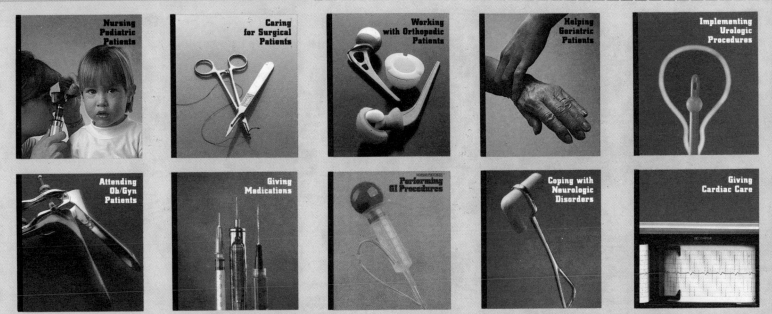

© 1983 Intermed Communications, Inc.

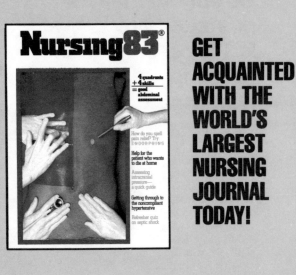
Keep your nursing skills growing... with *Nursing83*.®

Keep up to date on the latest breakthroughs in nursing care every month in *Nursing83*. With *Nursing83*, you'll be the first to learn about the new techniques and procedures that will mean more skills and knowledge for you... better care for your patients. All in a magazine that's easy to read, easy to understand, and colorfully illustrated to show *you* how to improve your nursing care.

☐ Send me 1 year (12 issues) of *Nursing83*. My check for $16 is enclosed, saving me $4 off the regular $20 price.

☐ Please bill me later for $16.

Name _____

Address _____

City _____ State _____ Zip _____

I am an: ☐ RN ☐ LPN ☐ Other   Do you work in a hospital? ☐ Yes ☐ No

7P83

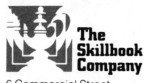
Introduce yourself to the brand-new NURSING PHOTOBOOK™ series

…the remarkable breakthrough in nursing education that can change your career. Each book in this unique series contains detailed *Photostories*… and tables, charts, and graphs to help you learn important new procedures. And each handsome PHOTOBOOK offers you • 160 illustrated, fact-filled pages • brilliant, high-contrast photographs • convenient 9"x10½" size • durable, hardcover binding • carefully chosen bibliography • complete index. Watch the experts at work showing you how to… administer drugs… teach your patient about his illness and its treatment… minimize trauma… understand doctors' diagnoses… increase patient comfort… and much more. Discover how you can become a better nurse by joining this exciting new series. You can examine each PHOTOBOOK at your leisure… for 10 days *absolutely free!*

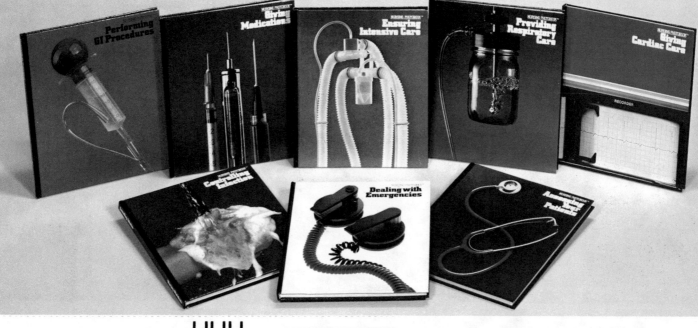

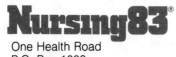
Be sure to mail the postage-paid card at left to reserve *your* first copy of *Nursing83.*

Nursing83 gives you clear, concise instruction in "hands-on" nursing. Every issue brings you in-depth clinical articles about the newest developments in nursing care—what's being discovered, researched, treated, cured. You'll learn about the new procedures, new techniques, new medications, and new equipment that will mean more skills and knowledge for you…better care for your patients!

Order your subscription today!

Home care

Protecting your toddler from burns

Dear Parent:
As a parent, you know how quickly an active toddler can get into trouble. You also know that few injuries are as painful and frightening to a child as a bad burn. To protect your child, take these simple—but very important—precautions.

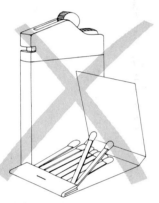

Keep matches and lighters out of your child's reach.

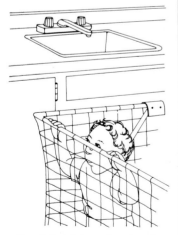

Don't let him play in the kitchen, unless he's in a playpen. You may trip over him or his toys, spilling hot food on him.

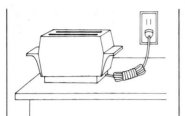

Make sure electrical cords don't hang over counters, tables, or ironing boards. The child may pull a hot toaster, iron, or crock pot on himself.

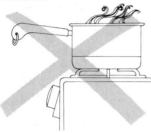

Don't let pot handles stick out over the edge of the stove. The child may grab at them.

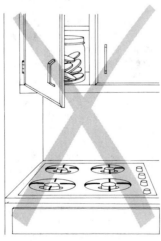

Don't store candy or cookies on the stove or behind it—the child may try to climb on the stove to find them.

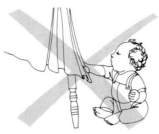

Don't use tablecloths. A toddler may try to pull himself up by grabbing a tablecloth and pull everything on the table on top of him.

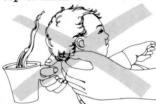

Don't hold the child while drinking hot coffee or tea—or any hot drink. If he bumps your arm, you may splash him with hot liquid.

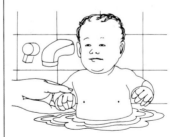

Don't leave any child alone in the bathtub—even for an instant. Remember, a child likes to turn knobs. He may turn on the hot water faucet and burn himself. As an extra precaution, make sure your hot water heater is set no higher than 130° F. (54.4° C.).

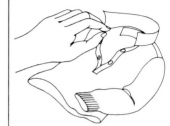

Check labels on the child's clothing and bedding. Make sure all clothing and bedding are nonflammable.

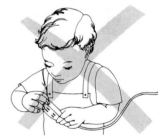

Don't let him play with—or chew on—electrical cords, including extension cords.

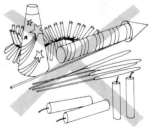

Be especially careful during holidays. Keep your child away from Christmas tree lights and cords. Don't allow him to play with fireworks or sparklers. And keep him away from flames, including candle flames, when he's dressed in a Halloween costume, especially a homemade costume.

Special problems

SPECIAL CONSIDERATIONS

Coping with frostbite

You're working in a clinic one winter day when 4-year-old Ricky Thompson comes in, accompanied by his mother. Ricky's fingers are blanched and without sensation. You immediately recognize the problem—frostbite. Although you may see many frostbite victims each winter, you never take the problem lightly. Left untreated—or treated improperly—frostbite can lead to tissue ulceration, necrosis, and gangrene.

Frostbite occurs when ice crystals form in the tissues and expand into extracellular spaces. The cell membranes eventually rupture, releasing histamine and causing red blood cell clumping and microvascular occlusion. As the tissue thaws, edema develops, further compromising blood supply to the injured tissue.

Superficial frostbite affects skin and subcutaneous tissue, most commonly of the face, ears, and other exposed body parts. Deep frostbite affects deeper tissues, commonly of the feet and hands.

A child suffering from superficial frostbite may not notice the condition while he's outside playing. But when he goes inside and his skin begins to warm, he may experience burning, tingling, numbness, skin mottling, and a grayish skin color. (If he's black, the affected skin becomes darker than the surrounding skin.) If deep tissues are affected, his skin will be white until thawed; then, it will turn purplish-blue (or very dark, if he's black). Deep frostbite also produces pain and skin blisters.

To prevent further injury, take these immediate steps:
• Remove constrictive clothing, and gradually rewarm the affected part in tepid water (100° to 105° F.; 37.8° to 40.6° C.). If the affected part's on his face, apply warm, moist towels. Also, give him warm fluids to drink. *Important:* Never rub the injured area, since this aggravates tissue damage.
• When the affected part begins to warm, the child will feel a tingling sensation and may complain of severe pain. His skin will look flushed and feel warm. Remove the affected area from the tepid water, and gently but thoroughly pat it dry. Check for a pulse. (If you don't detect one, notify the doctor at once.) Then, wrap the area in a bulky sterile dressing. If the injury is on the foot, place cotton or gauze pads between the toes to prevent maceration. To prevent pressure on injured feet, instruct the child not to walk.
• If possible, elevate affected parts to reduce edema.
• Give analgesics, as ordered, for pain. If the injury has caused vesicles, protect them so they don't burst. If they do (or if any type of open wound develops), give antibiotics and tetanus toxoid prophylactically, as ordered. (Of course, first make sure the child's not allergic to the medication.)
• Frequently assess circulation in the affected limb by feeling for pulses and checking blanching time. If pulses don't return, the doctor may perform a fasciotomy to reduce pressure from limb edema and maintain existing circulation. Severe damage or infection may make amputation necessary.

Document the condition and treatment, including the size and color of the affected area. Also, note the circumstances causing the injury. (If your patient developed frostbite because his parents are unable to provide adequate clothing or housing, refer him and his family to an appropriate social agency.)

Because the full extent of damage from frostbite may not be evident for several days, the doctor may hospitalize the child for further observation. If so, send a copy of your notes to the hospital.

Inform parents that the child may suffer some long-term effects; for example, increased sensitivity to cold and burning or tingling sensations. A deep frostbite injury may damage epiphyseal plates at the end of long bones, causing orthopedic deformity as the child grows. Warn them that permanent tissue damage may result if previously frostbitten skin refreezes.

Preventing cold injuries

Take this opportunity to teach the child's parents how to protect him from cold. Offer these suggestions:
• Dress him in mittens, not gloves, and provide many-layered clothing. Dress him in water-resistant fabrics, if possible.
• Provide at least two pairs of socks: cotton socks next to his skin, and wool socks over them. But don't apply so many socks that circulation's impaired.
• Cover the child's neck and head (including his ears) with a ski mask or a scarf and hat. Inform parents that a child loses significant amounts of body heat through his head, unless it's adequately protected.
• Encourage the child to come inside and change his clothes if he gets wet.

Assessing a patient for multiple traumatic injuries

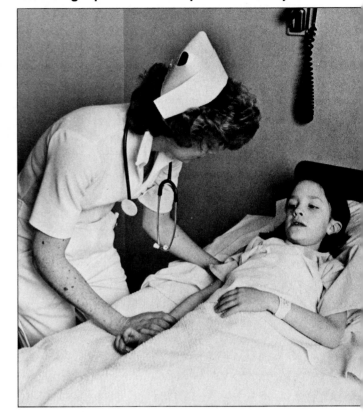

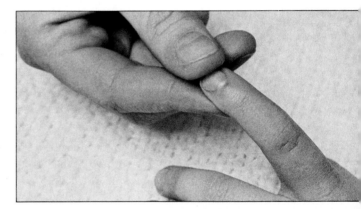

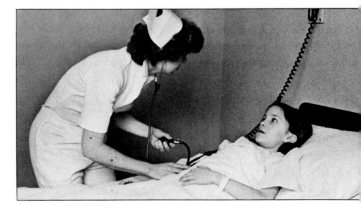

1 *You've just come on duty when Sandra Curnow, age 8, is admitted to your unit for observation following an automobile accident. Although Sandra had a complete assessment in the emergency department (ED), the doctor orders a head-to-toe assessment every hour for the first 4 hours to identify any developing signs or symptoms of multiple trauma. Here's how to proceed with your initial assessment:*

Before you start, review the assessment data and history gathered in the ED. Particularly note the patient's level of consciousness right after the accident. You'll want to watch carefully for any suspected complications noted in the ED.

Now, begin your assessment by determining Sandra's level of consciousness. For example, is she awake and alert? If she isn't awake, try calling her name.

When your patient's awake, explain the assessment procedure to her and encourage her to ask questions. Does she understand what you're saying? Are her answers appropriate? If everything's okay, she'll be oriented as to person, place, and time. To help reduce Sandra's anxiety, continue to talk to her as you continue with the assessment.

2 Suppose you can't awaken your patient by calling her name or shaking her arm. Apply firm fingertip pressure to her nailbed, as the nurse is doing here. Document how she responds—and how quickly.

3 Next, check Sandra's blood pressure in both arms. If possible, check her blood pressure while she's sitting up and lying down.

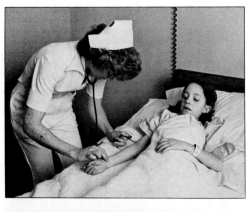

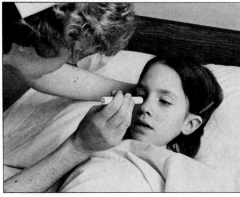

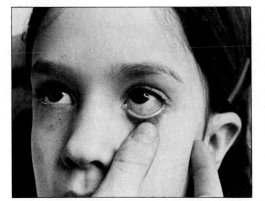

4 Take Sandra's radial, femoral, popliteal, and pedal pulses bilaterally. Compare for rate, rhythm, and equality. Remember, loss of a pulse may indicate tissue or vessel damage proximal to the lost pulse.

5 Now you're ready to assess Sandra's pupils. If all's well, they'll appear round, and equal in size and shape.

Then, darken the room slightly, and check Sandra's pupillary response to light. To do this, shine a penlight into one eye, then the other. Expect each pupil to constrict in response to the light. Sandra's pupil constriction should be consensual: when one pupil constricts in response to light, the other should constrict, too. Be sure to document the speed of pupillary response.

6 Next, gently pull down on her cheek as shown here, and observe the color of her conjunctiva. Repeat the procedure for the other eye. Also, closely examine each eye for lacerations, contusions, excessive tearing, or dryness. Keep in mind that excessive tearing or reddened conjunctivae may indicate irritation from a foreign body or infection. Dryness or pallor may suggest hypovolemia or a sympathetic nerve lesion.

7 Now, check Sandra's ears, nose, and mouth for drainage, bruises, abrasions, and edema. Suspect a facial fracture if you see periorbital edema. If drainage is present, note the color, amount, and consistency. Document the size and location of any bruises, abrasions, or edema. Then, examine her face for symmetry and color.

Important: If your patient's dark-skinned, note the color of her conjunctivae, palms, and the soles of her feet before evaluating any facial color changes.

Check for swelling around your patient's mouth and nose. If you see any, be alert for a possible airway obstruction.

Special problems

Assessing a patient for multiple traumatic injuries continued

8 Carefully examine Sandra's head and scalp for lacerations and tissue injuries. If you feel soft areas on her skull, suspect a depressed skull fracture.

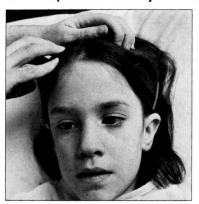

9 Now, ask her to open her mouth. Use a penlight and tongue depressor to check inside, as the nurse is doing here. Look for cyanosis, bleeding, missing teeth, or edema. Is edema present? Then monitor her closely for an airway obstruction.

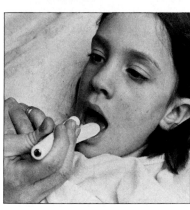

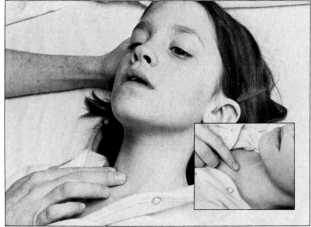

10 Unless contraindicated (for example, because of back injury), elevate the head of the bed to a 45° angle. Examine Sandra's neck, and palpate her jugular veins, as shown in this photo. If they're distended, pulsating, or collapsed, she may have a pulmonary or right-sided heart complication.

[Inset] Then, slide your finger over her suprasternal notch. If the trachea's shifted from midposition, check her breath sounds. She may have tension pneumothorax, hemothorax, or a pleural effusion.

Suppose you feel crepitus on palpation? Suspect subcutaneous emphysema from a damaged trachea, or pneumothorax.

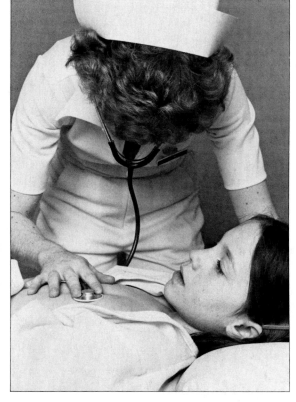

11 After lowering the bed, open Sandra's gown so you can see her chest. Carefully assess her chest for lacerations, deformities, rashes, or scars. Also, note whether her chest movements are symmetrical, and if her sternum retracts during inspiration.

Using a stethoscope, listen to Sandra's breath sounds, as shown here. Observe the rate and rhythm of her respirations and document any abnormal patterns. Then, count her apical heart rate and note any rhythm irregularities.

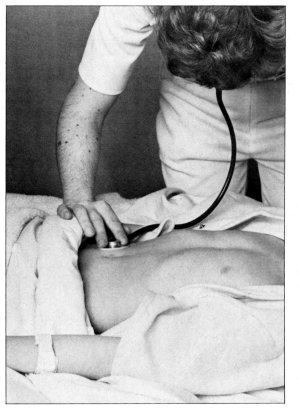

12 Now, assess Sandra's abdomen for masses, lacerations, and distention. Is her flank bluish (Turner's sign), or the skin around her umbilicus purplish? If so, blood may be collecting in her abdomen from internal injuries. Notify the doctor.

Suppose everything's okay. Then, listen for bowel sounds *before* you palpate her abdomen (see page 26 for information on this procedure). Count her peristaltic sounds, as the nurse is doing here. Expect to hear 15 to 34 sounds per minute. If you hear fewer sounds, suspect internal injury.

13 Gently percuss her entire abdomen. If you note a fixed area of dullness when you percuss her left upper abdominal quadrant, suspect a subcapsular or extracapsular hematoma of Sandra's spleen. Notify the doctor immediately.

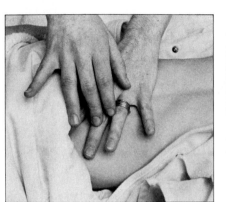

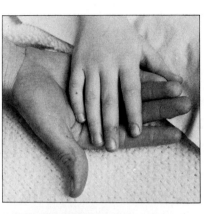

16 Now, check Sandra's nailbeds, as the nurse is doing here. Look for signs of cyanosis and pallor.

14 Next, gently palpate her abdomen for tenderness, bladder distention, and unusual masses. As you work, try to distinguish between local and referred pain, spasm rigidity, and rebound tenderness. Ask your patient to describe the location and type of pain she's experiencing. For example, ask her if the pain's shooting, constant, or intermittent, and whether she's felt the pain before. Does anything make it better or worse?

Next, check Sandra's genitals and perineum. Look for avulsed tissue, scars, or discharge. If there's discharge, note the color, amount, and consistency. Look for ecchymosis on her labia, which may indicate a fractured pelvis. If present, notify the doctor.

Note any urinary or fecal incontinence or bloody urine. These may indicate kidney or bladder damage.

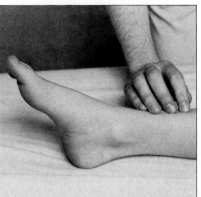

17 Closely observe Sandra's ankles. Do they appear swollen? If they do, gently depress the skin directly over her lower tibia, as shown here. Does the depression made by your finger remain? If it does, your patient may have pitting edema from an injury. Also, look for abrasions, bruises, and evidence of fracture.

15 Have Sandra perform range-of-motion movements of her arms and legs, unless contraindicated. Does she experience pain when she moves them? Note any impairment in sensation, skin color changes, bruises, or abrasions.

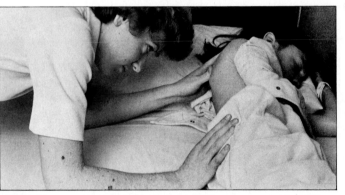

18 Now, position Sandra on her side, so you can check her back. Look for lacerations, hematomas, and other abnormalities. Remember, a hematoma at the patient's lumbar spine area may indicate an internal hemorrhage, probably from a fractured pelvis or vertebra. Notify the doctor immediately.

When you complete your assessment, document your findings in your nurses' notes. Notify the doctor immediately if you noted any inconsistencies with the data gathered in the ED, found any previously uncharted damage, or observed any change in your patient's level of consciousness.

Your next hourly assessment will probably take less time. Why? Because you've already established a data baseline. As you perform the next assessment, continue to look for drainage, hematomas, and changes in the patient's skin color and level of consciousness. Thoroughly document each assessment, and notify the doctor of any changes.

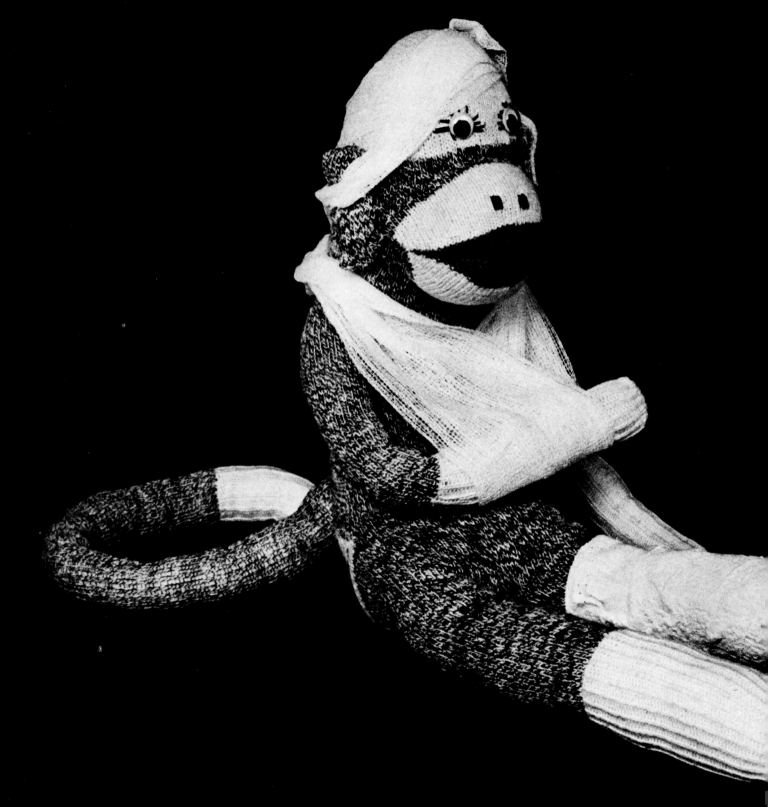

Providing Special Care

Cleft lip and palate

Orthopedics

Special challenges

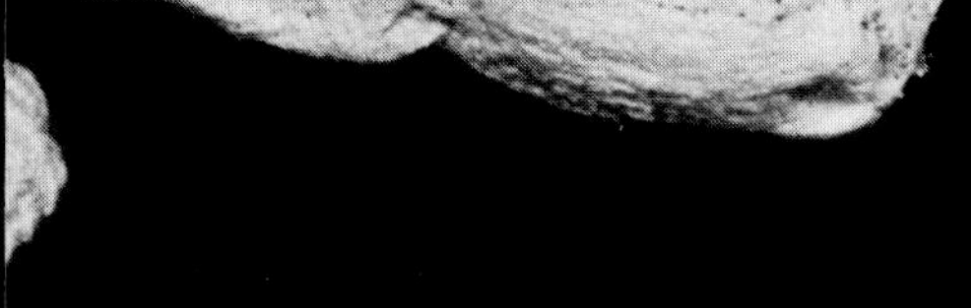

Cleft lip and palate

Would you be surprised to learn that cleft lip and cleft palate are common birth defects? About one out of every 700 infants has a cleft lip, with or without a cleft palate. Because these defects handicap the child physically and emotionally, you need to give him special care and support. And, of course, you must provide extra emotional support and teaching for the child's parents, too.

On the following pages, we'll discuss the information you'll need to perform these tasks. For instance, you'll learn:
• the various types of cleft lip and cleft palate and how they may be corrected through surgery.
• how to feed an affected child before and after surgery.
• how to prepare the parents to care for their child.

Learning about cleft lip and cleft palate

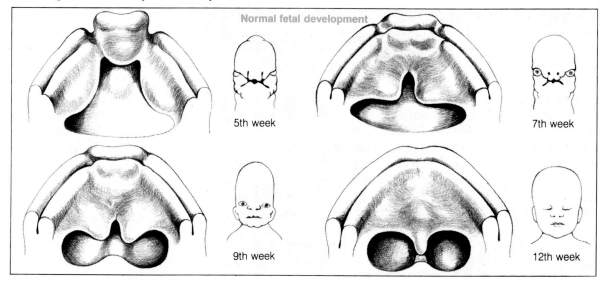

Normal fetal development

5th week

7th week

9th week

12th week

Although cleft lip and cleft palate are common birth defects, their precise cause remains a mystery. What's known is that between the seventh and twelfth weeks of gestation, the mouth and facial features of the fetus don't form properly.

For a look at normal mouth development, examine the above illustrations. The cleft lip defect probably originates at about the seventh week. Normally at that time, two horseshoe-shaped swellings appear on each side of the face and slowly move toward the middle; they eventually form the nostrils. Tissue just below the nostrils also moves together to form the upper lip. When this fusion doesn't take place, a cleft lip results.

Cleft palate may occur a few weeks later in gestation. As the neck and jaws of the fetus are formed, the tongue separates the two sides of the palate. Normally, the tongue moves downward, and the two sides of the secondary palate fuse together above it. If this movement's delayed, or the tongue doesn't descend, the palate won't fuse.

Since the lip and the palate develop separately, a child can have a cleft lip, a cleft palate, or both.

Clefts of the lip can appear on one side of a child's mouth (unilateral), or on both sides (bilateral).

The severity varies; the cleft may involve only the vermilion (darkened) tissue of the lip, or it may extend to the nose.

Cleft palate also varies in severity. It may affect only the uvula and the soft palate (the rear of the mouth); or it may extend from the soft palate into the hard palate. A cleft that stretches into only one nasal cavity is called a unilateral cleft palate; a bilateral cleft palate affects both nasal cavities.

About one child out of every six born with a cleft lip—either with or without cleft palate—has at least one other birth defect. The most common of these defects are fusing together of the child's fingers and toes (syndactyly), extra fingers or toes (polydactyly), malformed ears, spina bifida, congenital heart disease, clubfoot (talipes), and absence of external genitalia.

Helping the parents

The cleft lip defect can be seen at birth. And, because it's so obvious, parents may be shocked when they first see their new child. Emphasize positive aspects of the child's appearance to the parents, and remind them the defect can probably be surgically corrected.

The cleft palate defect, without cleft lip, isn't as noticeable. The cleft's usually detected by the doctor when he examines the child shortly after birth. Or, the cleft

may be discovered when the child has difficulty sucking or swallowing during his first feedings.

As a nurse, you'll help prepare the parents for the long-term health care their child will need. Most children with cleft lip or cleft palate will have some degree of impaired speech, and may need the help of a speech therapist to correct speech problems.

Because the defect causes the child to breathe through his mouth more than a normal child does, the shape of his mouth will change. Advise parents that the child will have dental problems related to the defect, and recommend that they seek special dental care to straighten the child's teeth and correct the shape of his jaw.

Also tell parents that a child born with a cleft palate is more susceptible to upper respiratory tract infections. He's also more susceptible to ear infections, primarily because the eustachian tube can't drain the middle ear properly. Recurring middle ear infections may result in hearing loss. To prevent hearing loss, he'll need frequent assessment and treatment by an otolaryngologist and an audiologist.

Emphasize to parents that in addition to surgery, their child will need a lot of special care, love, and understanding to overcome the defect. On the following pages, we'll show you how to help them.

Using special feeding techniques

Because an infant with a cleft lip and/or cleft palate can't suck properly, you can't feed him with a normal nipple device. And, because he must suck to compress the areola, his mother won't be able to breast-feed him. He'll need the special nipples and feeding devices shown at right to help him obtain nutrition and encourage him to use his sucking muscles, which are important in later speech development.

In general, feeding techniques are the same as for any infant. But do remember to follow these special guidelines:

• Allow extra time to feed the infant. You may need as long as 90 minutes for each feeding.

• Always position him upright for feeding. Remember, an infant with a cleft defect swallows a lot of air during feedings and vomits easily. By keeping him in an upright position you reduce the risk of aspiration.

• If you're feeding him milk, thicken it by adding a small amount of cereal. By doing so, you'll make the milk easier for him to swallow.

• If the mother was planning to breast-feed the infant, teach her how to remove milk with a breast pump. Then, she can feed him her own milk using the special device chosen.

• If you're using a nipple device, gently press it well into his mouth. By putting as much of it as possible into his mouth (without choking him, of course), you make sucking easier for him.

• Don't remove the feeding device from the infant's mouth unnecessarily, even though he may make unusual noises during the procedure. If you frequently remove the device, he may start to cry, making feeding more difficult.

• Frequently burp the infant, to expel the air he'll swallow during the feeding and reduce the risk of vomiting.

• Give him water after each feeding, to rinse away milk that adheres to his tongue and mucous membranes.

• Using a cotton-tipped applicator, apply cold cream or baby oil to the infant's lips to prevent drying and cracking. But, only use a small amount so his lips don't become too soft. (Soft lips may not hold sutures well following corrective surgery and may decrease the limited sucking strength he has.)

• Use a damp washcloth to gently wipe away any milk or other food that may have entered the child's nose and drained from it. Pat his skin dry.

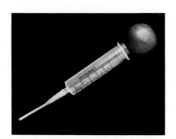

Rubber-tipped bulb syringe
Bulb syringe with rubber tubing on the end

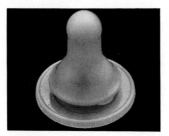

Preemie nipple
Nipple with an enlarged hole, allowing liquid food to drip out slowly; infant doesn't have to suck as hard

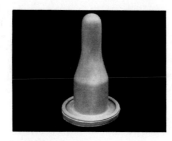

Lamb's nipple
Long, soft nipple delivers food to the back of the throat, making swallowing easier

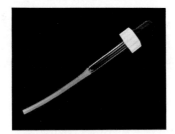

Rubber-tipped medication dropper
Ordinary medication dropper with rubber tubing on the end; good for administering small amounts of medication or fluid

Caring for a child with a cleft palate

Susan Moore's worried—even a little scared. She'll soon leave the hospital with her new son, Christopher, who was born with a cleft palate. And, since the doctor's decided to wait until after Christopher's first birthday to perform surgery, Mrs. Moore will have to provide special care for the next 12 months.

You can help Mrs. Moore prepare. Before she leaves the hospital, set aside plenty of time to teach her how to care for her son.

In addition, provide as much emotional support as possible. Assure her that surgery will correct the defect. Encourage her to express her feelings, and remain supportive if she expresses negative feelings.

Chances are, she'll feel more comfortable with her son when she's confident about caring for him. To teach her, use the following guidelines.

• Help her choose the best method for feeding her child. Choose a method she's comfortable with, so she can easily feed Christopher by herself. But, no matter what device she chooses, ask her to periodically feed him with a bulb syringe with rubber tubing attached. For a short time after surgery, he'll eat with this device. If possible, give Mrs. Moore the equipment to take home with her.

• Encourage Mrs. Moore to teach him to eat from a wide-bowl spoon, such as a soup spoon, and drink from a glass, as soon as he's old enough to sip. After surgery, Christopher may feed from these devices, too.

• Stress the importance of adequate nutrition for Christopher. Tell her to call her doctor for advice if she has any problems feeding him.

• Tell her to frequently position the child on his abdomen, so he becomes accustomed to this position. After surgery, he may be positioned this way.

• Also, ask her to periodically restrain Christopher's arms, since restraints are necessary following surgery. If possible, give her arm restraints to take home. Make sure she knows how to safely use them.

• Warn her that because of his defect, Christopher won't be able to speak properly until after his surgery. But tell her to encourage him to make sounds anyway.

• Urge Mrs. Moore to discourage him from sucking his thumb. He may alter the shape of his mouth, making surgical repair more difficult.

• Inform her that Christopher's very susceptible to upper respiratory infections, and advise her to keep him away from anyone who has a contagious disease, such as a cold or flu. Tell her to contact the doctor immediately if he develops an infection.

• Also inform her that the defect makes Christopher susceptible to ear infections and that recurring infections may affect his hearing ability. Advise her to have his hearing ability assessed by the age of 6 weeks, and once a month thereafter.

• Remind her that Christopher needs the same amount of stimulation, contact, and affection as any child.

Note: If Mrs. Moore wonders if other children she may have will be similarly affected, advise her to consult her doctor. For further assistance and support, refer her to an appropriate community agency or to the American Cleft Palate Educational Foundation, Inc., 331 Salk Hall, Pittsburgh, PA 15261.

Cleft lip and palate

Learning about surgical repair

Is one of your patients scheduled for surgical repair of a cleft lip or palate? Most likely, his parents need help understanding the procedure. Prepare yourself to answer their questions by reviewing the following.

Repairing a cleft lip

When will the doctor schedule cleft lip repair? That depends on the child's condition, the parents' ability to adjust to his appearance, and the doctor's own preference. For example, some doctors prefer to perform surgical repair shortly after the child's birth, to make his appearance less upsetting to the parents and to minimize any embarrassment or shame they may feel. But other doctors prefer to wait until the child's 2 or 3 months old, when he's stronger and better able to withstand surgery. Also, the delay gives the doctor a chance to identify other possible anomalies accompanying the cleft defect.

To repair a cleft lip, the doctor will probably stagger suture lines, as shown below, to lessen the risk of a notch in the

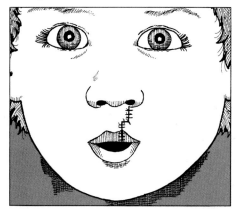

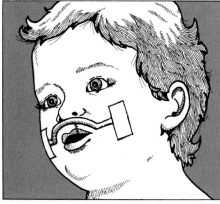

lip from scar tissue retraction. To reduce strain on the suture line, he may tape a curved metal device called a Logan Bow (see illustration above) over the child's

lip, for the first 24 postoperative hours.

Tell parents that the resulting scar will eventually fade, but will always be slightly visible. Further surgery (primarily cosmetic) may be indicated as the child gets older.

Repairing a cleft palate

Under most circumstances, the doctor will repair a cleft palate when the child's between ages 1 and 2—although the child may be as young as 9 months or as old as age 5. The precise time chosen for surgery depends on the severity of the cleft, the child's growth and development, and the doctor's preference.

To repair a cleft palate, he'll make incisions that release the soft tissues on both sides of the hard and soft palates. Then, he'll join together the tissues in the middle (see illustration below).

If the defect's severe, the doctor may try to keep the cleft from widening before surgery. He'll do this by wiring the two sides of the palate together. Then, the corrective surgery's easier to perform.

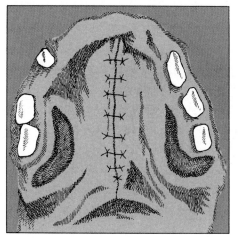

If the palate can't be repaired while the child's young, the doctor may decide to insert an artificial palate. This device blocks off the cleft, enabling the child to eat normally and develop near-normal speech patterns.

The doctor may also use an artificial device if the child doesn't have enough tissue available to close off the cleft. Or, he may take some tissue from another part of the child's throat, creating a graft over the site.

The child with a cleft palate may face cosmetic and other additional surgery, particularly on his nose and jaw. Cosmetic surgery on his nose will probably be delayed until he's a teenager, when bone growth's nearly complete.

Caring for a child after surgery

A child who's just undergone surgical repair of a cleft lip or cleft palate needs special care. Do you know how to provide it?

As you'll see from the information below, care varies somewhat, according to the type of surgery performed. But these specific guidelines apply to all your patients:
• Following surgery, position the child on his side until he's fully recovered from the anesthetic. This position allows oral secretions to drain out of his mouth, reducing the risk of aspiration. If necessary, gently aspirate excessive secretions with a small, soft catheter.
• To prevent injury to the surgical site, restrain the child's arms with arm restraints (see pages 47 and 48). But don't use restraints as a substitute for personal attention. Frequently reposition the child. Remove the restraints at least once every 2 hours, and examine his skin for signs of irritation.
• Whenever possible, hold him in your arms, or prop him up in an infant seat; encourage his parents to hold and play with him, too. These measures help stimulate him, without risking injury to the surgical site. In addition to making him happier, the activity helps prevent secretions from accumulating in his respiratory tract.
• After feeding the child, position him on his *right* side, to reduce the risk of vomiting.

What special considerations must you keep in mind for each of the two types of surgery? Let's first consider a child who's undergone cleft lip repair.

Providing care after cleft lip repair

During the postoperative period, focus your care on these areas.
Protecting the site:
After the child's fully recovered from the anesthetic, place him on his back. This position prevents him from rubbing his lip on the bed. To keep him from rubbing his mouth with his upper arms, pin the arm restraints to his gown or bed linen. If he's old enough to roll over, also apply a jacket restraint. (For more on jacket restraints, see page 49.) *Note:* When you place the child on his back after feeding him, remember to elevate his head.
Cleansing the site:
The child probably will have a small adhesive bandage strip in place. To keep the surgical site clean, change the bandage about 2 hours after the child

returns from surgery, and about every 6 hours thereafter, for 24 hours. (After 24 hours, the doctor will probably order the bandage removed.)

To remove the bandage, grasp each end, and simultaneously pull them toward the middle, as shown below. Be gentle. This way, you won't stretch the suture line.

Nursing tip: If the bandage is hard to remove, moisten it with sterile water or sterile normal saline solution.

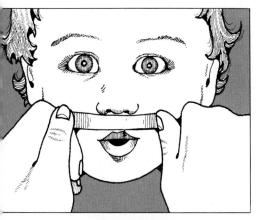

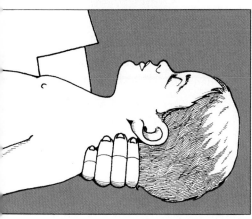

Next, use a cotton-tipped applicator dipped in sterile normal saline solution or hydrogen peroxide solution to cleanse the surgical site. After cleansing, rinse the site and pat it dry with clean applicators. Also cleanse the child's nostrils with an applicator dipped in sterile water or saline solution.
Feeding the child:
After the child's recovered from the anesthetic, begin feeding him clear liquids. To prevent him from sucking before his lip heals, use a bulb syringe with rubber tubing (see page 137). Direct the tubing toward the side and back of his mouth. When the surgical wound has healed, resume regular bottle feedings.

Providing care after cleft palate repair
Because cleft palate repair may involve the hard and soft palates, you'll need to take some additional precautions to prevent postoperative complications.
Preventing respiratory complications:
To prevent airway obstruction from edema, the doctor may insert a nasopharyngeal airway. If your patient has one in place, suction it every 2 to 4 hours, using a small, soft catheter.

Suppose, despite your best efforts, his airway becomes obstructed. Try to clear his airway by positioning his head and neck as shown in the lower illustration at left. Then, notify the doctor, and prepare to intubate the child by inserting a small endotracheal tube in his nose or mouth. *Important:* The child may have a small suture that holds his tongue in place. If so, you may have to cut the suture and pull his tongue forward to relieve the obstruction. Keep a suture set at the child's bedside.

Expect to see moderate oozing from the site for several days postoperatively.
Protecting the site:
Since the surgical site's internal, you may position the child on his abdomen without risking injury to the site. Also, although you'll still apply arm restraints, you may not have to pin them to his gown or bed linens.
Cleansing the site:
To cleanse the surgical site, fill a medication syringe with sterile normal saline solution, and remove the needle. Place the syringe inside the child's mouth, and carefully irrigate the suture line. Cleanse the site before and after each feeding, and as needed. Take care not to put anything else that's hard inside the child's mouth for 3 weeks following surgery.
Feeding the child:
Initially, use a bulb syringe with rubber tubing to feed the child, as you would for feeding a child following cleft lip repair. After 24 to 48 hours, however, an older child may resume using whatever feeding equipment he's familar with; for example, a cup or wide-bowl (soup) spoon. But don't let him use a nipple; sucking may damage the surgical site.

Let the child set the pace for the feeding, but allow plenty of time. Remember to frequently burp him, since he'll probably swallow a lot of air.
Note: Don't give the child milk for at least 24 hours after surgery, or until ordered by the doctor. Milk increases mucus secretions, making cleansing the site more difficult.

Teaching home care after corrective surgery

If your patient's recovering from cleft lip or cleft palate surgery, you'll have to teach his parents how to care for him at home. If necessary, review the preceding guidelines for postoperative care. (Keep in mind that some guidelines are specifically for either cleft lip or cleft palate repair.) Then, carefully explain all aspects of care to his parents, including special instructions and precautions for feeding and using restraints. Also, make sure they have all the equipment they'll need at home.

As you teach, emphasize that they must perform all procedures *gently*, to avoid injuring the surgical site. Then, depending on the type of surgery performed, give them these additional special instructions:
• If your child's recovering from cleft lip surgery, cleanse his lip two or three times a day. Gently wipe the area with a cotton-tipped swab dipped in mild soap and warm water. Also use a swab dipped in water to remove crusted material from around his nostrils. Rinse the skin with a clean swab dipped in water, and pat the skin dry.

To keep the skin around his lip and nostrils from becoming dry, gently apply a small amount of cold cream or oil. But, wipe off excess cream or oil, so his skin doesn't become too soft. Soft skin may cause his stitches to become loose.
• If your child's had cleft palate surgery, he'll probably have little feeling on the roof of his mouth for several months following surgery. Because of this, you may accidentally hurt the palate without realizing it. To avoid doing so, make sure you don't place anything hard into his mouth, such as your fingers, hard candy, or a toothbrush, fork, knife, or spoon.

During the first week he's home from the hospital, give him only liquids and very soft foods, such as gelatin, ice cream, and custard. After that first week, you can add other soft foods, such as well-cooked vegetables, cooked fruits without skins, cooked cereals, and strained or pureed meats. Then, ask the doctor when your child can resume his normal diet.

Orthopedics

Every day, a child performs all sorts of vigorous activities: climbing, running, and jumping. Unfortunately, these activities also make the child a candidate for an injury—such as a fractured arm or leg—that requires orthopedic care. Or, a child may require orthopedic care because of a birth defect, such as congenital hip displacement or clubfoot.

Because of a child's greater nutritional needs, plus the fact that his bones are continuing to grow, you'll need to give special care to a child who has an orthopedic injury or disorder. On the following pages, we'll give you the information you'll need; for example:
• how to prepare a child for wearing a cast.
• how to teach parents to care for their child's cast at home.
• how to prevent common immobility complications.
• how to prevent regression in the development of a child who's immobilized.

(For more information on giving orthopedic care, see the NURSING PHOTOBOOK WORKING WITH ORTHOPEDIC PATIENTS.)

PATIENT PREPARATION

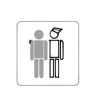

Preparing your patient for cast application

Ten-year-old Billy Semple walks into the hospital emergency department with his mother one morning, looking frightened. His mother, clearly upset, says she thinks Billy may have broken his arm when he fell off his bicycle.

After X-rays of Billy's arm confirm that it's fractured, the doctor decides to place a cast on it. Hearing this, Billy asks if the cast is punishment for injuring his arm. He also asks if the cast will ever be removed.

Help put Billy's mind at ease by telling him the cast is a hard bandage he'll have to wear for a short time. Explain that the cast will help his arm heal properly by holding the broken part of his arm very still.

Emphasize to Billy that the cast isn't punishment, and that he'll be able to do most of the things he did before he hurt his arm.

Tell him that his friends and family will be able to draw pictures on his cast, or sign their names on it. But, warn Billy's parents against painting over large areas of his cast. Doing so would make it nonporous, increasing the risk of skin breakdown.

Note: If your patient has a condition such as Osgood-Schlatter disease, you may have more opportunity for patient teaching before a cast's applied. In such a circumstance, consider helping him place a cast on a doll. By using this teaching technique, you can help him better understand the casting procedure.

For details on your role during and after cast application, read the information that follows.

Assisting with cast care

As you know, you'll assist the doctor when he applies a cast to a child's arm or leg. But the extent of your participation depends on many factors, including the extent of the injury, hospital policy, and the doctor's preference.

In most cases, you'll start by gathering the equipment needed for the procedure. Explain to the child why he must sit still; allow him to sit on his parent's lap if it reassures him. But don't have his parents assist if you feel they'll only upset him more. If your patient's an infant, encourage him to hold still by giving him a bottle during the procedure. A toddler may be more cooperative if you give him a toy or doll.

After the doctor's finished applying the cast, wait about 15 minutes for it to partially harden. Then, check the fit by trying to slip two fingers into the cast. If you can fit more than two fingers, the cast's too loose. Consider the cast too tight if you can't get two fingers into it. Tell the doctor if the cast doesn't fit properly, so he can make another cast.

You can also assess the cast's fit by:
• checking your patient's nails for capillary refill. If color return is sluggish, the cast may be too tight.
• checking pulses distal to the cast. As you know, a diminished or absent pulse also suggests

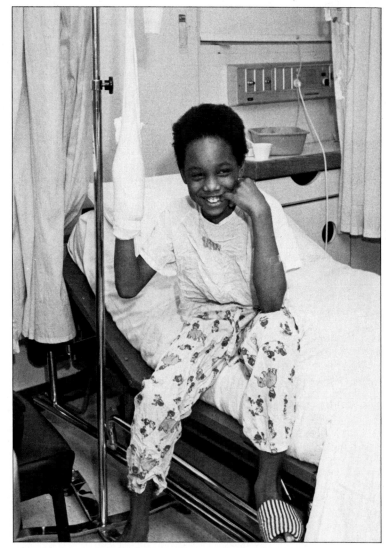

that the cast's too tight.
• feeling the temperature of the arm or leg affected by the cast. If the limb feels cold, the cast may be too tight, or the child may have damaged a blood vessel.
• asking your patient to move his fingers (if the cast's on his arm) or his toes (if the cast's on his leg). If your patient can't move them, the cast may be too tight, or he may have suffered nerve damage.
• asking the child if he can feel you touching his fingers or toes on the affected limb. Also, ask him whether the limb feels like it went to sleep or has a pins-and-needles sensation.

Notify the doctor of any problems you discover.

While the cast dries, take these measures to reduce and prevent pressure ridges from forming on the cast's inside. First, stack two regular-sized pillows, and cover them with a bed-saver pad. Then, using your palms, lift the casted limb onto the pillows. *Important:* Don't place the cast on plastic, since this inhibits drying. And don't handle the cast with your fingertips until it's completely dry, or you'll cause fingertip indentations in the plaster.

Make sure the cast is elevated above the child's heart level and that the pillows extend above and below the cast. After 2 hours, reposition your patient's cast on the pillows, alternating between the supine, side-lying, and prone positions. Doing so allows the cast to dry evenly. Repeat this procedure about every 2 hours, or as ordered.

· Suppose the doctor wants to keep your patient's casted arm or leg elevated to increase drainage and keep an infection from spreading. To do so, cut a piece of stockinette that's about 4' long and 4" wide (120 cm x 10.2 cm). Place the stockinette over the child's cast, and tape it to the cast. Tie the other end of the stockinette to the top arm of an I.V. pole, as shown at left. This procedure helps prevent edema and allows the child to move around.

Trimming a cast

1 *After your patient's cast is completely dry, check for rough cast edges, and finish any that you find by smoothing or trimming them. This precaution helps prevent skin irritation and breakdown. Also, a finished cast will hold cotton cast padding or stockinette better, if* either is applied. For details, read on.

Suppose one edge of your patient's cast is extremely rough. Carefully smooth or trim the edge with a cast knife or scissors, as shown here. Or, pull rough edges away from the skin, using duck bill forceps.

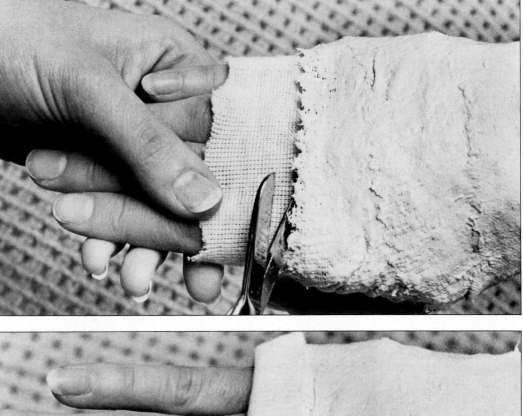

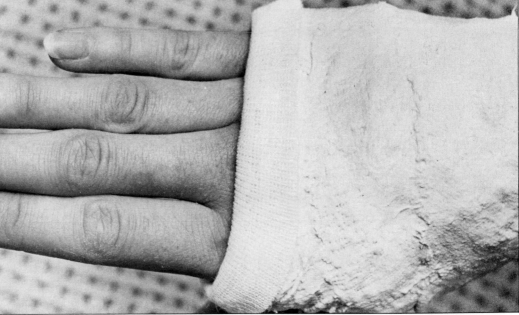

2 When you're finished, grasp the edge of the stockinette resting between the child's arm and the cast. Pull the stockinette's edge over the cast edge, as shown, and tape it in place. If you can't do this for any reason (for example, because the doctor didn't apply enough stockinette under the cast), petal the edge, as instructed in the following photostory.

If your patient's old enough, teach him how to assess his cast. Tell him to routinely check for rough edges and petal any that he finds. If he's too young, teach his parents.

Orthopedics

Petaling and protecting a cast

1 *To cover an edge you've trimmed (or a rough edge that can't be trimmed), petal it with moleskin. Here's how:*

First, cut several 4" x 2" (10.2 x 5.1 cm) moleskin strips. To keep the strip corners on the outside of the cast from catching on clothing and peeling off of the cast, round off the corners on one end of the strip, as the nurse has done here.

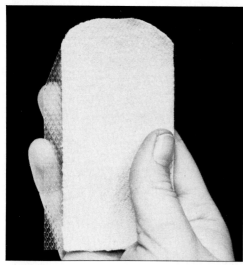

2 If your patient's old enough, show him how to apply the moleskin strips to his cast. Doing so may help the child adjust to the cast and give him some feeling of involvement in his care. If he's too young, show his parents, so they can perform the procedure at home.

Tuck the moleskin strip's unrounded end just inside the cast, so its sticky side is against the cast, and the rounded end protrudes from the cast. Avoid creasing the moleskin, to prevent skin irritation and breakdown under the cast. Fold down the rounded end over the cast's edge, as shown here, and press it in place so it adheres firmly to the cast.

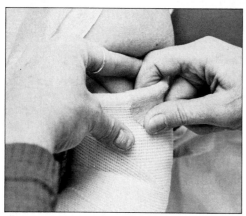

3 Repeat the procedure, applying overlapping pieces to the cast edge until all rough edges are covered. Or, allow the child or his parents to complete the petaling.

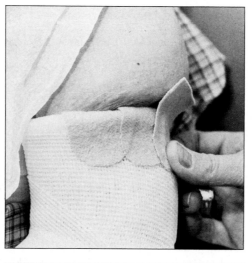

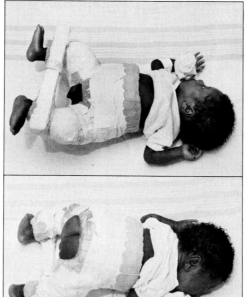

4 If your patient's wearing a spica cast like the one shown above, you'll have to keep the cast edges surrounding the perineal area from becoming soiled. To do so, cover the cast with clear plastic wrap, and secure the wrap with adhesive tape, as shown.

🔊 *Nursing tip:* Instead of clear plastic wrap, you may use Op-Site™, a clear plastic wound dressing with an adhesive backing.

Remember to document everything in your nurses' notes

Sending the child home with a cast

Remember Billy Semple who suffered the fractured arm? Within a few hours, Billy will go home, wearing a cast. To teach Billy and his mother how to care for the cast, use the following home care aid.

Although the cast will disrupt Billy's normal routine, reassure him and his mother that he still can do most of the things he did before the injury. For at least 48 hours, however, Billy will have to take special precautions to protect the cast while it dries. Encourage him to aid drying by elevating the uncovered cast on two pillows as much as possible. Remind Billy and his mother to frequently change the cast's position, using their palms, not their fingers.

If the doctor applied a plaster cast, warn Billy that the wet cast will feel heavy, but will get lighter as it dries. Also, tell Billy not to poke at the wet cast with his fingers.

Emphasize to Billy and his mother that the instructions and precautions you'll teach them are important to ensure his comfort and prevent complications. Teach them how to perform special exercises ordered by the doctor that will help prevent complications.

Also emphasize to Billy and his mother that they must continue cast care, as directed in the following home care aid, for as long as he's wearing the cast.

Finally, give Billy's mother a copy of the home care aid, and review the instructions with her and Billy.

Home care

Caring for your child's cast

Dear Parent:
The doctor's immobilized your child's broken bone with a cast. To make sure the bone heals properly, follow the instructions on this checklist.
• Reduce swelling in your child's arm or leg by elevating it above his chest level as much as possible.
• Several times a day, check for swelling above and below the cast. (Compare his casted arm or leg with the other one.) A little swelling's normal. But if it doesn't go down after you've elevated the cast for 1 hour, call the doctor. Apply ice to the swelling.
• Several times a day, touch the skin above and below the cast. Ask the child to tell you if he feels your touch, or if he feels a tingle or increase in pain. He may feel some pain, even when you're not touching him. But if his arm or leg feels numb, tingly, or like it's asleep, call the doctor.
• At least 3 times a day, ask your child to perform the exercises shown below (depending on the location of his cast). If he can't move his fingers or toes, or complains of pain, call the doctor.
• At least 3 times a day, check his circulation by pressing briefly on his middle fingernail (on a casted arm), or large toenail (on a casted leg).

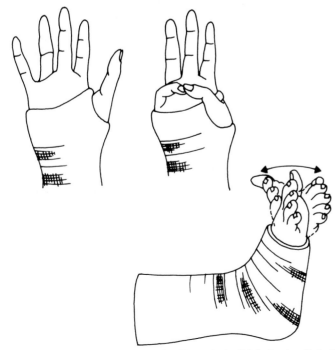

Release pressure when the skin under the nail turns white. If the normal pink color doesn't return quickly, call the doctor. Also call the doctor if the skin above or below his cast changes color, or if his fingers or toes feel cold and don't warm up when you cover them.
• Every day, wash the skin along the cast's edges. But first, protect the cast's edges with plastic wrap. Then, wash the skin with mild soap and water. Using a damp cloth, wipe the skin you can reach under the cast, but don't wet the cast itself. Thoroughly dry the skin. Finally, using a towel or a pad saturated with rubbing alcohol, massage the skin under and along the cast's edges.
• Although your child may occasionally complain that the skin under his cast itches, don't let him try to scratch it by inserting anything under the cast. He might damage his skin, causing an infection. You may prevent some skin irritation by removing loose visible plaster particles. Just reach an inch or two inside the cast, and pull them out. (But never try to trim or remove the cast yourself.)
• Call the doctor if you notice: any object stuck in the cast; a weakened, cracked, loose, or tight cast; or a bad smell, warm, damp area, or fresh stain coming from inside the cast.
• When your child's cast becomes dirty, clean it with a damp cloth and dry cleaner, such as Comet®. Wipe off any excess moisture when you're done. Or, follow these special instructions: _____
_____
• Bring him back to have his cast checked or removed on this date: _____

If your child's wearing a plaster cast:
Protect the cast against wetness. When he's bathing or going outside in wet weather, wrap the cast in a plastic bag. *Tie* the bag securely above the cast, using gauze or fabric strips—but don't use rubber bands. If the cast becomes wet, let it dry naturally (for example, let the child sit in the sun). Don't cover it unless it's completely dry and hard.

If your child's wearing a fiberglass (or other non-plaster) cast:
Ask the doctor if the child can swim or shower with it. If so, the doctor will probably tell you to let it dry naturally, without using a fan or dryer. Follow his instructions.

Orthopedics

Preventing immobility complications

Like an adult, the child who's immobilized while recovering from an orthopedic injury is susceptible to respiratory, muscular, and metabolic complications. In fact, because of his distinctive anatomy and physiology, he may be at even *greater* risk than an adult.

We've already described a child's susceptibility to respiratory complications (see pages 88 through 90). A long period of immobilization increases that risk.

Immobilization also increases the risk of metabolic complications. A growing child normally needs more nutrition than an adult; add to that the stress of an injury and subsequent immobilization, and the requirement increases. Why? Because immobilization causes increased protein and nitrogen breakdown, requiring increased protein intake for bone and tissue healing.

Finally, since a child continues to develop his muscle coordination until late adolescence, a long period of immobility will delay it.

The following chart presents possible immobility complications involving these three body systems and shows what steps you can take to prevent them. (For more information on common immobility complications, see the NURSING PHOTOBOOK PROVIDING EARLY MOBILITY.)

System
Respiratory

Complications
• Pooling of respiratory secretions
• Respiratory infections
• Hypostatic pneumonia
• Atelectasis
• Respiratory acidosis
• Pulmonary emboli

Nursing interventions
• Turn and position your patient regularly, according to his needs.
• Make sure his body is well aligned and his joints and muscles are properly supported.
• Encourage him to cough and deep breathe to fully expand his lungs and clear secretions.
• Observe and assess his respiratory patterns and breath sounds.
• Encourage the use of incentive spirometry and deep breathing exercises, as needed; be prepared to administer intermittent positive-pressure breathing (IPPB) treatments, if ordered.
• Perform chest physiotherapy at least once every 8 hours.
• Carefully explain all procedures to your patient and his family, and emphasize their importance.

System
Muscular

Complications
• Contractures
• Decreased muscle tone
• Muscle atrophy

Nursing interventions
• Turn and position your patient regularly, according to his needs.
• Make sure his body's well aligned, and his joints and muscles are properly supported.
• Perform complete range-of-motion exercises at least three times a day.
• Use supportive devices, as needed, such as footdrop stops, splints, trochanter rolls, and hand rolls.
• Whenever possible, reduce edema by elevating his arms and legs.
• Hyperextend your patient's hips at least three times a day, unless contraindicated.
• Explain all procedures to your patient and his family, using words they understand.

System
Metabolic

Complications
• Increased protein and nitrogen breakdown
• Hypercalcemia (calcium is released from bones and absorbed by the blood)

Nursing interventions
• Perform complete range-of-motion exercises to help slow the rate of calcium loss from your patient's bones.
• Give him cranberry juice to increase the acid level of his urine. Doing so lessens the risk of kidney stone development.
• Administer a diet high in protein and calories.
• To increase his appetite, try to give him foods that he likes. Offer frequent, small meals.
• Make sure he gets adequate rest. Perform several of your nursing duties at one time to minimize interruptions.
• Encourage him to maintain a high-protein diet for several weeks after he's no longer immobilized, to help replace lost protein.

Psychosocial care of the immobilized child

Sally Carruthers, age 12, has been active her entire life. Her mother jokingly refers to her as a perpetual-motion machine. But recently, Sally was struck by a car while riding her bicycle. Her right leg was fractured in the accident. Because her leg isn't healing properly, the doctor's decided to immobilize it with a spica cast, as shown at right. As you probably know, a spica cast immobilizes *both* legs, in order to keep the injured leg extra still.

Sally will be in the hospital for nearly 2 weeks, and will have to wear the cast for about 3 months. For the first time in her life, she won't be able to enjoy the freedom of movement she cherishes. Her ability to use activity as an outlet for her feelings is severely impaired. The prospect can make even a friendly, happy child such as Sally become shy and sullen.

Combating the psychological and emotional effects of immobilization presents a special nursing challenge. Degrees of immobility vary—obviously, a child wearing only an arm or leg cast can be more active than one who's in traction. And a child's reaction to immobilization can vary as well. For example, the immobilized child may feel frustrated and angry at her sudden lack of freedom. She may lash out with uncontrolled rage, giving way to temper tantrums punctuated by cursing and screaming.

The child may also feel isolated, since she has less contact with children her own age. She'll have to rely on you and her family for social interaction.

A child may view immobilization as the loss of her independence. She'll feel helpless and vulnerable, and may worry about her own safety. And, if your patient's a toddler, a long period of immobilization may delay development of her learning and musculoskeletal skills.

What you can do
Through nursing care, you can help the child overcome these difficulties. Above all, try to stimulate her and keep her mind active; by doing this, you help prevent any stagnation or regression in her intellectual development.

Now, here are some points to remember:
• Use dolls to explain immobilization procedures to a younger child. Then, the child can express herself through the doll, giving you insight into her feelings.
• Allow the child to participate in her own care as much as possible; for example, let her help plan her daily routine, choose the clothes she's going to wear, or select her favorite foods.
• Try to place the child in a room with other children her own age. Plan activities for the entire group, such as a sing-along.
• Give the child a chance to express herself through artwork. Coloring, drawing, and finger painting are good ways for a child to release her emotions and develop fine-motor coordination.

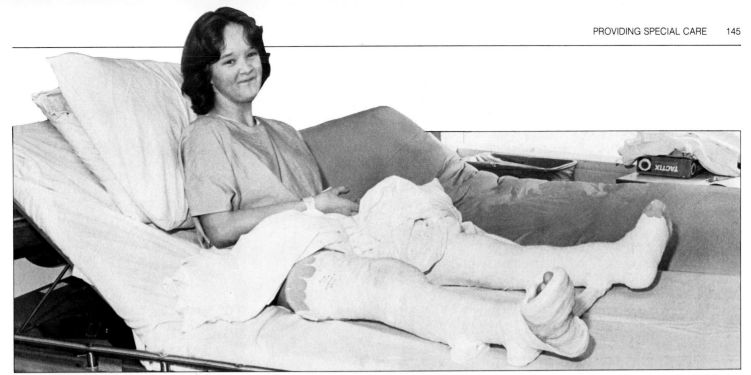

• Unless the doctor orders otherwise, encourage the child to be as mobile as she can possibly be. Provide her with a wheelchair, stretcher, or creeper, if appropriate. Doing so allows the child to move around by herself, giving her a greater feeling of independence.

• If your patient can't leave her bed, have her bed periodically moved into the playroom so she can talk to other patients. Also, give her a soft, sponge-like ball to play with. By bouncing the ball off the wall, she can release frustration without causing any damage. In addition, if your patient's in traction (see photo below), encourage her to lift herself with a trapeze, if possible. This will help her feel more independent.

• Make sure the child has a radio and television available for entertainment. But don't let that become her *only* form of entertainment. Provide and encourage other pastimes too.

• If your patient's school age, encourage parents and friends to help with her studies.

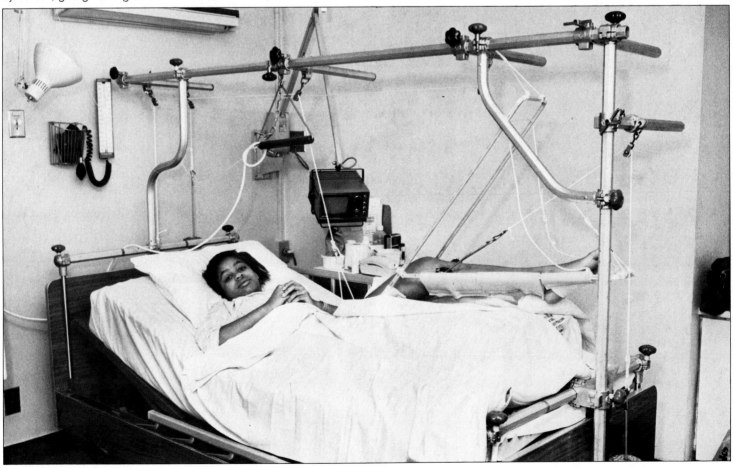

Special challenges

Whenever you care for an abused child or a child who's dying, you've accepted one of the greatest challenges nursing has to offer. Coping with these special patients—and their families—requires clinical skill, emotional strength, compassion, and diplomacy.

You'll need to work closely with the child and his family to establish a supportive and trusting relationship. And, in addition to providing quality care, you may also need to refer the child and family for help as needed.

The next few pages will help prepare you for these challenges.

Understanding child abuse

When we talk about child abuse, we're actually referring to a worldwide problem that crosses continental, cultural, racial, sexual, and socioeconomic boundries. In fact, in the United States alone, over 500,000 cases of suspected abuse exist each year.

A child abuser isn't easy to identify. Don't assume he'll fall into a stereotype. For example, he may *not* be a teenage parent, live-in lover, or drug user. He may, in fact, be a community activist, teacher, church leader, or doctor. And most likely, he's someone the child knows— a parent, another relative, an older child, or a family friend. And keep in mind that he may abuse the child emotionally or psychologically, rather than physically.

But what makes someone abuse a child? Usually a triad of factors: the child's temperament (he may be hyperactive, highly intelligent, chronically ill, or very demanding); environmental stresses (the abuser may be facing financial difficulties, an unwanted pregnancy, a divorce, or family pressures); or the abuser's own background. For example, the abuser may have come from a family where he was abused and view child beating or neglect as the proper way to control inappropriate behavior. He may also feel that sexual abuse is his right as an adult.

What about the child? Usually, an abused child's torn by conflicting feelings. Naturally, he resents the treatment he receives—but he still feels ties of affection for those who abuse him. Remember, he's been conditioned to believe he deserves abuse or neglect. And, in cases of sexual abuse, he may be led to believe the abuse is a privilege.

As a nurse, you may be the first person to see the abused child, or to monitor his behavior over a period of time (for example, during hospitalization). Of course, when you see signs that may indicate abuse (see the following information), you have a legal responsibility to report your suspicions.

Child abuse: Recognizing signs and symptoms

Do you think your patient may be abused? You can't always be sure, because abuse injuries may resemble accidental injuries. But, by gathering detailed information about the accident and obtaining a careful history, you'll know when to become suspicious. Ask yourself:
• Is the reason for his injury unexplained or implausible?
• Does he have a large number of injuries in different stages of healing?
• If he's under age 1, does he have a long-bone fracture?
• Does he seem accident-prone?
• Has the child been in your emergency department before? Or, is your hospital a long way from the child's home? (Remember, an abuser may switch from one emergency department to another to avoid suspicion.)
• Who brought the child to the emergency department? Does his story seem consistent with the child's story? Is he vague about the details? Does he blame someone else for the accident? Does his version of the story change each time he tells it?
• Does the child look like he's had an accident? Is his hair tousled, face smudged, or clothing dirty?
• Was the child brought in with a complaint other than the abuse? For example, did you discover a broken arm while treating him for a cold?
• Is the parent or guardian's concern appropriate for the injury? Or, is his response exaggerated or absent?
• Does the parent or guardian appear uncomfortable with your questioning?
• Does the child seem afraid of adults?

Recognizing abuse

As you perform your head-to-toe assessment of the child, be alert for these specific signs of abuse.
If you suspect the child may be physically abused, watch for:
• circular abrasions around the ankles and wrists from tying down the child.
• whiplash injuries such as muscular tension and swelling of the child's neck from vigorous shakings.
• muscle or subcutaneous tissue damage from floggings with a wet towel.
• radiologic findings such as healed or new fractures or dislocations (especially in the shoulder).
• human bite or fingernail marks.
• bald spots.
• injury to oral mucosa or frontal dental ridge (such as from having a bottle

forced into the mouth).
• loop marks from beatings with a belt; multiple or clustered bruises on trunk or buttocks.
• bloody urine, or a purplish color on flank or around umbilicus (may indicate internal injuries).
• old or new cigarette burns.
• burns with unusual patterns.
If you suspect the child may be physically neglected, watch for:
• signs of malnutrition, including wasting of subcutaneous tissue, abdominal distention, dull eyes, and sore gums.
• inadequate clothing in cold weather.
• parasitic infections.
• signs of inadequate medical attention, such as uncorrected eyesight or hearing, or tooth decay.
If you suspect the child may be emotionally neglected, watch for:
• apathy, hyperexcitability, or other behavior problems.
• emotional or developmental immaturity, depression, neurosis, or psychomotor illness.
• parental role playing among siblings. When all children in a family are neglected, older children may mother younger ones.
If you suspect the child may be sexually abused, watch for:
• genital or rectal injuries.
• bloody or painful urination or bowel movements.
• symptoms of venereal infections, such as gonorrhea, trichomoniasis, herpes, or moniliasis.
• signs of secretions in mouth or pharynx, or on hair or skin.
• pelvic hematomas discovered during a rectoabdominal exam.

Finally, closely observe the interaction between the child and the parent or guardian. Does the parent verbally abuse the child? Does the parent seem more concerned about how the accident affects him, rather than the child? Also keep in mind that an abused child may cling to the abusive parent.

Be sure to carefully document your findings, based on your physical assessment and observations—not on your opinions or suspicions. Remember, your nurses' notes may be introduced as evidence in a court hearing. Be sure to document any lesions, bruises, or healing wounds. Also, describe the child's behavior, as well as conversations you have with family members or friends. Document exact quotes when possible.

Suspicious burns: Recognizing signs of abuse

When you examine a child who has small, multiple burn marks on his skin, suspect cigarette burns, an easily recognizable form of child abuse. But also suspect child abuse when you encounter *any* burn injury that doesn't fit the explanation given for it.

Suppose, for example, Mrs. Taylor brings her 4-year-old son Donny into the emergency deparment. Donny has nearly identical, socklike burns on both feet. If Mrs. Taylor tells you that Donny stepped into a bathtub that he'd accidentally filled with hot water, think twice. Common sense tells you that a child steps into a tub one foot at a time and immediately withdraws the foot if the water's too hot. Although he might accidentally burn *one* foot, he probably wouldn't burn both.

Likewise, keep in mind that accidental scalding caused (for example) when a child tips a pot of hot coffee on his hand, will have a splash pattern. Suspect burns that resemble mittens, or any burn with an unusual shape or pattern, such as a coil or grid pattern.

Note: Take care to closely examine scald burns. Remember, what looks like a burn may actually be scalded skin syndrome, which is a staphylococcal infection.

Identifying child abuse

Quietly clinging to his mother, 4-month-old Jack Warren arrives in your hospital's emergency department. Maria Warren, Jack's mother, tells you her son has a cold and needs a prescription for medication.

As you gather the background information you need for Jack's history, you notice that Mrs. Warren has become edgy. "Are all these questions really necessary?" she asks. After you assure Mrs. Warren they are, you realize that her question has made you uncomfortable. In fact, it continues to nag at you as you begin Jack's head-to-toe physical assessment. Suddenly you spot several bruises on Jack's left arm. When you ask Mrs. Warren about the marks, she explains curtly, "Jack fell down the steps at the babysitter's last week." With surprise, you notice that Mrs. Warren avoids eye contact as she speaks.

As you continue your examination, you're struck with how quiet and subdued Jack is—in fact, he seems groggy. But when you mention your observation to Mrs. Warren, she shrugs it off: "Well, he has a cold. I guess it's made him sluggish."

You begin to wonder. How could a 4-month-old infant accidentally fall down the steps? Why is he so groggy? Jack's injuries and behavior, coupled with Mrs. Warren's apparent discomfort with your questions, make you suspicious. Could Jack be an abused child?

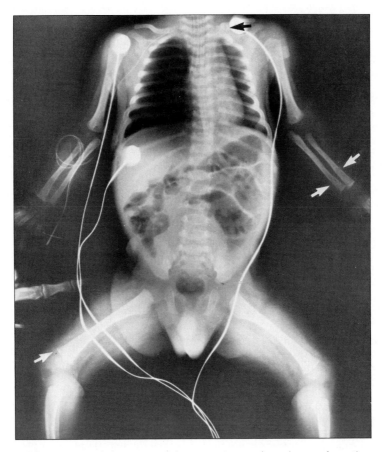

When you explain your suspicions to the doctor, he orders an X-ray (shown above). As you see, it reveals multiple fractures in various stages of healing—strong evidence of a history of abuse. Here's how to interpret the X-ray, starting with the most recent injury:

• Take a look at Jack's right knee. You'll see a chip fracture, resulting from jerking the limb with such force that the ligaments are ripped away from the bone, carrying a bone chip with them. Since you didn't observe bruising in the area, this injury is probably very recent.

• Now, examine Jack's left ulna and radius, where you observed bruising. You'll see healing spiral fractures, caused by a twisting injury. In an infant, this type of fracture nearly always signals abuse. In fact, *any* type of long-bone fracture in a child younger than age 1 suggests abuse.

By comparing his arms, you see that his left arm's ulna and radius lack sharp definition from periosteal elevation. This periosteal elevation is caused by fibrin collection around the broken bones.

• Study Jack's upper chest, and compare his left clavicle to his right. Notice the formation of calcium deposits in the area. Within 10 days after a fracture, these deposits begin to fill the fibrin network.

What about Jack's grogginess? Consider these possibilities: a head injury and drug or alcohol abuse. Closely examine his head for bruises (especially behind his ears), soft spots, and cuts or abrasions—all may indicate battering. Also, observe him for any signs of increased intracranial pressure (for example, abnormal pupillary responses to light). If you see any indications of head injury, the doctor may order a head X-ray, too.

Suppose you don't observe any such indications. Now, consider the possibility that Mrs. Warren gives the infant small amounts of alcohol to keep him quiet. Your tactful questioning may confirm this.

In Jack's case, consider the accumulated data reason to suspect child abuse. Document all your findings, including the child's history, the mother's responses to your questions, your observations, and all X-ray findings.

Special challenges

Child abuse: Taking action

If your observations and clinical findings indicate your patient's abused, take prompt action to get immediate help for the child and family. Here's how to proceed:

• Inform the doctor of your suspicions. If he feels your suspicions are justified, he may hospitalize the child—even if the injuries are minor. By doing so, he removes the child from the home, allowing time to further evaluate the family environment.

• Follow your hospital's policy on reporting child abuse. You may be required to notify your medical director or the hospital's legal advisor. In any event, be sure to keep your supervisor advised, so she can be prepared to help you.

• Report your suspicions to the proper agency by phone and then by written report. The agency may be the child welfare office, the district attorney's office, a social service agency, or the police, depending on state law.

• Speak to the parent (or guardian), and assess his attitude. To gain his confidence, avoid these judgmental gestures: turning your back to him, avoiding eye contact, directing your questions away from him, ignoring or belittling his comments, or standing over him when he's sitting.

• After assessing the parent's attitude, explain what you've done, and tell him you want to help. If the parent reacts negatively and tries to take the child home, you may need to get an order from legal authorities to retain the child.

• Inform the parent that the appropriate agency will review the facts and decide on further action. This action may range from obtaining professional counseling for the family to initiating legal proceedings. Explain that through counseling, he may find ways to deal with his anger other than by attacking or neglecting his child.

• Stress that child abuse requires treatment for the family as well as for the child.

• Try to help the abuser identify situations that may precipitate an abusive act.

• Prevent abuse recurrence by coordinating a team effort to continually evaluate the child's progress. If you work in a hospital, flag the child's hospital file. That way, if he's brought to the hospital again with suspicious injuries, your co-workers will know what follow-up action to take. If you're a school or public health nurse, actively look for signs of continued abuse or neglect.

• Refer the abuser to Parents Anonymous, or another support group in your community.

Assessing your feelings

Let's face it—coping with child abuse is emotionally draining. Be fair to yourself—and your patient—by evaluating your own feelings in each situation. In order to help your patient and his family, you must remain open-minded, nonjudgmental, and supportive, even if their values and practices differ from your own. If you feel uncomfortable discussing child abuse with the family, or aren't sure you can do so calmly, ask a co-worker to step in.

A child's view of death

How does a child perceive death? To some extent, that depends on his previous experience and religious upbringing. But you can make some generalizations about his attitudes and opinions based on his age and developmental level, too. Use these guidelines to help you understand what your young patient's thinking.

Toddler. A child this age is very dependent on his family. So, because death means separation from his family, he may be terrified by the idea of death. But at the same time, he can't conceive of death's permanence. To him, death is a temporary state, like sleep. During play therapy, a child this age may pretend that a doll dies and then comes back to life.

Keep in mind that many parents describe death as "like going to sleep." If so, a toddler may be frightened of sleep, because he associates it with death and separation from his family.

Preschooler. After age 3 or 4, a child begins to fantasize about death, and views it as almost magical. At the same time, he considers death temporary. He may be confused by his parents' grief and assume that their unhappiness is directed toward him. As a result, he may consider death to be a punishment for some real or imagined misbehavior and feel guilty. Encourage parents to give continuing reassurance to a child this age.

School age. At this age, a child begins to develop an intellectual understanding of death. He probably believes in spiritual immortality, regardless of his religious upbringing. Because he still has difficulty grasping the nearness and permanence of death, he may focus his concern on his parents and their distress, rather than on himself.

Adolescent. An adolescent may romantasize about life and death, and place more importance on acting bravely than on expressing his true feelings. You can help him by encouraging him to express himself in private, away from his peers.

Providing support

Regardless of your patient's age, you can take these steps to help him express and resolve his feelings:

• Visit him as often as you can—especially when you *don't* have to perform any nursing care. This conveys your concern for him as an individual, not just a patient.

• Don't lie or try to evade the child's questions. If he's old enough to ask a question, he's old enough to get an answer. (Suppose the child asks for information his parents don't want him to know? Read the text at right for suggestions.)

• Use words and concepts he's familiar with. For example, if your patient's a toddler, don't speak about death in abstract terms—he won't understand you.

• Encourage the child to express himself in words, pictures, or by playacting.

• Explain all procedures and treatment to him and his family. This will reassure him and may open communication about his feelings.

• Make the child as comfortable as you can. Use pain control and comfort measures, as needed. In addition, express your concern for him as often as possible by touching, hugging, or holding him (if he enjoys physical contact), or by just sitting with him.

What to tell the child

"I'm dying, aren't I?" Five-year-old Joey Lukas has cancer, and his doctor doesn't expect him to live more than 3 months. Every day he seems to get weaker. Yet, his parents don't want to tell him the truth about his condition. They feel the truth will upset him, preventing him from enjoying what little time he has left.

As a nurse, you face a dilemma. You probably believe in being straightforward with your patients and answering their questions as best you can. But at the same time, you recognize an obligation to the parents of your patient. Certainly you don't want to add to their pain by defying their wishes.

What do you say to a patient like Joey, who knows that something's seriously wrong? How can you be fair to him without betraying his parents?

Try responding to his question with an open-ended question like this: "Why do you feel that way, Joey?" or "What makes you think so?" Encourage him to express his feelings. Is he frightened? Angry? Does he feel that everyone's deceiving him? Or perhaps he just wants reassurance that his suspicions aren't correct.

Use your insights from your conversation with Joey to open a dialogue with his parents. If you believe that Joey knows the truth and is suffering because no one will discuss it with him, encourage them to speak frankly with him. But don't belittle their reluctance to do so—acknowledge how difficult speaking about death is for everyone. At the same time, reinforce the need for openness and communication among family members. Emphasize that Joey needs their love and support now more than ever—and that lack of communication will only keep them apart.

Of course, if you've worked with terminally ill patients before, you know that support between patient and family can be a two-way street. An older child may be ready to accept his impending death sooner than his parents are. If so, he may extend to them the support *they* need at this time.

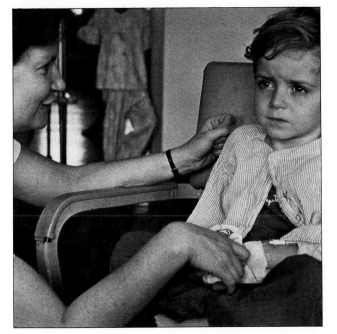

SPECIAL CONSIDERATIONS

Learning about sudden infant death syndrome (SIDS)

Picture this: It was about midnight when Lorna Soranno tiptoed over to the crib to check on 4-month-old Tommy. Earlier this week, she had called the doctor about Tommy's runny nose and cough; the doctor told her not to worry about it. And, anyway, Tommy seemed much better that evening. When Lorna peeked into the crib, Tommy was lying quietly, just as she'd left him—too quietly, she thought in alarm. When she picked him up, he felt lifeless. She called the ambulance.

When help arrived, Tommy was dead. The doctor told Lorna that he suspected sudden infant death syndrome (SIDS), and suggested an autopsy.

Sound familiar? If you've ever talked to a family after a SIDS death, you've probably heard a similiar story. SIDS, as you know, is associated with two factors: age and sleep. The syndrome is the leading cause of death in infants between ages 1 week and 1 year; premature infants are at greater risk than full-term infants. And, SIDS almost always occurs while the infant's asleep. Generally, SIDS is more common in overcrowded environments and during the winter months.

Autopsy findings usually include:
• minor respiratory tract infection
• petechiae over the lungs, pericardium, and thymus
• lung congestion and edema.

The cause and treatment of SIDS still remains unknown. But careful infant screening helps identify high-risk infants, such as those with a low birth weight, hyaline membrane disease, history of sleep-induced apnea, and a family history of SIDS. In most cases, the doctor will order an apnea monitor for these infants. The monitor sounds an alarm when the infant stops breathing for a preset length of time. Prompt action, ranging from simply providing tactile stimulation to giving cardiopulmonary resuscitation, may help the infant regain spontaneous respiration. (For more information on apnea monitors, see the NURSING PHOTOBOOK USING MONITORS.)

Helping the family

As a nurse, you may be the first person the parents encounter after their child's death. Speak to them in a gentle tone, and let them know you care. In easy-to-understand terms, explain SIDS. Assure family members that they did nothing to cause the infant's death and nothing they could have done would have saved him. Reinforce your verbal messages by touching their hands. Prepare them for the questions the coroner will ask, and the adjustments—both physical and psychological—they'll have to make in the days, weeks, and months to come. Remember, this situation causes extreme stress for the family. Carefully assess what they understand, and reinforce your emotional support, as necessary.

Before the family leaves the hospital, give them the name, address, and telephone number of the local SIDS association. They'll be able to answer additional questions and provide continued emotional support. (If the family is accompanied by a friend, relative, or clergyman, give this information to him too.)

Note: For more on helping parents cope with a child's sudden death, read the information on page 151.

Special challenges

Helping parents face a child's death

Last week, 14-year-old Robin Gottshall was admitted to your unit suffering from unexplained, persistant low-grade fever, fatigue, heart palpitations, nosebleeds, and recurrent infections. After testing, the doctor's ready to give Robin's parents the diagnosis: acute myeloblastic leukemia (AML).

You know that Robin faces a long-term, probably fatal illness. You'd like to help her and her family. But you're not sure of yourself—you wonder if you're really qualified to help them.

The fact is, no one's uniquely qualified to provide emotional support to others—especially virtual strangers—at such a time. But if you *want* to help, you can.

To your patient and her family, your concern alone can be immensely comforting. Sensitivity and compassion are the only qualifications you really need.

On these two pages, we'll give you some guidelines you may find helpful. But remember, no advice is appropriate in every instance. Consider your own good judgment, based on your assessment of the people involved, to be your most reliable guide.

Confronting terminal illness

To a parent, losing a child is unnatural—even if the child is an elderly adult. Perhaps this explains why the death of a child is so devastating. Even anticipating such a loss can create overwhelming emotions—including fear, anger, hostility, and disappointment—that can affect the child and even tear apart the family. In order to support their child, Robin's parents need continuing help in dealing with their own powerful emotions.

If you're a busy floor nurse, you may not be able to provide as much time as you'd like to comfort and support Robin and her family. And, because hospital schedules change, you may not always be available when they need you most. That's why every hospital should have at least one person whose full-time job is providing such support.

Whether or not you're that full-time support person, try to follow these basic guidelines:
• Ask to be present when the doctor gives the parents the diagnosis. Chances are, they'll be too upset to absorb many details. By listening to what the doctor has to say, you can later reiterate and clarify the information. Your presence also gives the family a chance to get to know you.
• Follow up with personal contact or a telephone call within several days. Give your name and phone number (or those of another support person or agency), and

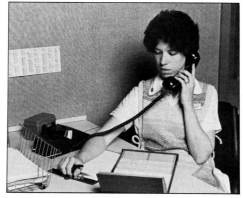

urge them to call if they need any kind of help. Keep in mind that while friends and family will initially be very supportive, support tends to melt away when illness is prolonged. Even if the family doesn't need outside help now, they may appreciate it in the future.
• Encourage parents to express their feelings. For example, they may feel angry at the hospital staff for hurting the child, or for being unable to cure her. But they may be reluctant to express this anger, for fear it will affect the child's care. Assure them that the emotions they feel—even the most negative ones such as anger at the child herself—are normal reactions. Use open-ended questions to encourage them to express themselves, and remain supportive and nonjudgmental, no matter what they say. They may be able to share feelings with you, an outsider, that they'd be ashamed to express to a relative.
• When the patient's hospitalized, include her family in her care. Chances are, family members will resent being asked to leave the room while you care for the child. Also, remain receptive to suggestions they give, even those relating to nursing care. Remember, if they care for the child at home, they may know as much about indwelling (Foley) catheter care or nasogastric tube

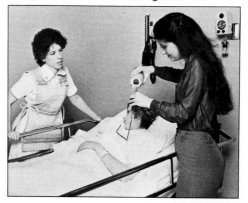

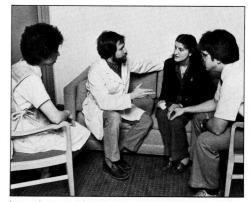

insertion and feeding as you do.
• Encourage the doctor to discuss all important matters, such as prognosis and treatment, with both parents at once—and do so yourself. Informing only the mother, for example, forces her to relay the information to the father—placing an additional burden on her. In addition, she may be tempted to shield her husband from some information, reducing open communication between them.
• Modify your nursing priorities to meet the patient's most important needs. For example, encourage family members to hold the child—even if it means bending some rules about sitting on the bed.
• Don't overwhelm the family with your presence. Part of support is knowing when to step back.
• If parents face difficult choices, such as whether to turn off a respirator or whether to donate one of the child's kidneys, avoid contributing your personal opinion. Focus instead on making sure they know everything necessary to make an informed decision. Then, no matter what they decide, be supportive.
• Recognize that the child's illness places extraordinary stress on the family. If necessary, encourage parents to spend more time with their other children at home, and assure them that it's okay if both parents don't visit the sick child all the time. The patient herself can help by thanking her brothers and sisters for allowing their parents to stay with her—this gesture helps siblings feel they're making a contribution, too. Also keep in mind that long-term illness may strain the parents' marriage. They may need additional counseling to maintain an open, supportive relationship.
• Tell parents what signs indicate impending death, so they can prepare themselves. If the child dies while they're holding her, reassure them that they did nothing to hasten her death.

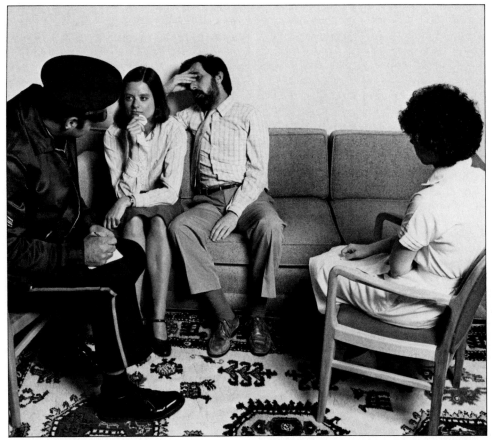

Coping with sudden death

If your patient has a long-term illness, you have a chance to become acquainted with the child's family before she dies. But if a child dies suddenly, and you've never even met her parents, your job becomes even more difficult.

Consider this situation: Marcy Odom, age 6, is pronounced dead on arrival at the emergency department (ED)—the victim of a hit-and-run driver. Her parents are on the way to the hospital, unaware that their daughter is already dead. What can you do to help them cope with this crisis?
• First, don't try to anticipate what their reactions will be. Remember, no two people react alike. Prepare to be accepting and supportive, even if the parents' reactions aren't what you consider appropriate.
• If necessary, clarify any information the doctor gave them, and answer their questions. They may take comfort from knowing that the child died in a hospital and that everything possible was done for her.
• Prepare the family for police questioning by informing them that the police routinely investigate accidental deaths. Otherwise, they may be shocked when suddenly

confronted by a police officer. Also, gently prepare them for the types of questions they'll have to answer. Keep in mind that even a simple question like, "Where were you when the accident happened?" can trigger overwhelming guilt feelings.

If you work in the ED, you can ease stress on bereaved parents by encouraging police and ED staff to work together. Through cooperation, you may be able to avoid asking painful questions more than once.
• Prepare the body for the parents to see. Remember, viewing the body is an important step towards accepting death—which is especially difficult in cases of sudden death. Remain with the family or leave them alone, according to their preference.
• Inform them that the coroner must be notified of the accidental death and that he may decide to perform an autopsy.
• Make sure someone (a family friend, if possible) accompanies the parents home.
• Several days later, follow up with a phone call and ask if you can do anything for them. Chances are, family members will remember exactly who you are—most people remember someone who's been kind to them in a crisis.

After a death: What not to say

Like most people, you probably feel at a loss when confronted with someone else's grief. What can you possibly say to ease their pain?

The fact is, not much. But you *can* avoid some common cliches that may add to their distress; for example:
• "I understand," or "I know just how you feel." Even if you yourself have experienced a similar loss, you can never know exactly how someone else feels. Such a statement may make parents feel that you're trivializing their feelings.
• "Things will soon get back to normal." Bereavement may last a year or more—and for a parent, life won't ever be exactly the same.
• "How many other children do you have?" Don't diminish the loss of one child by pointing out that the parents have others— or that they may have other children in the future. Remember, each child is unique and irreplaceable.

Don't feel you must fill every silence with words. Sometimes just your physical presence, combined with an attitude of concern, is best.

Beware, too, of using prepared speeches to comfort bereaved parents. As always, warmth, sincerity, and spontaneity are the best policy.

Recognize your feelings

If you've developed a relationship with a dying child and her parents, you, too, will grieve when the child dies. In such a situation, don't try to maintain an artificially professional demeanor. If you feel like crying with the family, do so—it's an honest expression of your feelings.

But always remember that the family's needs come first. Don't allow yourself to fall apart, placing them in the position of supporting you.

Also, don't force yourself to work with parents you can't sympathize with. For example, suppose the parents of a dead child are suspected of child abuse. If you feel angry at them, acknowledge how you feel— and ask someone else to step in. In order to be supportive, you must genuinely *want* to help. Family members will know if you're forcing yourself, no matter what the reason.

Finally, recognize your limitations. For one reason or another, you won't be able to help everyone. Ask someone else to help, when appropriate. And never underestimate the value of support by others who've suffered similar losses. If a support group for bereaved parents doesn't exist in your community, consider organizing one.

Appendices

Assessing growth and development

As a nurse, you're skilled at recognizing physical problems, such as a vision or musculoskeletal defect. But as a *pediatric* nurse, you must be equally skilled at recognizing abnormalities in a child's growth and development.

Use the following chart as a general guide to some major developmental milestones. (The illustrations accompanying each age group show how a child's body is proportioned at different stages of development.) If you suspect that your patient has a developmental problem, refer him for further testing with a screening tool such as the Denver Developmental Screening Test (DDST). For more details on normal height, weight, and vital signs measurements at different ages, see page 154.

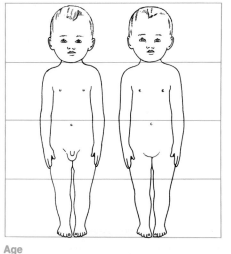

Age
1 year
Physical development
- Weight since birth triples
- Length since birth increases about 50%
- Head and chest circumferences are equal
- Can breathe through mouth when nose is occluded
- Rooting, Moro's and tonic neck reflexes disappear
- May have 6 to 8 teeth

Motor activity
- Occasionally attempts to stand alone
- Walks with someone holding one hand
- Uses thumb and forefinger to pick up objects; pokes at things with one finger
- Sits up for prolonged time without support
- Places one object after another into a container

Sensory ability
- Makes body adjustments to aid in dressing
- Responds to name
- Localizes sounds; listens for sounds to recur
- Eyes follow rapidly moving objects

Social skills
- Is afraid of strange surroundings; clings to mother
- Enjoys playing simple ball games
- Shows emotions such as jealousy
- Appears affectionate; hugs and kisses when asked to do so
- Plays simple interactive games such as peek-a-boo
- Explores objects by chewing and biting on them

Communication skills
- Understands simple commands such as *wave bye-bye*
- Says one or two other words besides repetitive *momma* and *dadda*
- Recognizes objects by names
- Imitates animal sounds
- Shakes head to signify *no*
- Stops activity when told to do so

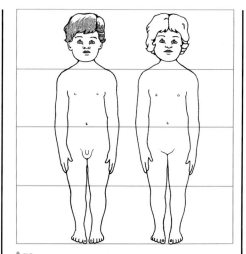

Age
1 to 3 years (toddler)
Physical development
- Anterior fontanel is closed
- Able to control anal and urinary sphincters
- Height and weight increase at slower rates
- Birth weight quadruples by age 30 months
- Arms and legs lengthen from ossification and long-bone growth
- Primary dentition complete

Motor activity
- Goes up and down stairs alone, by placing both feet on a step before climbing to next step
- Jumps down steps without losing balance
- Kicks ball forward without losing balance
- Turns door knobs
- Rides tricycle
- Holds crayon with fingers; copies crosses and circles

Sensory ability
- Vision is 20/40; accommodation is complete
- Hearing ability (including ability to localize sounds) fully developed

Social skills
- At 15 months, feeds self with little difficulty, tolerates some separation from mother, begins imitating parents
- At 24 months, feeds self well, helps undress himself, becomes possessive of toys. Has daytime elimination control.
- At 36 months, engages in parallel playing (playing in close proximity to others but without interaction), puts things away, pulls people to show them something, wants and displays increased independence from mother, begins to recognize sex differences, and knows his own sex. May achieve nighttime elimination control.

Communication skills
- From 15 to 18 months, uses his own jargon—sounds that he understands but that aren't real words
- By 24 months, uses 2- to 3-word phrases, and correctly pronounces vowels. Has a 270- to 300-word vocabulary.
- By 3 years, has a 900-word vocabulary and uses 4- to 5-word sentences

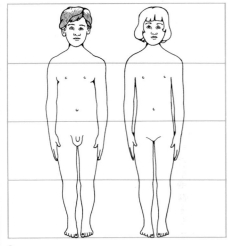

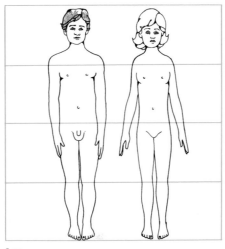

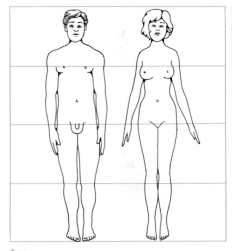

Age
4 to 5 years (preschooler)
Physical development
• Pulse and respiratory rates and blood pressure decrease
• Height and weight gains remain constant
• Height since birth doubles
• First permanent teeth erupt
• Right- or left-handedness established
Motor activity
• Walks down stairs, alternating feet
• Throws and catches ball well
• Ties shoelace in bow by age 5
• Hops on one foot
• Uses scissors well
Sensory ability
• Visual acuity approaches 20/20
Note: Amblyopia most often develops at age 4.
Social skills
• At age 4, is very independent and aggressive; shows off and tattles on others. May have imaginary playmate; may live in fantasy world.
• At age 5, is less rebellious, ready to accomplish tasks at hand. Cares for himself; is independent but trustworthy. Starts to understand rules and conformity; may notice prejudices; identifies with parent of same sex.
• Egocentric
Communication skills
• At age 5, can follow three commands given in a row, asks meanings of new words, has vocabulary of 2,100 words, counts and identifies coins, uses sentences of 6 to 8 words, describes drawings in detail

Age
6 to 12 years (school age)
Physical development
• By age 6, growth and weight gains slow, dexterity increases; child is very active
• By age 7, grows at least 2″ (5.1 cm) per year, posture becomes more tense and stiff
• By age 8, grows 2″ (5.1 cm) per year, lateral incisors erupt, movement becomes more graceful
• By ages 10 to 12, growth slows, weight gain increases; child may become obese at this age. Pubescent changes begin to appear; a girl's body lines start to become soft and rounded
Motor activity
• At age 6, is aware of using hand as a tool; draws, prints, and colors well
• At age 7, repeats activities to become proficient at them; uses table knife
• At age 8, fine motor control well developed; able to use tools such as hammers and screwdrivers
Sensory ability
• Fully developed
Social skills
• May become highly self-critical. Subject to depression, if unable to live up to others' expectations
• Develops a strong sense of industry
• May assume independent duties and chores
• Has defined ideas and attitude towards sex
• Enjoys hobbies, physical activity, and sports
Communication skills
• Has a 2,500- to 2,600-word vocabulary
• Capable of producing all the sounds in his native language (any articulation problems present at this age need special evaluation)
• Uses complex sentence structure
• Uses tone and new vocal patterns to express ideas
• Uses words to express feelings, desires and attitudes

Age
13 to 18 years (adolescent)
Physical development
• Experiences significant changes in bones, muscle, and adipose tissue. Hormonal changes cause shoulder breadth, arm and leg length increases in boys; hip, pelvis, and breast development in girls. *Note:* Approximately 99% of adult height is reached by age 18.
Motor activity
• All gross and fine motor skills are developed. Activities now serve to refine motor skills.
Sensory ability
• Fully developed
Social skills
• Explores emotional needs. Frequent testing of parents' authority may cause barrier between child and parents.
• Explores sexuality
• Feels strong need to conform with peers
• May romanticize about daily life, or fantasize about death
• Begins making long-range plans
Communication skills
• Has an adult's proficiency with language, but may frequently use slang or jargon to communicate with peers

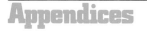

Height and weight measurements: Some guidelines

As part of any routine assessment, you weigh your patient, measure his height, and take his vital signs. But can you tell immediately whether your findings are within normal limits for his age and sex? This chart and the one below provide guidelines.

Height distribution among girls (by percentile)

Percentile	3		50		97		3		50		97	
Age	inches	cm	inches	cm	inches	cm	inches	cm	inches	cm	inches	cm
Birth	18.5	47.1	19.8	50.2	21.1	53.6	18.2	46.3	19.9	50.6	21.5	54.6
6 months	24.0	61.1	25.7	65.2	27.1	68.8	24.8	63.0	26.1	66.4	27.7	70.4
12 months	27.1	68.9	29.2	74.2	31.0	78.8	28.1	71.3	29.6	75.2	31.6	80.3
18 months	29.5	74.9	31.8	80.9	34.1	86.7	30.5	77.5	32.2	81.8	34.7	88.2
2 years	31.5	80.1	34.1	86.6	36.7	93.3	32.6	82.7	34.4	87.5	37.2	94.6
3 years	34.8	88.4	37.7	95.7	40.7	103.5	35.7	90.6	37.9	96.2	40.5	102.8
4 years	37.5	95.2	40.6	103.2	44.2	112.3	38.4	97.5	40.7	103.4	43.5	110.4
5 years*	39.4	100.0	42.9	109.1	46.8	118.8	40.2	102.0	42.8	108.7	46.1	117.1
5 years*	40.4	102.6	43.2	109.7	46.5	118.0	40.2	102.1	43.8	111.3	47.0	119.5
6 years	42.5	108.0	45.6	115.9	49.4	125.4	42.7	108.5	46.3	117.5	49.7	126.2
7 years	44.9	114.0	48.1	122.3	51.9	131.7	44.9	114.0	48.9	124.1	52.5	133.4
8 years	46.9	119.1	50.4	128.0	54.1	137.4	47.1	119.6	51.2	130.0	55.2	140.2
9 years	48.7	123.6	52.3	132.9	56.5	143.4	48.9	124.2	53.3	135.5	57.2	145.3
10 years	50.3	127.7	54.6	138.6	58.8	149.3	50.7	128.7	55.2	140.3	59.2	150.3
12 years	54.3	137.8	59.8	151.9	64.8	164.6	54.4	138.1	58.9	149.6	63.7	161.9
14 years	58.3	148.2	62.8	159.6	67.2	170.7	57.6	146.4	64.0	162.7	69.7	177.1

Height distribution among boys (by percentile) — columns 3, 50, 97 as above

Weight distribution among girls (by percentile)

Percentile	3		50		97		3		50		97	
Age	pounds	kg	pounds	kg	pounds	kg	pounds	kg	pounds	kg	pounds	kg
Birth	5.8	2.63	7.4	3.36	9.4	4.26	5.8	2.63	7.5	3.4	10.1	4.58
6 months	12.7	5.76	16.0	7.26	20.0	9.07	14.0	6.35	16.7	7.58	20.8	9.43
12 months	16.8	7.62	21.5	9.75	27.1	12.29	18.5	8.39	22.2	10.07	27.3	12.83
18 months	19.4	8.80	24.5	11.11	30.9	14.02	21.1	9.57	25.2	11.43	31.5	14.29
2 years	21.6	9.80	27.1	12.29	34.4	15.60	23.3	10.57	27.7	12.56	34.9	15.83
3 years	25.6	11.61	31.8	14.42	41.8	18.96	27.0	12.25	32.2	14.61	39.2	17.78
4 years	29.2	13.25	36.2	16.42	48.2	21.86	30.1	13.65	36.4	16.51	44.3	20.09
5 years*	32.1	14.56	40.5	18.37	52.8	23.95	33.6	15.24	40.5	18.37	50.4	22.86
5 years*	33.7	15.29	41.4	18.78	51.8	23.50	34.5	15.65	42.8	19.41	53.2	24.13
6 years	37.2	16.87	46.5	21.09	58.7	26.63	38.5	17.46	48.3	21.91	61.1	27.71
7 years	41.3	18.73	52.2	23.68	67.3	30.53	43.0	19.5	54.1	24.54	69.9	31.71
8 years	45.3	20.55	58.1	26.35	78.9	35.79	48.0	21.77	60.1	27.26	79.4	36.02
9 years	49.1	22.27	63.8	28.94	89.9	40.78	52.5	23.81	66.0	29.94	89.8	40.73
10 years	53.2	24.13	70.3	31.89	101.9	46.22	56.8	25.76	71.9	32.61	100.0	45.36
12 years	63.6	28.85	87.6	39.74	127.7	57.92	67.2	30.48	84.4	38.28	124.2	56.34
14 years	81.1	37.69	108.4	49.17	150.8	68.40	79.8	36.20	107.6	48.81	150.6	68.31

Weight distribution among boys (by percentile) — columns 3, 50, 97 as above

* The differing figures for 5 years reflect two separate study populations.

Modified from Studies of Child Health and Development, Department of Maternal and Child Health, Harvard School of Public Health; and from studies by Howard V. Meredith, Iowa Child Welfare Research Station, The State University of Iowa. In Vaughan, Victor C. III, et al. NELSON TEXTBOOK OF PEDIATRICS, 11th ed. Philadelphia: W.B. Saunders Co., 1979.

Vital signs measurements: Knowing what's normal

Age	Temperature	Pulse	Respiratory rate	Blood pressure
Under 1 year	99.1° F.* (37.3° C.*)	80 to 160/minute (*Newborn:* 70 to 170/minute)	20 to 40/minute (*Newborn:* 30 to 80/minute)	63 mean (using flush technique)
2 years	98.8° to 99.1° F.* (37.1° to 37.3° C.*)	80 to 120/minute	24 to 25/minute	96/30
4 years	98.5° to 98.9° F. (36.9° to 37.2° C.)	80 to 120/minute	22 to 24/minute	98/60
6 years	98.4° to 98.5° F. (36.9° C.)	75 to 115/minute	21 to 22/minute	105/60
10 years	98.0° to 98.2° F. (36.7° to 36.8° C.)	70 to 110/minute	19/minute	112/64
14 years	97.6° to 97.9° F. (36.4° to 36.6° C.)	65 to 100/minute	18/minute	120/75

*Rectal temperature

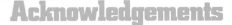
Using a nomogram

One way to calculate appropriate drug doses for your pediatric patient is according to his body surface area (see page 53). To determine body surface area, use the nomogram below.

If the child has normal height for his weight, just locate his weight (in pounds) in the column boxed in green. His body surface area (in square meters) is printed beside his weight.

For a child whose height *isn't* normal for his weight, locate his height in the left-hand unshaded column, and his weight in the right-hand column. Connect the two measurements with a straight line. The point at which the line intersects the S.A. (surface area) column identifies the child's surface area.

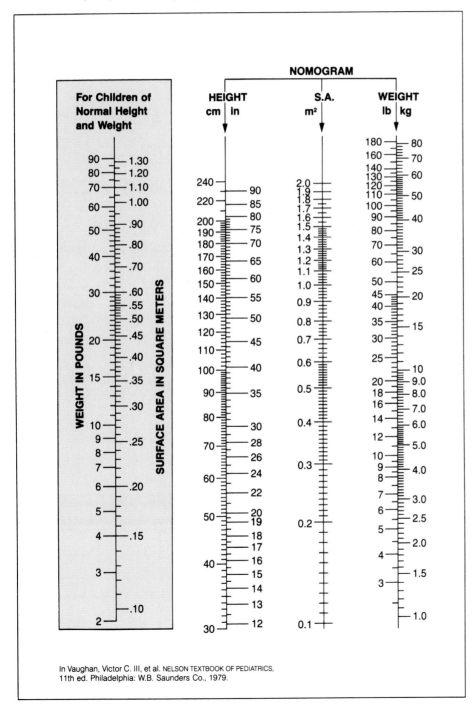

In Vaughan, Victor C. III, et al. NELSON TEXTBOOK OF PEDIATRICS, 11th ed. Philadelphia: W.B. Saunders Co., 1979.

We'd like to thank the following people and companies for their help with this Photobook:

ACCURATE MEDICAL SERVICE
Willow Grove, Pa.
Chuck Hepler, Manager

AMERICAN HOSPITEX
Division of American Hospital Supply Corporation
Evanston, Ill.

AMERICAN MEDICAL INSTRUMENT CORPORATION
Subsidiary of Vernitron Corporation
Flushing, N.Y.
Grace Giordano, General Manager

ANGELICA UNIFORM GROUP
St. Louis, Mo.

W.A. BAUM CO., INC.
Copiague, N.Y.

DITTMAR
Philadelphia, Pa.

DYNAREX CORPORATION
Elmsford, N.Y.

FAIRHOPE FABRICS, INC.
Fall River, Mass.
Irving Gross, Vice President

MARK-CLARK PRODUCTS
Division of M-C Industries, Inc.
Topeka, Kan.

NATIONAL CATHETER CO.
Argyle, N.Y.
J. Thomas Burns, Director of Marketing

OHIO MEDICAL PRODUCTS
Division of Airco, Inc.
Madison, Wis.

PEDICRAFT, INC.
Jacksonville, Fla.

PORTEX, INC.
Wilmington, Mass.

SEAMLESS HOSPITAL PRODUCTS COMPANY
Wallingford, Conn.
Ben Brausen, Product Manager—Urological

J. SKLAR MFG. CO., INC.
Long Island City, N.Y.

SUGAR BABE, INC.
Princeton, N.J.
Lory M. Needelman, President

3M COMPANY
Medical Products Division
Eagan, Minn.

WATERLOO INDUSTRIES, INC.
Medical Division
Waterloo, Iowa
John J. Robert, Sales Manager

WELCH ALLYN
Skaneateles Falls, N.Y.
Douglas Hufnagle, Advertising Manager
Anna Naff
Wilmington, Del.
Charlotte Sheehan, RN
Wilmington, Del.

Also the the staffs of:
BERKS VISITING NURSE HOME HEALTH AGENCY
Reading, Pa.

CHILDREN'S HOSPITAL OF PHILADELPHIA
Philadelphia, Pa.
Karen E. Roper, RN, BSN, MSN

COMMUNITY GENERAL HOSPITAL
Reading, Pa.

Selected references

Books

Azarnoff, Pat, and Sharon Flegal. PEDIATRIC PLAY PROGRAM: DEVELOPING A THERAPEUTIC PLAY PROGRAM FOR CHILDREN IN MEDICAL SETTINGS. Springfield, Il.: Charles C. Thomas, Pub., 1975.

Barnard, Martha Underwood. HANDBOOK OF COMPREHENSIVE PEDIATRIC NURSING. New York: McGraw-Hill Book Co., 1981.

Bates, Barbara. GUIDE TO PHYSICAL EXAMINATION, 2nd ed. Philadelphia: J.B. Lippincott Co., 1979.

Brown, Marie S., and Mary A. Murphy. AMBULATORY PEDIATRICS FOR NURSES, 2nd ed. New York: McGraw-Hill Book Co., 1980.

Chinn, Peggy L., and Cynthia J. Leitch. CHILD HEALTH MAINTENANCE: A GUIDE TO CLINICAL ASSESSMENT, 2nd ed. St. Louis: C.V. Mosby Co., 1979.

DEALING WITH EMERGENCIES. Nursing Photobook™ Series. Springhouse, Pa.: Intermed Communications, Inc., 1980.

DeAngelis, Catherine. PEDIATRIC PRIMARY CARE, 2nd ed. Boston: Little, Brown and Co., 1979.

Farrell, Jane. ILLUSTRATED GUIDE TO ORTHOPEDIC NURSING. Philadelphia: J.B. Lippincott Co., 1977.

GIVING CARDIAC CARE. Nursing Photobook™ Series. Springhouse, Pa.: Intermed Communications, Inc., 1981.

GIVING MEDICATIONS. Nursing Photobook™ Series. Springhouse, Pa.: Intermed Communications, Inc., 1980.

Graef, John W., and Thomas E. Cone, Jr., eds. MANUAL OF PEDIATRIC THERAPEUTICS, 2nd ed. Boston: Little, Brown and Co., 1980.

Hardgrove, Carol B., and Rosemary B. Dawson. PARENTS AND CHILDREN IN THE HOSPITAL: THE FAMILY'S ROLE IN PEDIATRICS. Boston: Little, Brown and Co., 1972.

Hilt, Nancy E., and E. William Schmitt, Jr. PEDIATRIC ORTHOPEDIC NURSING. St. Louis: C.V. Mosby Co., 1975.

Howry, Linda Berner, et al. PEDIATRIC MEDICATIONS. New York: J.B. Lippincott Co., 1981.

Jones, Dorothy, et al. MEDICAL SURGICAL NURSING: A CONCEPTUAL APPROACH. New York: McGraw-Hill Book Co., 1978.

Leifer, Gloria. PRINCIPLES AND TECHNIQUES IN PEDIATRIC NURSING, 3rd ed. Philadelphia: W.B. Saunders Co., 1977.

Levin, Daniel L., et al. PRACTICAL GUIDE TO PEDIATRIC INTENSIVE CARE. St. Louis: C.V. Mosby Co., 1979.

McFarlane, Judith, et al. CONTEMPORARY PEDIATRIC NURSING: A CONCEPTUAL APPROACH. New York: John Wiley and Sons, Inc., 1980.

Malasanos, Lois, et al. HEALTH ASSESSMENT. St. Louis: C.V. Mosby Co., 1977.

Marlow, Dorothy R. TEXTBOOK OF PEDIATRIC NURSING, 5th ed. Philadelphia: W.B. Saunders Co., 1977.

Oremland, Evelyn K., and Jerome D. Oremland, eds. THE EFFECTS OF HOSPITALIZATION ON CHILDREN: MODELS FOR THEIR CARE. Springfield, Il.: Charles C. Thomas, Pub., 1973.

Pagliaro, Louis A., and Robert H. Levin, eds. PROBLEMS IN PEDIATRIC DRUG THERAPY. Washington, D.C.: Drug Intelligence Publications, 1979.

Petrillo, Madeline, and Sirgay Sanger. EMOTIONAL CARE OF HOSPITALIZED CHILDREN: AN ENVIRONMENTAL APPROACH, 2nd ed. Philadelphia: J.B. Lippincott, Co., 1980.

Plank, Emma N., et al. WORKING WITH CHILDREN IN HOSPITALS, 2nd ed. Chicago: Year Book Medical Pubs., Inc., 1971.

PROVIDING RESPIRATORY CARE. Nursing Photobook™ Series. Springhouse, Pa.: Intermed Communications, Inc., 1979.

Roberts, Kenneth B. MANUAL OF CLINICAL PROBLEMS IN PEDIATRICS. Boston: Little, Brown and Co., 1979.

Russell, Helen. PEDIATRIC DRUGS AND NURSING INTERVENTION. New York: McGraw-Hill Book Co., 1979.

Saunders, William, et al. NURSING CARE IN EYE, EAR, NOSE, AND THROAT DISORDERS. St. Louis: C.V. Mosby Co., 1979.

Scripien, Gladys, et al. COMPREHENSIVE PEDIATRIC NURSING. New York: McGraw-Hill Book Co., 1975.

Smart, Mollie, and Russell Smart. CHILDREN: DEVELOPMENT AND RELATIONSHIPS, 3rd ed. New York: MacMillan Pub. Co., Inc., 1977.

Stone, L. Joseph, and Joseph Church. CHILDHOOD AND ADOLESCENCE: A PSYCHOLOGY OF THE GROWING PERSON, 4th ed. New York: Random House, Inc., 1979.

USING CRISIS INTERVENTION WISELY. Nursing Skillbook® Series. Springhouse, Pa.: Intermed Communications, Inc., 1979.

Vaughan, Victor C. III, et al. NELSON TEXTBOOK OF PEDIATRICS, 11th ed. Philadelphia: W.B. Saunders Co., 1979.

Wass, Hannelore, et al. DEATH EDUCATION: AN ANNOTATED RESOURCE GUIDE. Washington, D.C.: Hemisphere Publishing Corp., 1980.

Whaley, Lucille F., and Donna Wong. NURSING CARE OF INFANTS AND CHILDREN. St. Louis: C.V. Mosby Co., 1979.

Periodicals

Bunch, W.H. *Common Deformities of the Lower Limb,* PEDIATRIC NURSING, 5:18-22, July-August 1979.

Chee, C.M. *Symposium on Central Nervous System Disorders in Children. Seizure Disorders,* NURSING CLINICS OF NORTH AMERICA, 15:71-82, March 1980.

Farrell, Jane. *Symposium on Orthopedic Nursing. Nursing Care of the Patient in a Cast Brace,* NURSING CLINICS OF NORTH AMERICA, 11:717-724, December 1976.

Fitzgerald, Robert T. *Prehospital Care of Burned Patients,* CRITICAL CARE QUARTERLY, 1:13-24, December 1978.

Gross, R.H., and M.S. Hitch. *Screening of Newborn Infants for Hip Dysplasia—The Role of the Orthopedic Nurse,* ONA JOURNAL, 6:186-189, May 1979.

Harrell, J., and P.L. Meehan. *School Screening for Spinal Deformity,* ONA JOURNAL, 6:203-208, May 1979.

McGuire, Andrew. *Prevention of Burns,* CRITICAL CARE QUARTERLY, 1:1-11, December 1978.

Piercy, Sharon. *A Care Plan that Really Works for Children on Long-Term I.V. Therapy,* NURSING81, 11:66-69, September 1981.

Santilli, N., et al. *Screening for Seizures,* PEDIATRIC NURSING, 7:11-15, March-April 1981.

Voyles, J.B., et al. *Pulmonary Problems in Infants and Children,* AMERICAN JOURNAL OF NURSING, 81:509-532, March 1981.

Selected references for pediatric patients

Berger, Terry. I HAVE FEELINGS. New York: Human Sciences Press, Inc., 1971.

Clark, Bettina, and Lester L. Coleman. GOING TO THE HOSPITAL. New York: Random House, Inc., 1971.

Rey, H.A., and Margaret Rey. CURIOUS GEORGE GOES TO THE HOSPITAL. Boston: Houghton Mifflin Co., 1966.

Stein, Sarah B. HOSPITAL STORY. New York: Walker and Co., 1974.

Watson, Jane W., et al. SOMETIMES I'M AFRAID. New York: Western Publishing Co., Inc., 1971.

Weber, Alfons. ELIZABETH GETS WELL. New York: Thomas Y. Crowell, Co., 1977.

Available from Let's Talk About It™, Family Communications, 4802 Fifth Avenue, Pittsburgh, PA 15213:
GOING TO THE HOSPITAL
HAVING AN OPERATION
WEARING A CAST

Index

Index